T0369660

INCOMMUNICABLE

INCOMMUNICABLE

Toward Communicative Justice in Health and Medicine

CHARLES L. BRIGGS

Duke University Press *Durham and London* 2024

© 2024 Duke University Press
All rights reserved
Printed and bound by CPI Group (UK) Ltd, Croydon, CR0 4YY
Project Editor: Michael Trudeau
Designed by Courtney Leigh Richardson
Typeset in Warnock Pro by Westchester Publishing Services

Library of Congress Cataloging-in-Publication Data
Names: Briggs, Charles L., [date] author.
Title: Incommunicable : toward communicative justice in health
and medicine / Charles L. Briggs.
Other titles: Communicative justice in health and medicine
Description: Durham : Duke University Press, 2024. | Includes
bibliographical references and index.
Identifiers: LCCN 2023028150 (print)
LCCN 2023028151 (ebook)
ISBN 9781478026006 (paperback)
ISBN 9781478025788 (hardcover)
ISBN 9781478059240 (ebook)
Subjects: LCSH: Communication in medicine. | Communication
in public health. | Physician and patient. | Medical anthropology. |
Language and medicine. | BISAC: SOCIAL SCIENCE /
Anthropology / Cultural & Social | MEDICAL / Public Health
Classification: LCC R118 .B625 2024 (print) | LCC R118 (ebook) |
DDC 610.1/4—DC23/ENG/20231211
LC record available at https://lccn.loc.gov/2023028150
LC ebook record available at https://lccn.loc.gov/2023028151

Cover art: Untitled, from the series *Lingering*, 2020–2021.
Archival pigment print on silk charmeuse. © Pato Hebert.
Courtesy of the artist.

For Dick Bauman
friend, interlocutor, coconspirator

CONTENTS

ACKNOWLEDGMENTS

Books are strange beasts. They grow out of so many conversations, collaborations, obstacles, dead ends, and dreams. I am always terrified when I begin to write an acknowledgments section. Sure, there is the fear that I will overlook someone who made a crucial contribution. It is, however, the task itself that creates angst, reducing all of these entanglements to a hundred variations on the phrase "thanks to. . . ." If I were an artist, I would draw a picture that would include my interlocutors and a few crucial scenes. For want of a better approach, here goes.

This book emerged when I finally felt ready to present a full statement of the ways I have been wrestling with age-old divides between work on language and communication, health and medicine for decades. Never a loner, I have been in conversation with many scholars and practitioners who also tackle these issues, each in their own way. Starting in 1983, conversations with Aaron Cicourel have always been inspirational and formative. Also at the University of California, San Diego (UCSD), colleagues in Ethnic Studies and other departments deepened my understanding of race, racialization, and racism; conversations with Steve Epstein, Natalia Molina, and Nayan Shah regarding medicine and Otherness and with Ana Celia Zentella on the politics of multilingualism and linguistic racism helped push the project along. Howard Waitzkin's reflections on more than half a century of seeing patients, his trenchant critiques of how capitalism infects medicine and public health, and his efforts to build alternatives have stimulated productive conversations over decades. Jaime Breilh and Eduardo Menéndez have taught me immensely about critical epidemiology and Latin American social medicine. Mohan Dutta's leadership in challenging dominant approaches to health communication has afforded crucial insights. Some ten years ago, Paja Faudree and I struck up a conversation that sparked several American Anthropological Association sessions, an essay in *Anthropology News*, visits between Berkeley and Brown, and collaborative efforts to mentor graduate students attempting to bridge linguistic and medical anthropology. Emily Avera has sustained a group that grew out of these conversations right through the present.

In thinking through the COVID-19 pandemic, a number of collaborations were crucial. Building on work with the Latinx Research Center at the University of California (UC), Berkeley, Clara Mantini-Briggs MD MPH and I organized the Latinx COVID-19 Autoethnography Collective in January 2021. The group included Gabriel Cesena, Yadira Hernández Figueroa, Ryann Hirt, Joyce Huchin, Cameron Johnson, Gisselle Rosales, Brandon Rubio, and Nate Tilton. Our weekly meetings provided a powerful sense of how the pandemic was greatly increasing educational, economic, health, and other equities for students from racialized minority communities, and they helped all of us feel less isolated during difficult times. Rosales and Rubio subsequently participated in a podcast project directed by Mantini-Briggs and sponsored by Berkeley's Latinx Research Center and the Institute for the Study of Societal Issues (ISSI). Rosales generously allowed me to use part of her contribution to the podcast project in chapter 8.

I participated in the Humanities Research Institute seminar "How We Make It: Disability Justice for the Long Haul" in the spring of 2022. Organized by the incomparable Megan Moodie, it included Sharon Daniel, Pato Hebert, Tammy Ho, Alexandra Juhasz, Cynthia Ling Lee, Rachel Lee, Marina Peterson, and Nikita Simpson. In a series of remarkable discussions, I learned a great deal about struggles with long COVID and disability and how art provided a powerful matrix for individual and collective efforts to keep going and to remember. As readers will see in chapter 7, I am deeply indebted to Hebert for an interview that brought these issues, literally, into focus and for the stunning photograph that graces the cover.

Sarah Ramírez shared her deep knowledge of and commitment to the people of the San Joaquín Valley and generously made my work on COVID-19 there possible. Between July 2021 and the present (January 2023) I have interviewed physicians, psychiatrists, nurses, dentists, public health officials, journalists, community-based organizations, elected officials, judges, educators, religious professionals, firefighters/paramedics, police officers, long-term care facility operators, and a wide range of laypeople. Although I cannot, alas, thank you by name, I want to acknowledge your tremendous generosity in sharing time with me and your deep and moving reflections on how your lives were affected by COVID-19. They were some of the most astounding conversations I have ever experienced. I also had the opportunity to join some of you as you worked, preached, healed, tended to livestock, fixed cars, flipped through and commented on what appeared on your cellphones, and much more. Thanks for all that you taught me. I hope that this book gives you the sense that I listened carefully.

This book and the COVID-19 project could never have emerged if it were not for a partial sabbatical from UC Berkeley in 2021–22. I thank fellow participants in the Cultural Logic of Facts and Figures: Objectification, Measurement, and Standardization as Social Processes project at the Norwegian University of Science and Technology in Trondheim, especially principal investigator Tord Larsen, for years of conversation and helpful research support. I have also benefited greatly from fascinating discussions with John Ødemark and Eivind Engebretsen occasioned by the Body in Translation project at the University of Oslo, where I was honored to serve as a professor II in 2022–23. Plans for a residency there were, alas, thwarted by COVID-19. The Latinx Research Center and the ISSI's Berkeley Center for Social Medicine provided a stimulating and supportive context, and I benefited from conversations with colleagues at UC Berkeley, particularly—in the present context—Lawrence Cohen, Seth Holmes, Karen Nakamura, Stefania Pandolfo, and Nancy Scheper-Hughes. I owe a debt of gratitude to a funky old RV parked in the woods next to our driveway. As I was living in a household with four adults and two wonderful grandchildren, Brielle and Ian, it provided a quiet and contemplative space that, fortunately, lies beyond the reach of telephones and the internet. It also afforded a safer way to do fieldwork in October–November 2021. Graduate students at UC Berkeley and UCSD challenged my thinking and shared their wide-ranging knowledge of scholarship and insights derived from their own work and life experiences. The UC Berkeley undergraduates Nicole Carrasco, Leslie Ceciliano, Leslie Correa, Emily De Arman, Phoebe Douvan, Kartal Kaya, Anai Ramos, and Miyah Saeyang helped with research on social media and transcription and in several cases participated in interviews. I thank audiences at UC Berkeley, UCSD, and UC Los Angeles; at Brown University, the University of Chicago, Hong Kong University, the University of Massachusetts, Amherst, York University, Rutgers University, Ghent University, the University of Oregon, Pennsylvania State University Medical School, the University of Oslo, University College London, Beijing Normal University, and the Colegio Médico del Perú; and at academic meetings and conferences.

Mark Nichter gave generously of his time to read the manuscript and offer extensive and very helpful comments. I thank Dick Bauman for what he called an "hortatory" critique and a number of valuable suggestions and for decades of friendship, collaboration, and support. At Duke University Press, Ken Wissoker provided seasoned encouragement and advice, Michael Trudeau was extraordinarily painstaking as project editor, and Courtney Leigh Richardson conveyed the book's spirit splendidly in designing the cover. Two anonymous reviewers for Duke University Press provided a model of critical and insightful commentary, and I thank them deeply. Jasmine Cancino and Jasmine Valenzuela helped with the index. Conversations and collaborations with Clara Mantini-Briggs, MD MPH, continue to provide the inspiration that keeps me going, as does my never-ending love for Feliciana.

I write amid the COVID-19 pandemic. To say that COVID-19 is a communicable disease would seem to traffic in the obvious. On 11 January 2023, the Johns Hopkins University Coronavirus Resource Center reported 665,378,952 confirmed cases and 6,713,334 deaths worldwide. The figures for the United States, where I reside, were 101,409,175 confirmed cases and 1,098,304 deaths. How the virus achieves its communicable capacity has also often overreached the ability of epidemiologists to capture it. After initial projections of the importance of surface contact—leading to an emphasis on hand washing, hand sanitizing, and spraying disinfectant—attention shifted to how human beings share space and at what distance and how long infected individuals offer their unwanted viral companion species to other humans through airborne residues. Projecting COVID-19's communicability through unilinear temporalities and spatialities, the promise that mitigation measures today will lead to "normal" times and spaces tomorrow, proved to be epidemiologically problematic and to induce uncertainty and distrust among public health's "publics," particularly as even more frightful additional "waves" emerged. Tying communicability to a totalizing figure of SARS-CoV-2 gave way to concern with the fractured communicabilities of new variants. Rochelle Walensky, director of the US Centers for Disease Control and Prevention (CDC), declared, "The Delta variant . . . is one of the most infectious respiratory viruses we know of." Still, the subsequent omicron variant was even more communicable, so transmissible that it crowded out Delta in the viral race to infect human bodies, and then XBB.1.5 outcompeted previous omicron variants.[1]

Full stop. I have just exploited and simultaneously naturalized the second dimension of COVID-19's communicability. Felicitously, the term *communicability* also points to the circulation of discourse. To be communicable, a semiotic entity must be capable of traveling and invoking a response in others; COVID-19 could not be more communicable in this sense, either. People avidly searched the drumbeat of COVID-19 statistics, even as they were often reminded that figures fell far short of capturing the communicability of the SARS-CoV-2 virus: its circulation far outpaced the ability—and, in many cases, the willingness—of nation-states to provide adequate testing. News about COVID-19 dominated the "mainstream media" starting early in the pandemic. The *New York Times* published some three to five articles daily on H1N1 (or "swine flu") in 2009 (Briggs and Hallin 2016, 1). For COVID-19, by contrast, I counted thirty-five articles in the 16 March 2020 edition (selected because it was the last day I received a paper copy), with business, international, sports, arts and entertainment, travel, politics, advertising, metropolitan, and editorial sections all infected by the pandemic. Apart from obituaries, which were not yet dominated by COVID-19 deaths, I counted only thirteen articles in which the pandemic was not featured. The massive avalanches of discourse about COVID-19 on social media and the internet significantly shaped people's experience of the pandemic—and often what actions they took or refused to undertake.

Thus, COVID-19 brings into focus two senses of communicability: the circulation of pathogens and discourse about them. The promise of communicability is that if health authorities create a sufficiently persuasive, clear, and convincing avalanche of "messages" about COVID-19 and mitigation measures and laypeople heed what they say, the circulation of discourse will impede the movement of SARS-CoV-2 viruses. How public health professionals attempt to "control" epidemics posits separate discursive and viral circuits, even as they entangle the two by projecting an intrinsic and inverse relationship between them. Communicability accordingly lives a dual existence. On the one hand, it consists of cultural models that construct their referents, affording particular ways of imagining the circulation of viruses and discourse and mapping their interrelations, even as it impedes other imaginaries. On the other hand, representations of epidemics invite us to assimilate fevers, headaches, and feelings of fatigue as much as masks, spatial gaps, bottles of hand sanitizer, crowds, vaccination needles, and epidemiological statistics through affordances they offer. These terms are far from purely ideological or linguistic artifacts. If we take them in their familiar and narrow senses, this dimension of communicability is also produced by vast arrays of actors (including health officials, journalists, social media "influencers," and clinicians), practices (such as staging press conferences, producing podcasts and social media posts, talking with patients, and discrediting "misinformation" and "conspiracy theories"), and infrastructures (such as schools of medicine, schools of public health and journalism, websites, YouTube channels, pandemic "exercises" or scenarios, and the communications or public relations wings of health-related institutions). Epidemic communicability is also deeply rooted, however, in the more-than-human, the movement of viruses among and inside bodies, as well as immune systems, vaccines, and ventilators.

This book is not primarily a study of COVID-19. Rather, extending efforts to decolonize anthropology by challenging how it has been "complicit if not in fact collusive with the prevailing forces of neocolonial domination" (Harrison, [1991] 1997, 1), I seek to decolonize the fundamental understandings of language and communication and health and medicine that make such projections of communicability possible.[2] The argument traces a three-hundred-year history of efforts to cast science and medicine as both separate from and more fundamental than language and communication. A common conception shared by both professionals and laypeople casts medical and public health knowledge as produced in leading laboratories, clinics, and epidemiologists' offices and then converted into "communication" through translation into lay registers by physicians in speaking with patients, health educators, journalists, and advertisers. Communicative objects are then conveyed to lay audiences. This book offers a countergenealogy. I trace how conceptions of medical knowledge and of communication were coconstructed in the seventeenth century, infusing medical logics into conceptions of language, perceptions of language's precarity as a basis for communication and social relations, and remedial programs for imposing linguistic order. By the same token, communicability similarly shaped what could count as medical knowledge, what would be excluded, and who would be authorized to claim it. I go on to make the more radical claim that how these seemingly opposing and autonomous discursive regimens were connected has placed white supremacy and the colonial production of categories of others at the center of conceptions of language and communication, health and medicine, right through the present.

Communicability is both imaginary and far too real at the same time. It involves what linguistic anthropologists refer to as language ideologies (Kroskrity 2000a; Schieffelin, Woolard, and Kroskrity 1998), cultural models that project particular, partial, and interested ideas about what language and communication are and how they are entwined with individuals, populations, places, and politics. Communicable models cast some words, texts, images, and communicative practices as intrinsically mobile, as imbued with the ability to travel and generate increased knowledge. Discourses excluded from dominant communicable models get cast as intrinsically *im*mobile—or, at least, not worthy of traveling. Formulations classified as conspiracy theories provide a striking example. One way that communicable models exercise power is by naturalizing the perspectives they project, thereby making others seem unnatural, inferior, or even unthinkable. Like forms of knowledge, communicabilities are always multiple and often competing. Some communicabilities gain widespread circulation and aspire to exercise the panoptic power of shaping what counts as knowledge, who gets to make it, how it can legitimately travel, and how it becomes a deus ex machina that should pervasively structure materialities and natural-cultural relations. This effect should come as no surprise. Particular communicabilities become implicit emblems of race, class, sexual, and national hierarchies, invested with power through epistemological and ontological frameworks, infrastructures, and realms of practice. In such arenas as education and medicine, they create hierarchies and imbue them with material consequences by casting individuals and entire racialized populations as failed communicators.

Moving beyond pandemics, this book focuses primarily on how communicability provides a foundational basis for the immense power of biomedicine and global health and a key locus of the daily work of creating new forms of authority and recruiting patients and populations as crucial collaborators in sustaining its dominance. I trace how particular communicable models are so deeply woven into the fabric of biomedicine that they have become—in ways both minute and largely invisible and as major objects of attention—the manifestation that mostly directly enters into the eyes and ears of laypeople. Daniel Hallin and I have thus used the term *biocommunicability* to refer to forms of communicability that carry the authority of biomedicine (Briggs and Hallin 2016). Juxtaposing what are projected as medical and communicative practices in a single term challenges three centuries of efforts to make science and medicine, language and communication seem like autonomous spheres. Biocommunicability suggests that such "communicative" forms as public health pronouncements, conversations between clinicians and patients, and pharmaceutical advertisements are not only caught up with viruses; health infrastructures; medical technologies; health inequities; and broader social, political, and material inequities but are also partially constitutive of them.[3]

Rather than projecting a self-confident, unified, and pervasive hegemonic force, however, I tell a different story by tracing how communicability has also infused medicine and communication with anxieties and precarities. Ironically, communicability becomes a privileged site for representing and ameliorating failures, contradictions, and challenges that emerge within bio-medicine and from refusals to be interpellated by dominant forms of and efforts to assert competing communicabilities. I trace how laypeople, particularly members of racialized populations that get stereotyped as biocommunicable failures, critically engage dominant models in spaces that range from encounters with physicians to efforts by social movements to create alternative perspectives on and forms of providing health care. I am also interested in ways that biocommunicability falls short of dominating the words and actions of physicians and other health professionals, either when its gaps, contradictions, and effects accumulate to such a degree that they cannot be brushed aside or when solidarity with patients and populations denigrated as communicable failures drive them to collaborate in crafting more equitable forms. Indeed, creative and courageous efforts by some physicians and public health professionals to challenge dominant communicabilities and join underserved and stigmatized communities in forging alternatives are also important parts of this story.

The final two chapters of the book provide a striking example of this juxtaposition of power and precarity by focusing on a biocommunicable train wreck: the COVID-19 pandemic in the United States. Even after COVID-19 vaccines were widely available and government agencies at all levels launched massive efforts to urge people to get vaccinated, the unvaccinated accounted for most COVID-19 hospitalizations and deaths in 2021. Early in the pandemic, the CDC and World Health Organization (WHO) linked viral and communicative dimensions of COVID-19 in decrying an "infodemic." The circulation of so-called misinformation and disinformation was blamed for why the United States, an immensely wealthy country that has hoarded a massive quantity of the world's COVID-19 vaccines, has one of the lowest COVID-19 vaccination rates among rich countries. And by 2022, even vaccine- and mask-friendly US audiences had grown weary of COVID-19 public health discourse, citing "pandemic fatigue." Hospital physicians were frustrated with unvaccinated patients who filled emergency rooms (ERs) and intensive care units (ICUs), angry that they seemed to trust "misinformation" more than health professionals' advice.

I argue here that biocommunicability lies behind this massive erosion in trust in the United States in COVID-19 public health discourse and widespread rejection of masking, COVID-19 vaccination, and other prevention and treatment measures. Such statements generally lead to criticisms of the content of "messages" crafted by public health authorities and the role of journalists in disseminating them. I reject this approach for several reasons. One is that the roots of this dilemma in the United States lie in shifting trends in biocommunicability over the past eighty years, particularly in the clash between two competing forms. One projects laypeople as passive recipients of unilinear, hierarchically ordered transmissions of biomedical knowledge from health professionals. The other, more recent variety portrays agentive, self-interested individuals who actively seek knowledge about their health from multiple sources. These two models of communicability are racialized in both implicit and explicit ways due to how they imbricate forms of medical profiling (Briggs and Mantini-Briggs 2003) that stereotype and often stigmatize nonwhite patients and are coproduced with forms of linguistic profiling (Baugh 2003) that project Black, Latinx, and Native American populations as communicatively defective. I demonstrate how these trajectories clashed catastrophically in the pandemic, partly due to the way they got entwined with racial politics during a period in which white supremacy, violence against nonwhite people, and protests against anti-Blackness all intensified.

Racial inequities are crucial here for many reasons. Black, Latinx, and Native Americans in the United States were vastly more likely to be hospitalized and die from COVID-19 than white people, drawing attention to deep, persistent racialized inequities of health. The brutal murder of George Floyd by Minneapolis police officers on 25 May 2020 and the ensuing focus on racism partially de-medicalized these statistics, positioning the differential impact of COVID-19 within broader structural inequities and forms of racialized violence that predate the pandemic.[4] Nevertheless, the implications of my argument are not limited to the United States or to the complex nexus of racializing ideologies and practices that unfortunately still flourish there. A number of examples are drawn from outside the United States, including from nearly four decades of ethnographic work in Venezuela and from research conducted by other scholars around the world. Moreover, the effects of racialization and racism are a global phenomenon, affecting the distribution of resources, rights, and political power worldwide.[5] Crucially, the scientific and communicative imaginaries that feed into dominant communicabilities and help imbue them with power are also racialized: their foundation lies in the elevation of white, elite, European men in the seventeenth century to the status of universal embodiments of rationality, enlightenment, and modernity. I suggest that racialized ideologies of communicability and attendant ways of constructing, classifying, and disciplining individuals and populations shape people's access to rights and resources worldwide.

Responding to demands that scholars reflect on how racial inequities are hardwired into anthropology and other disciplines and into white scholars' own perspectives and practices, I came to see that using dominant communicabilities as a starting point in much of my work on language (Bauman and Briggs 2003) and health (Briggs 2005a) was grounded in white, elite, male, ableist, Euro-American privilege. Although my goal was to dislodge them through documentation and critical analysis, I had not yet adequately appreciated that biocommunicability is fundamentally colonial, deeply connected to whiteness, and constitutes one of the ways that racial violence is inflicted on a daily basis on populations targeted by structural racism. I realized that I needed to unlock my thinking and find a radically new way to begin.

Over two pandemic years, these unsettling sources of discomfort began to come together as I reread Hortense Spillers's remarkable essay "Mama's Baby, Papa's Maybe: An American Grammar Book." Spillers (1987, 67) connects the violent "hieroglyphics of the flesh" of slavery to the social-scientific and political violence of the so-called Moynihan Report's efforts to blame the effects of racism on the "matriarchal" pattern supposedly evident in Black families (Moynihan 1965). Tracing the legacy of slavery, colonialism, and conquest through the present, Spillers sees difference not as springing from culture or ethnicity but, rather, as the reduction of subjugated Black flesh to objects whose violent treatment can be justified as necessary. I was struck by her account of Equiano, who was captured in what is now Nigeria, and taken to England, and who wrote an autobiography. Spillers draws attention to the passage in which Equiano describes his European captors on the slave ship: "Their complexions, too, differing so much from ours, their long hair, and the language they spoke (which was different from any I had ever heard)" (Equiano 1969, 27, quoted in Spillers 1987, 69). Spillers comments: "We are justified in regarding the outcome of Equiano's experience in the same light as he himself might have—as a 'fall,' as a veritable descent into the loss of communicative force." I am interested in locating this "loss of communicative force" beyond the issue of a "strange" language. I see it as connected to the total violence of slavery and its legacy in carceral and other dimensions of anti-Black violence and racism in the contemporary United States.

Spillers's essay and other texts that it inspired helped me come to grips with my sense that focusing on communicability was dangerously incomplete. Savannah Shange insightfully brings together Spillers's concern with the "hieroglyphics of the flesh" and attention to racialized perceptions of the materiality of voice in analyzing how gentrification, race, social death, and the afterlives of slavery shaped the politics of race and multiculturalism in a San Francisco high school.[6] Shange (2019, 96) additionally draws on work by Frank Wilderson (2010, 59) in suggesting that "Black (girl) flesh spills forth in excess of the discourses that seek to locate it, to know it, to translate its 'noncommunicability.'" Shange's ethnography opens up other angles that enlarge this concept. One was the refusal of some "ordinary Black girls" to perform the disciplined voices of educational aspirational demanded by the school, even as they created artifacts (homework, tests, etc.) that met its standards. Shange carefully traces how race enters into assessments of the materiality of voices and flesh, into complaints by teachers that particular Black girls spoke too loud and too often. One student engaged in ethnographic refusal, telling Shange (2019, 119): "You can follow me, but I'm not gonna talk to you." Shange extends this "epistemology" by quoting John Jackson's critique of the ethnographic *"will to know everything"* and its connection to the *"will to disclose everything"* (Jackson 2013, 158, quoted in Shange 2019, 121). Shange frustrates what she sees as her readers' wish that she might end the girl's silence through a final act of disclosure.[7]

Reflecting on Shange's refusal thus opened up the possibility of repositioning myriad phenomena construed as pathological failures to perform dominant communicabilities. Here I am drawn back to sites I have often examined in my work that get identified as communicable trouble zones. They include what are deemed to be forms of "resistance," "ignorance," or noncompliance in clinical settings and discrepancies in case definitions and other refusals to fit epidemiological modes of classification. These projected failures are built into the design of health education and communication programs and journalists' interpretations of health inequities as caused by cultural barriers to biomedical knowledge. In school settings, parents are often blamed for educational inequities of race and class. They are depicted as not speaking or reading to their children enough or in the proper ways.[8] Youth are also blamed for embracing communicative practices that purportedly block their ability to learn. When individuals or entire populations get characterized as failing to align themselves with dominant communicabilities, they are held responsible for health, educational, and other inequities, following a rather bizarre cause-and-effect logic that renders invisible shifting relations between language and capital.[9] Adding to Spillers's list of agents who, in Shange's words, "operationalize key nodes in the state apparatus," Shange includes "teachers and principals and police and social workers and anthropologists" (2019, 96).[10]

Building on how Shange disrupted my thinking, I develop here the concept of *incommunicability*, which is productive in three crucial ways. First, it captures how some individuals and populations are banished from communicability, deemed incapable of performing utterances and actions that demonstrate their status as modern, rational, liberal subjects. Even as incommunicability is projected as encompassed by communicability, the subjects it produces are expelled to exterior, distanced, often stigmatized realms. Incommunicability thus becomes a pathological outside that comes after dominant communicabilities are in place—and in charge. Second, Shange's "Black girl ordinary" gestures toward how incommunicability can be inhabited productively, thereby refusing communicability's positioning as the primordial grounds for defining and evaluating subjects, subjectivities, and positionalities. This response both acknowledges how communicability and incommunicability are coproduced and turns its back on the binary. It also plays on "in-community," suggesting how finding ways of occupying spaces of incommunicability can turn forms of totalizing repression into collective ways of being, a point I develop later in the interlude, "Social Movements and Incommunicability-Free Zones."[11] Finally, incommunicability invites us to reject communicability as the taken-for-granted starting point, presenting *incommunicability as an alternative analytic*. The term thus turns the tables by repositioning communicability *within* incommunicability, thereby dislodging communicability from its ideological dominance in defining language, medicine, and other domains and challenging hegemonic practices.[12]

The term also helps extend Audra Simpson's insights into refusal in her powerful book *Mohawk Interruptus*. She details how the Mohawks of Kahnawà:ke often refused the culturalist and subordinating forms of multicultural recognition that denied the sovereignty that rightfully belong to "a precontact Indigenous polity" (2014, 2). Multicultural recognition constitutes a matrix of communicable strategies, purporting to offer subjects projected as incarcerated by culture (Appadurai 1998) the possibility of being granted status as communicable subjects in exchange for disidentifying with stigmatized forms of incommunicability. Turning away from offers of communicable redemption opens up spaces of refusal marked by performing forms of incommunicability associated with what is projected as the inability to claim the rights of Canadian citizenship. Embracing incommunicability "understands the terms of bondage, and chooses to stay within them" (Simpson 2014, 24). This refusal provides critical perspectives on how settler colonialism ties communicability to white supremacy, thereby rendering any alternatives incommunicable. As an ethnographer, Simpson (113) embraces this "theoretically generative" space of refusal, thereby incorporating tactics of refusal into her own work in ways "that can both *refuse* and also take up *refusal* in generative ways." Accordingly, refusal opens up possibilities for embracing incommunicability as an analytical point of departure and for supporting efforts to unseat dominant forms of communicability.

Reflecting on Spillers's, Shange's, and Simpson's provocations made me realize that biocommunicabilities produce constructions of incommunicable voices, flesh, forms of knowledge, and practices and tie them to sites where bodies are deemed problematic. Health professionals attempt to monopolize the agency required to define, classify, surveil, and discipline ways of talking about health; in doing so, they create incommunicabilities, assessing perceived failures of communicability and stigmatizing articulations that lie outside authorized registers, sites, and channels as incommunicable. Like the positioning of "Black girl ordinary" in educational settings, subjects who actively refuse the social, political, educational, and medical promises of communicability expose the claims to transparency, causality, and authority on which communicability rests, including its underpinnings in white supremacy, thereby opening up possibilities for creating or enacting alternatives. Such insights, I argue, challenge us to decolonize fundamental understandings of language and communication, health and medicine and join efforts to craft alternatives.

Bridging the Divide between Medical and Linguistic Anthropology

In pursuing this goal, I find myself up against ways that anthropology is subdisciplined, structured in such a way that medical and linguistic anthropologists generally inhabit separate, sometimes opposing, analytical frameworks, research practices, curricular trajectories, American Anthropological Association sections, and journals. The bibliographies of works in linguistic, medical anthropology, and social/cultural anthropology, even those focusing on the same objects of research, often show little overlap. When graduate programs recruit faculty and graduate students, the processes are often separate and sometimes are guided by a zero-sum logic: if more resources are allocated to that other field, ours will be shortchanged. Even when advanced graduate students and new PhDs coming from different fields are investigating the same phenomena, they often do not know that researchers in other subdisciplines have productively and radically revised our understanding of the objects they are analyzing. Medical anthropologists sometimes do not realize that linguistic anthropologists have critically engaged the commonsense notions of multilingualism, translation, meaning, and embodiment that medical anthropologists often employ. Linguistic anthropologists sometimes embrace commonsense definitions of diseases, forms of care, and medical technologies that medical anthropologists have critically engaged.

At the same time, there is a long research tradition—sometimes reflected in graduate training and even more in ways that graduate students and recently trained scholars explore alternative routes—that offers important synergies between linguistic, medical, and social/cultural anthropology and adjacent fields. A major goal of this book is to question the foundational divides that have often marginalized this research and expand on efforts to offer productive bridges. Let me begin by picking up on the insights offered by Shange and Simpson in pointing to how recent work by linguistic anthropologists can extend their insights. The field has been transformed by Black, Latinx, and Native American scholars and others who argue that understandings of race, racism, and racialization will remain analytically and empirically fragmented and incomplete without "viewing race through the lens of language and language through the lens of race to better understand them as co-constitutive processes" (Alim, Reyes, and Kroskrity 2020, 2). Linguistic anthropologists trace how whiteness and white supremacy are authorized by equating them with communicability, with what is projected as a homogeneous, dominant speech code (the Monoglot standard, in Michael Silverstein's [1987] 1996 terms) that purportedly provides unique access to rational, modern ways of thinking and acting. As communicability gets implicitly—and deeply—connected to whiteness, nonwhite bodies get stereotyped as incapable of performing these purportedly superior forms of language and subjectivity.[13] People racialized as white are thus simply presumed to be communicable subjects unless disqualified by stigmas associated with the working class, sexuality, and disability. However, the default status for individuals and populations classified as nonwhite is incommunicability; middle- or upper-class and professional status provides racialized individuals with only partial, temporary escape from the presumption of incommunicability. Rethinking earlier work (Bauman and Briggs 2003), I analyze the role of John Locke in establishing and naturalizing these relations among race, communicability, and rationality; inscribing them into how medical knowledge is created and communicated;

and both equating communicability with whiteness and obscuring its links to white supremacy.

Linguistic anthropologists have denaturalized these tight entanglements of race and language by demonstrating how they often rest on constructions of stigmatized speech that bear little or no relation to people's actual utterances and actions. A crucial reference is Miyako Inoue's analysis of critical commentary by Japanese male intellectuals at the turn of the twentieth century regarding how women's speech seemingly challenged Japanese values and violated standards of acceptable language. Inoue (2003) brilliantly demonstrated that a highly visible and stigmatized class of incommunicable subjects can be performatively constructed by inventing what are claimed to be ways that its members actually speak, even when the semiotic markers of incommunicability are fictive. She argued that the Meiji male intellectual thereby constructed himself "as a particular historical subject" by becoming the "auditory double" of the schoolgirl. The power of models of incommunicability is thus revealed by how they can create communicable authority and incommunicable stigma in ways that bring categories of subjects into being and attach them to people, even when their correspondence to actually existing bodies, subjectivities, and modes of communication is thin or nonexistent.[14]

Parallel to how medical anthropologists and others have investigated health inequities, linguistic anthropologists have focused much attention on mapping communicative inequities and identifying the structural forces that produce them. Two recent research trajectories have much to contribute. Extending debates about white supremacy, racism, and racialization, an emerging group of scholars has carved out a field of "raciolinguistics" that seeks to "enhance our understanding of the processes of racialization by highlighting language's central role in the construction, maintenance, and transformation of racial and ethnic identities" (Alim, Rickford, and Ball 2016, 7). Jonathan Rosa and Nelson Flores (2020, 90) focus their analysis on how categories of language and race "have been co-naturalized in particular societal contexts." They draw on Inoue's (2013, 93) work in tracing the centrality of a "white listening subject" that constitutes its racial privilege by imagining incommunicable subjects and communicative practices. They examine how "raciolinguistic ideologies" stigmatize the linguistic practices of racialized populations. Much of this work seeks to go beyond documentation and analysis to contribute to efforts to confront white supremacy globally and promote justice.

Influential work by Jane Hill (2008) has sparked a host of studies of linguistic racism. She drew attention not simply to overt acts of discrimination, which many white people would condemn, but also to covert forms that invisibly reproduce denigrating stereotypes of nonwhite people. A key mechanism here lies in dominant language ideologies, whose roots I trace back to the seventeenth century in chapter 1, that are referential, tied to stable relationships between sound and meanings, and personalistic, seen as expressing the beliefs and intentions of individual speakers. This language ideology positions individuals as the prime interpreters of their words, given that they alone can purportedly access their beliefs and intentions, and it directs attention away from the harm that racist speech inflicts on people and populations targeted by stereotypes. Work by Laura Graham (2011), Hill (2002), Paul Kroskrity (2015), Barbra Meek (2006, 2013), and Bernard Perley (2011) has demonstrated how centrally "language ideological processes of racialization" (Kroskrity 2021, 180; 2020) enter into making and naturalizing denigrating constructions of indigenous people; research by white scholars is sometimes complicit in this process.

Work on raciolinguistics and linguistic racism come together in an impressive recent volume, *The Oxford Handbook of Language and Race* (Alim, Reyes, and Kroskrity 2020). I find it interesting that none of the book's twenty-one chapters focuses on health, medicine, or health care.[15] Health—including limited access and poor quality of health care; medical profiling; and higher rates of illness, death, and maternal and child mortality—are principal sites in which racism is constructed and experienced. Clinical settings are crucial spaces in which linguistic profiling is enacted as patients, simply on the basis of their racial classification, are judged to be incommunicable, as speaking the wrong languages or language varieties, being less able to understand their providers, and less capable or willing to assimilate the biomedical knowledge they are provided and less capable of transforming it into "healthy behaviors." Media representations of how health, communication, and race intersect project denigrating forms of linguistic and medical racism to millions of viewers and readers, thereby continually infusing old stereotypes with new political and medical content (Briggs and Hallin 2016). As I detail in chapter 6, the health education components of global health programs transport North American and European racialized projections of health and communication around the world by embedding them in interventions that claim to alleviate health inequities through infusions of communicability, often without addressing their structural roots or providing better access to health care. When incorporated into clinical practices, health education, and media representations, these entanglements of linguistic and medical racism inform unhealthy health policies (Castro and Singer 2004), thereby amplifying the denigrating effects of these embodied inequities. This book argues that research on language, race, racism, and racialization is analytically and empirically limited if subdisciplinary boundaries push health off the map of linguistic anthropologists. It also suggests why linguistic anthropologists have much to offer in studying and confronting medical inequities. Indeed, if constructions of language, speaking practices, and speakers are important means of creating and policing racial hierarchies, even as medicine and health are some of the key ways that racial inequities are embodied—with crucial effects on who lives and who dies—the need for more research that systematically explores their connections seems crucial.

There are, moreover, countercurrents of research that fruitfully connect issues of language and health. Gregory Bateson (1972) used close studies of interaction in seeking social causes for psychiatric disorders. Aaron Cicourel (1992) made significant contributions to linguistic and medical anthropology based on decades of research in and on medical schools. Drawing on the ethnography of communication and other frameworks in linguistic anthropology, Michael Agar (1973) conducted decades of research on drug use and treatment. Elinor Ochs used interaction analysis and video ethnography to illuminate such conditions as agoraphobia and autism (Capps and Ochs 1995; Ochs 2015). Arthur Kleinman (1988) showed scholars and caregivers alike the value of "illness narratives" in providing insight into patients' experiences of illness and care and the "explanatory models" they use to make sense of them. Cheryl Mattingly and Linda Garro (2000) have emphasized the importance, complexity, and multiple ways that narratives shape illness and healing, and Mattingly (1998) drew our attention to how their plots can be enacted corporeally and verbally. Byron Good (1994) offered a semiotic analysis of medical knowledge and practice that attends to details of the language and aesthetics of patients' articulation of their complaints. In identifying "idioms of distress," Mark Nichter (1981, 2008) documented a broader semiotics that links referential and nonreferential dimensions of speech with somatic, material, and other modes of experiencing and expressing distress and deconstructed how biomedicine deems only particular ways of understanding health and disease and defining practitioners and patients to be legitimate. Charles Goodwin's (2010) sensitive studies of his father traced how aphasia patients collaborate with others in effecting interaction and creating meaning. David Parkin's (2013) work brings together extensive research on both language and healing modalities in eastern Africa. I have used critical linguistic and medical anthropological approaches to explore how communicative- and health-based types of profiling intersect during outbreaks and epidemics (Briggs and Mantini-Briggs 2003, 2016). Joel Kuipers (1989) and James Wilce (2009) crafted review articles that explore points of contact between linguistic and medical anthropology and scholarship that reaches across their boundaries.

Encouragingly, the past decade has witnessed an efflorescence of work that draws deeply on linguistic and medical anthropological perspectives and entwines them in diverse and creative ways. E. Summerson Carr (2011) carefully documents how communicable dimensions of recovery pedagogies imposed on addicts in need of food and shelter reveal connections between linguistic and medical inequities and how clients critically revise them. New analytics and research strategies are needed to grasp the complex and shifting imbrications of media ideologies (Gershon 2010), technologies, and practices, including but not limited to the looming specter of "anti-vaxx" social media networks that algorithms and public health officials cannot tame. Lynette Arnold (2020) documented how migrants use cell-phone conversations to impose biomedical discipline on their relatives back home. Juliana Friend (2022) tracked how sex, modesty, and pleasure circulate digitally in Senegal through both digital health education programs sponsored by non-governmental organizations and online pornography. Xochitl Marsilli-Vargas's (2022) work in Buenos Aires examined how mediatization helps extend psychoanalysis from dyadic clinical interactions into mass media and everyday encounters among laypeople. Mara Buchbinder (2015, 2021) explored the complex relational communicative practices used by adolescent patients, clinicians, and parents in grappling with pain and analyzed how debates and practices around assisted dying often hinge on linguistic as much as medical ideologies. T. S. Harvey (2013) traced the complexities of discursive, material, and embodied practices that unfold in Mayan healing practices and interface with biomedicine. Sonya Pritzker (2014) traced the diverse discursive practices involved in translating Chinese medicine as it moves between China and the United States. Linguistic anthropologists have provided examples of lay care and health communication initiatives that exceed the logics and channels prescribed by professionals. Anna Corwin (2021) assessed claims that Catholic nuns are less prone to dementia by closely following forms of care in interaction provided by other sisters. Bringing together linguistic and medical anthropology and ethnomusicology, Steven Black (2019) documented how HIV-positive members of a South African choir used songs, stories, and jokes in combining Christianity with HIV/AIDS activism and advocacy, thereby engaging audiences that ranged from global "experts" to relatives, neighbors, and other HIV-positive individuals.

In perhaps the most prominent area of overlap between linguistic and medical perspectives, sociologists, linguistic anthropologists, and other scholars, beginning in the 1970s, opened a broad research agenda focused on doctor-patient interaction (Heritage and Maynard 2006). It particularly sprang from work by sociologists building on conversation analysis and ethnomethodology perspectives who used tape recordings and, later, audiovisual recordings of "actual occurrences" of clinical encounters to produce transcriptions that afforded detailed analysis of, in the words of Emanuel Schegloff (1992, 106), "the details of actual occurrences of conduct in interaction." The physician and sociologist Howard Waitzkin (1991) scrutinized how doctor-patient interaction renders clinical medicine complicit in reproducing broader social inequities in clinical spaces and, simultaneously, in hiding their effects behind narrow biomedical logics. Close analysis of language and interaction have been developed for other arenas of care, such as Mattingly's (1998) careful analysis of narrative and healing in occupational therapy and Carr's (2011, 2021) analysis of language and interaction in social work, addiction treatment, and "motivational interviewing" approaches to behavioral intervention. Scholars trained in linguistic and medical anthropology have examined clinical interactions beyond biomedicine (see, e.g., Briggs 1994, 1996; Harvey 2013; Pritzker 2014). Doctor-patient interaction is a remarkable example in which academic research has transformed professional practices, as taken up by physicians, nurses, and the faculties who train them. Clinical training now includes videos that model how physicians should interact with their patients to maximize biocommunicability. Students gain practice in enacting biocommunicability through staged interactions in which they interview people trained to act as patients and through evaluations of audiovisual recordings of patient encounters.

One of the most fruitful areas in which synergy between the two fields can emerge lies in attention to issues of inequity and profiling. Researchers have demonstrated that Black and Latinx patients receive lower-quality health care than white patients, even after controlling for socioeconomic status and health insurance (Smedley, Stith, and Nelson 2003). Strong evidence of medical profiling emerged from work by Michelle Van Ryn and Jane Burke (2000), who found that US physicians assumed that Black patients abused drugs and alcohol more frequently and were less educated and intelligent, less attentive to medical guidance, and less likely to follow treatment guidelines. Systemic health inequities are often individualized as questions of communicative incompetence, bad behavior, lifestyle, ignorance, or noncompliance. Medical anthropologists have studied health inequities ethnographically. To name just a few examples, Dána-Ain Davis (2019) sensitively documented how medical racism positions Black female professionals—despite their apparent class privileges—as more likely to face premature and low-birthweight infants. Work on HIV/AIDS (Farmer 1992; Sangaramoorthy 2014) and diabetes (Doucet-Battle 2021; Moran-Thomas 2019) has analyzed how systemic health inequities are often individualized and misrepresented as questions of bad behavior, lifestyle, ignorance, or culture. Carolyn Rouse (2009) showed how doctors normalized requests by sickle cell patients for pain medications through a stereotype of Black patients as manipulating practitioners to satisfy drug addictions. Social justice perspectives have helped change conversations about health, locating scholars as part of broader efforts initiated by members of medically underserved populations and social movement organizations to confront inequities (see Krieger 2011).

To extend research that challenges linguistic-medical scholarly boundaries and suggest the importance of these efforts in addressing justice issues, I have used the concept of *health/communicative inequities*. The term uses a lexical juxtaposition to suggest how these seemingly discrete axes are deeply connected. A primary focus of this book is on the ideological labor that both coproduces communicative and health inequities and obscures their entanglements, including from scholars and practitioners.[16] Dominant strategies often project communication and medicine as separate, autonomous domains, even as they enmesh them in ways that naturalize health and communicative inequities. A central part of this ideological labor is crafting dominant communicabilities: understandings of how knowledge is made and who makes it, how it travels, who is required to receive it, and how this knowledge should be embodied. With reference to biomedicine, one way that dominant biocommunicabilities become powerful is by framing them as direct reflections of how communication and medicine work. Any gaps between these idealized, abstract, hierarchizing models and facts on the ground are deemed problematic, requiring a search for what seems to have gone wrong and who is responsible.

Here is where incommunicability comes in. Although gaps between ideological models and the pragmatics of how communication and medicine unfold are unavoidable, they usually get blamed on people with the least power and access to linguistic and medical resources. Judging an individual or population to be incommunicable reifies health and communicative inequities and blames patients for their health problems. The result is not only the stigmatizing of populations but a thwarting of the stated goals of improving health, empowering patients, and fostering cooperation between health professionals and patients. The impact of being judged incommunicable goes far beyond clinical and public health spaces. It not only renders entire populations expendable by obscuring the need to focus on and transform the structural factors that produce grossly inequitable distributions of health, disease, and death, but it defines a baseline of rationality and moral responsibility—stigmatizing members of racialized populations as incapable of saving, or unwilling to save, not only their own lives but those of their family members.[17] By critically engaging how established perspectives and practices systematically produce incommunicability through processes—such as doctor-patient communication and health communication and their institutional and global extensions—I hope to help remove one of the major roadblocks to fundamental changes and make a significant contribution to achieving justice. Far from condemning by fiat all health professionals as conspiring to advance this project, I try to highlight here how some clinicians and public health practitioners work with social movements to craft alternatives.

A Reader's Guide to the Book

This book moves through a wide range of issues, fields, and analytics and is in dialogue with multiple interlocutors. At the same time that I incorporate examples available in the published literature, as well as from a broad range of media sources, the argument draws on nearly four decades of research that brings together linguistic, medical, and media anthropology, mostly conducted in Venezuela and the United States. I have worked in many areas of Venezuela, but mainly in the Delta Amacuro rainforest on the country's eastern edge. People I met there in 1985 thought that studying the indigenous language, called Warao, might be of value to efforts to establish bilingual education programs and help improve health services. Racialized health inequities, including unconscionable levels of infant and child mortality, tuberculosis, and malaria, meant that issues of health, disease, healing, and death pervaded everyday life and conversation and emerged in a host of verbal and musical genres. These range from mythic narratives and gossip to healing songs and chants, funerary laments, and performances of political speech that advanced demands for an end to centuries of crushing colonial policies and practices. I witnessed outbreaks of cholera in 1992 and rabies in 2008, events that first led me to assist with public health and clinical efforts and then conduct research designed to figure out why so many people died from diseases that can be prevented, respectively, by clean water and vaccinations. In both of these cases, I collaborated with a remarkable Venezuelan public health physician, Dr. Clara Mantini-Briggs. A central focus throughout was linking perspectives and practices of nurses and physicians with those offered by healers. I also draw on research in other areas of Venezuela that documents how underserved communities and progressive professionals and political leaders crafted bold alternatives to unhealthy health policies (Castro and Singer 2004), as inspired by the Bolivarian socialist revolution led by President Hugo Chávez Frías.

Working in cholera and rabies outbreaks was, in a word, devastating. I promised myself that I would never investigate another epidemic. Then along came COVID-19 in 2020. Teaching and administrative duties were so overwhelming during the first year and a half that I had little time to think about research. My affiliation with the Latinx Research Center at the University of California, Berkeley, led me to collaborate with eight undergraduates, two graduate students, and Mantini-Briggs in launching the Latinx COVID-19 Auto-ethnography Collective, starting in January 2021. Dr. Mantini-Briggs and I wanted to support UC Berkeley undergraduates' efforts to reflect on and confront through activist interventions the effects of the pandemic in augmenting the impact of racialized inequities of education, health, housing, employment. Weekly, laterally organized meetings over Zoom enabled us to share our experiences of the pandemic. Their accounts of being displaced from their UC Berkeley dorms and apartments, losing jobs, caring for relatives, and trying to forge new futures after the pandemic led me to begin to think about the effects of COVID-19 and mitigation measures.

In July 2021, a sabbatical leave gave me time to look more broadly at how the pandemic affected people's lives, work, fundamental assumptions about the world, and visions for the future. I thus began interviewing physicians, psychiatrists, physician assistants, nurses, dentists, public health officials, journalists, community-based organizations, elected officials, judges, educators, religious professionals, firefighters/paramedics, police officers, and laypeople. I have conducted over eighty interviews, some by Zoom; others, in person. When possible, I have stayed in touch with interviewees, learning how their lives and reflections have changed since our conversations. I complemented interviews and observations in California with work in New Mexico and Montana. A month in Montana helped illuminate the complex worlds that people who embrace biocommunicability often reduce to stereotypes about people who are depicted as "anti-vaxxers," "anti-maskers," "conspiracy theorists," and circulators of "misinformation." Conversations with them suggested how they came to view scientists, health professionals, journalists, and public health officials as forming a category of arrogant, prevaricating Others. Complementing interviews with extensive observation enabled me to see how in/communicabilities circulate and how they have been woven into the details of ranching, building, worshipping, shopping, and relaxing—and what happens when people experience COVID-19 symptoms.

Nevertheless, this book is not an ethnography of language and health in a Venezuelan rainforest; nor does it focus entirely on the COVID-19 pandemic. One goal for this book is to upset ways of thinking about these topics that have been in place for some three hundred years. Equally important, I want to provide a resource for scholars and students who are more open to radically different perspectives on what it even means to say "language and health" or "communication and medicine." The book also seeks to assist clinicians, public health professionals, journalists, and community activists in developing new approaches and practices. I hope to contribute to efforts by academics, practitioners, and activists to counter monopolies over biocommunicability—over claims that there is only one legitimate way to produce health knowledge, promote its circulation, and receive and embody it. This process of decolonization must, I think, be designed and deployed in such a way as to effectively counter the projection of particular individuals and populations as unfit for communicability—as incapable or unwilling to assimilate biomedical content and transform it into healthy states, let alone to join in contributing knowledge of health and disease. Here's the crux: I want this book to help eliminate one of the primary excuses for blaming disadvantaged populations for the effects of racialized health, housing, employment, educational, economic, and other inequities and inspire collective efforts to achieve health/communicative justice.

This book is written in modular fashion. I invite you to approach its three working parts in whatever way makes the most sense to you. Part I attempts to provide a new philosophical and analytic base by creating dialogues with four interlocutors. You may know the work of three of them—John Locke, Frantz Fanon, and Georges Canguilhem—but you may not have met them in the guise in which I introduce them: as philosopher-physicians. Few of Locke's vast legions of readers know that he was trained and practiced as a physician. The reason, I suspect, is that he hid it. His *Essay Concerning Human Understanding* was a foundational attempt to cast science and medicine, on the one hand, and language and communication, on the other, as "separate provinces of knowledge." As a result, important connections between these two crucial arenas for the development of semiotics have warranted little attention.[18] Establishing himself as the patron saint of communicability, Locke decreed that only individuals who magically separate body and mind and speak in purely rational, disembodied, transparent, and disinterested fashion could save the world from confusion, discord, and disorder. I want to introduce you to a different Locke, one whose work was shaped by disability and who decreed that disorders of language and disease must be cured by similar reductionist, instrumentalist practices of diagnosis and intervention. By reading Locke against the grain by foregrounding his pervasive anxiety about incommunicability, we can begin to see how, in spite of himself, he can teach us how incommunicability can become a productive force rather than a stigmatizing plague to be stamped out.

Fanon's many readers know that he was both a doctor and a philosopher. His diagnosis of the colonial and racist roots of ill health and his careful presentation of political diagnosis uses the classic clinical method of closely examining details of particular cases, even as he jumped scale to analyze the structural underpinnings of mental illness engendered by colonialism. I connect Fanon as physician and as philosopher of language in exploring his insights into ways that colonialism and racism infect languages and language varieties and how they racialize patients as ipso facto communicable or incommunicable. Locating Fanon as the prophet-in-waiting of the field of doctor-patient interaction studies that would emerge decades later, I suggest that his trenchant, angry, and ironic critique of how colonial physicians speak to their patients holds the key to analyzing pedagogies that currently promise to teach providers how to be better communicators. Even as his focus is on highly racialized and denigrating examples, he opens up the possibility of taking a broader approach in analyzing how caregivers more generally can render patients incommunicable. Fanon also pinpointed how denigrating images of Blackness in media texts prefigure the violence sparked by anti-Black racism.

The transition from Locke to Fanon is bridged by a dialogue with W. E. B. Du Bois, especially his *The Souls of Black Folk*. He provides a powerful voice for countering Locke's claims for the universal primordiality of communicability and disrupting its implicit connections to whiteness. Writing decades before Fanon, Du Bois ([1903] 1990, 8) analyzed how racialized media forms and everyday racist acts, along with pervasive structural inequities, require Black people to practice double-consciousness, "this sense of always looking at one's self through the eyes of others," that induces a painful splitting of the subject. In discussing his concept of "the Veil," I follow his keen analysis of how racism produces white incommunicability vis-à-vis Black social worlds, thwarting the ability of white people to perceive them or to gain awareness of their own myopia. Du Bois layers his texts with stylistic and generic shifts in such a way as to move between analyzing and performing the entanglement of communicability with incommunicability. I sit uncomfortably with the powerful chapter that recounts the death of his eighteen-month-old child. The chapter leaves me with a troubling question. The figure of the doctor enters the story not through an analysis of racialized inequities but through a visit by a "gray physician," who arrives as the child is dying. I reflect on the racial health inequities that might have helped lead to the death, wondering that Du Bois did not work this element into the impressive mosaic he provides of the effects of anti-Black racism in *The Souls of Black Folk*.

My third philosopher-physician is Foucault's teacher, Georges Canguilhem. Alas, he does not join Du Bois and Fanon in shattering the illusion that bodies, minds, and patients are individual, deracialized, and universal. Canguilhem does, however, make a powerful contribution to the primary focus of the book: how health professionals' efforts to promote biocommunicability often systematically produce incommunicability. Canguilhem carefully reflects on how patients' experience with a chronic or prolonged illness forces them to reexperience their bodies and how they are situated vis-à-vis space, others, and the world. He shows that these new spaces are not interpretable through the lenses patients had used in negotiating their prior, "normal" lives. The pathological state instead becomes the only world that is experientially accessible. Physicians, in a nutshell, make things worse. In clinical encounters, doctors ask these patients to calibrate their world, point by point, in terms that spring from anatomy and physiology, from understandings of how organs are supposed to function. Physicians thus ask patients to use a lost language to describe corporeal worlds that seem alien and confusing. In the process, physicians not only impede what would later come to be known as doctor-patient communication but undermine patients' struggles to know and articulate the pathological worlds that are becoming "normal" for them. Canguilhem will later help us at various points, including sorting out why attempts to impose biocommunicability as the only legitimate foundation for confronting a complex, sneaky virus named SARS-CoV-2 ended up turning boundaries between communicability and incommunicability into social and political chasms.

Part I has a different structure than you might expect. The last thing I want to do is to turn these interlocutors into tools for constructing a single, overarching, tightly woven framework that purportedly flows from my own ideological labor. Mountains of writing focus on Locke, Fanon, and Du Bois, but I invoke them only sparingly. My reasons are twofold. First, I don't want to drown out their voices and or dilute how they can help us make a fresh start in rethinking in/communicability. Second, I try to avoid oversimplifying their interventions as bodies of content, as propositions that can be easily shuffled into the decks of existing scholarly literatures. This move permits an engagement with figural and formal (or poetic or rhetorical) features of their texts and dimensions of their lives. I have chosen these four figures because they highlight how communicability became a fundamental part of the infrastructure of white supremacy and racial hierarchy and, through the work of Du Bois, Fanon, and Canguilhem, how we can craft a philosophical and analytic base for dismantling it and crafting alternatives. I find reflection on the complex interplay between their lives and their written work provides a productive way to explore these issues.

Part II, however, requires a dialogue of a very different sort. There my dialogic partners are quite different, given that I jump some three hundred years ahead from Locke's foundational move to concentrate on two ways that clinical and public health professionals attempt to cross the divide between medicine and communication. Chapter 5 follows a body of social-science literature that has made a significant difference in how doctors and other health professionals are trained and the fine-grained, moment-to-moment dynamics of how they interact with patients. The ambition is lofty: helping caregivers listen more sensitively to their patients and increasing patients' engagement with their providers. Fanon's early warning sits on my shoulder, however, as I look closely at how this emphasis can enact biocommunicability in ways that can stigmatize patients as incommunicable failures, thereby affecting health outcomes and patients' confidence in providers and forms of care. Chapter 6 shifts to the field of health communication. Building on fieldwork in Venezuela, the chapter complements US-based examples, including some that focus on COVID-19. It traces how biocommunicability jumps scale as health communication programs are exported from the United States, Europe, and international agencies such as the World Health Organization to produce what are sometimes denigrating diagnoses of incommunicability in low- and middle-income countries. An interlude that follows the chapter discusses examples in which populations that face racialized health inequities grabbed hold of biocommunicabilities and used them to forge innovative health communication and healthcare programs.

Part III pivots toward ethnography. Engaging just a fraction of the remarkable conversations I was honored to undertake during the pandemic, I try to figure out what went so terribly wrong in the United States with COVID-19 health communication. Chapter 7 traces a remarkable situation in which research on severe acute respiratory syndrome (SARS) infections—fairly limited despite the major role of SARS viruses in such manifestations as the "common cold" and past epidemics—suddenly become the global priority. Rather than entering into the contested fray of efforts to trace SARS-CoV-2's global footprints, I focus on how health professionals declared a monopoly on the production of knowledge about a remarkably tricky microbe. Even as scientists, physicians, and public health professionals struggled to understand the virus and its effects, they clung to a long-standing communicable model that grants health professionals a monopoly over producing biomedical knowledge. Because laypeople were cast as passive recipients of emerging medical and public health knowledge and guidance, their potential contributions to addressing the pandemic's unanswered questions were dismissed in advance. Nevertheless, many laypeople used their own experience of the pandemic, the archives of health commonsense they had acquired over decades, and the tsunamis of material appearing in mainstream and social media to fill in remaining gaps. I use two ethnographic dialogues to provide depth here: an artist trying to figure out how post-acute sequelae of SARS-CoV-2 infection (PASC), or long COVID, was taking hold of his body and a retired package delivery driver and contractor in Montana whose negative view of COVID-19 communicability led him to reject masking, vaccination, and just about everything health professionals were saying about the disease. I place them in dialogue by exploring how—despite the incredible dissimilarity in their lives and political views—they both felt they were thrown by health professionals and journalists into a space of incommunicability.

Chapter 8 involves dialogues with a more extensive set of interlocutors in reflecting on a conundrum: even as health professionals claimed a monopoly on pandemic knowledge production, they largely passed along the burden of care to laypeople, except when severe symptoms required hospitalization. Undertaking this task, even in the absence of COVID-19 symptoms, required remarkable forms of creativity and collaboration that expanded notions of care far beyond narrow biomedical definitions of prevention and treatment. We listen to the challenges faced by grandparents, students, farmworkers, and people stereotyped as "anti-vaxxers" as they attempt to innovative forms of care and daily living. The very concept of "the pandemic" explodes as viruses, mitigation measures, and their seemingly constantly expanding effects get woven into the fine details of lives, mainly through ongoing relations of care. We also listen to caregivers—firefighters/paramedics, an ICU nurse, an ER doctor, an epidemiologist, and an infectious disease physician—to see what happens when patients do require acute care. Here dominant stereotypes—that of the heroes celebrated by pot-banging neighbors and of arrogant, distanced professionals—collapse as health professionals found themselves sinking into incommunicability even as they attempted to impose biocommunicable authority on patients and lay populations. We learn that many professionals got trapped by the same contradictions between insufficient knowledge and overwhelming burdens of care as laypeople. In the pandemic, biocommunicability was called on to perform the same task in the pandemic that Locke decreed for communicability more than three hundred years ago: locating what are deemed pragmatic failures of communicability, diagnosing their source, and intervening in such a way as to eradicate them. Chapters 7 and 8 demonstrate the continuing failure of the promise of communicability—how claiming monopolies on legitimate knowledge and stigmatizing anyone who challenges them—thwarts efforts to improve health and end health inequities.

I analyze in this book how communicability and incommunicability are relational, such that making seemingly new biocommunicabilities (perpetually required of medical schools and global health programs) and imbuing them with power requires producing new incommunicabilities. I fear that the process still requires making incommunicabilities seem so pathological that they undermine communicability, communication, rationality, and, according to Locke, social order. In short, we could paraphrase a comment that is attributed to Malcolm X about racism: communicability is like a Cadillac; they come out with a new model every year.

My goal in this book has been to help break this cycle. I suggest that it is time to bury the Lockean legacy, which decrees that communication requires diagnoses of miscommunication and interventions whose ethical value is ensured in advance by the claim that they are designed to fix things. One of the major things that went wrong in the United States with COVID-19 is that some 99 percent of the population was continually told that it had nothing worthwhile to contribute to making sense of a new, puzzling disease. On the contrary, I suggest that starting from the assumption that all parties have something significant to offer and then placing their perspectives in dialogue is far more likely to result not just in "buy-in" but in perspectives and actions that generate structural change. My concern in the pages that follow is not just to analyze the negative effects of imposing communicability and stigmatizing all those who are deemed to reject its authority or fail to embrace it. I also point out, particularly in the interlude, ways that groups classified as incommunicable have creatively crafted alternatives, not by denying the value of biomedicine, but by challenging its monopolistic claims. Given the stigmatizing and denigrating effects of classifying people as incommunicable, I end with a proposal that we should collaborate in creating *incommunicability-free zones* and in turning each encounter enacted in medical, educational, public health, and other institutional spaces into efforts to confront health/

communicative inequities and further health/communicative justice. If anthropology can play a leading role in breaking the cycle of the production of incommunicability and helping to end the pervasive role of dominant communicabilities in producing hierarchies, inequities, and stigma, this may be one of its most important contributions to countering a matrix of intellectual quagmires and to promoting health, justice, and dialogue.

PART I

*Philosophical Dialogues in Search
of Incommunicability*

1

THE INCOMMUNICABLE MENACE
LURKING WITHIN LOCKE'S CHARTER
FOR COMMUNICABILITY

It would seem hard to find a more confident communicability than John Locke's founding document of modern European understandings of language and communication, *An Essay Concerning Human Understanding*. Hans Aarsleff's (1982) influential history of linguistic thought is tellingly titled *From Locke to Saussure*, reflecting his positioning of Locke as bringing modern linguistic thinking into existence and thus paving the road that led to the twentieth-century foundational work of Ferdinand de Saussure ([1916] 1959). Locke declared that language had to decide between being the transparent and precise exchange of signs and the most pernicious cause of disorder, conflict, and civil war. As a reviewer pointed out, Locke was not alone in attempting to find ways to communicate with readers and interlocutors; René Descartes, David Hume, and Thomas Hobbes shared this preoccupation. Nevertheless, what is important about Locke's anxiety is the particular form he gave to his efforts, which sparked the larger significance of the *Essay*. In it, Locke brought language into being—that is, as a discrete object with boundaries that must be policed, subject to ways of knowing that are fundamentally different from those other foundational "provinces of knowledge": science and politics.[1] Locke positioned himself outside the ranks of the "master-builders" of the sciences, mentioning Robert Boyle, Christiaan Huygens, Isaac Newton, and Thomas Sydenham. Locke ([1690] 1959, 14) humbly suggested that he was "employed as an under-labourer" who could—by purifying language—help in "clearing the ground a little, and removing some of the rubbish that lies in the way to knowledge." Communicability's enemy, he argued, was the body—particular, positioned, affective, gendered, laboring, actually existing bodies. Ironically, it was Locke's insistence that language's core is pure communicability that enabled him to launch a project that continues to produce and naturalize social hierarchies and practices of subordination more than three hundred years later. Why, accordingly, turn to Locke in tracing histories of *in*communicability and thinking through language and medicine? How perverse, and yet, perhaps, how tantalizing.

After lavishly thanking his patron, Earl Thomas Herbert, then president of the Royal Society, Locke's *Essay* begins with the following lines in his "Epistle to the Reader":

READER,

I HAVE put into thy hands what has been the diversion of some of my idle and heavy hours. If it has the good luck to prove so of any of thine, and thou hast but half so much pleasure in reading as I had in writing it, thou wilt as little think thy money, as I do my pains, ill bestowed. ([1690] 1959, 7)

If we were to read the *Essay* subversively, we might wonder who the "I" might be here. If this "I" is taken as the author of a book that is deeply concerned with severing relations between bodies, knowledge, and language, this opening appeal to "diversion" and "pleasure" might seem rather strange. Locke (8) later argued that when knowledge is passed from one body to another, "taken upon trust from others," it is not truth. When language is tied to particular sorts of bodies (those of women, laborers, children, "illiterate people," and "savages") it cannot become genuinely communicable—that is, transparent, precise, and stable. In the opening lines, however, Locke projected an embodied, social relationship with me, his reader, as he puts the *Essay* in my hands, placing him alongside me in the many spaces I have read it. We face a double conundrum: an invitation to experience "pleasure" in reading a call to disembodiment and affective disengagement, one invested in bodily and material practices, all geared to establishing a regime for analyzing how such claims are produced.

Locke thus seems inadvertently to call into question his self-declared status as the patron saint of the disembodiment of language and knowledge. What, then, should we think about his standing as a "founding father" of

Eurocentric communicability? In another passage in the "Epistle," Locke tells us the story of how it came into being:

Were it fit to trouble thee with the history of this *Essay*, I should tell thee, that five or six friends meeting at my chamber, and discoursing on a subject very remote from this, found themselves quickly at a stand, by the difficulties that arose on every side. After we had awhile puzzled ourselves, without coming any nearer to a resolution of those doubts which perplexed us, it came into my thoughts that we took a wrong course; and that before we set ourselves upon inquiries of that nature, it was necessary to examine our own abilities, and see what objects our understandings were, or were not, fitted to deal with. This I proposed to the company, who all readily assented; and thereupon it was agreed that this should be our first inquiry. Some hasty and undigested thoughts, on a subject I had never before considered, which I set down against our next meeting, gave the first entrance into this Discourse; which having been thus begun by chance, was continued by intreaty; written by incoherent parcels; and after long intervals of neglect, resume again, as my humour or occasions permitted; and at last, in a retirement where an attendance on my health gave me leisure, it was bought into that order thou now seest it. ([1690] 1959, 9)

This passage is an origin story for the *Essay*; it enables Locke to sneak in crucial premises and a powerful teleology. Communicability requires a "course" that proceeds in unilinear fashion through constant motion toward a goal. When this trajectory was arrested by "difficulties that arose on every side," the participants found themselves "at a stand." The *Oxford English Dictionary* suggests that, in Locke's day, "stand" could refer to "a state of being unable to proceed in thought, speech or action; a state of perplexity or nonplus." When communicability is impeded in this fashion, it produces a crisis of incommunicability, one that requires an intervention.[2] Proximal, ad hoc remedial action could not repair the conversation's course: something much more drastic and foundational was required.

Rather than simply throwing up their hands and decrying the cursed nature of language, however, the company's first reaction to the "stand" seems to have been to embrace it, to share a space of puzzlement where doubts and perplexities could be the focus of collective reflection. Might "diversion" and "pleasure" have surfaced there, as well, had they been permitted? Inhabiting this realm of incommunicability might have unlocked assumptions and discursive practices, opening up novel ways of thinking and acting. Locke, being the occupant of the chamber in Shaftesbury's Exeter House in London (Woolhouse 2007, 98), the guiding force behind the meeting, and, crucially, the author of this account, cut off this process as soon as he realized it was taking place. He rejected the possibility of normalizing incommunicability as unavoidable or opening himself up to the space it created. Pathologizing incommunicability, he rather assigned himself the task of providing a diagnosis. Through an act of scalar magic, Locke turned the vignette into a quest to provide a nosology of pathologies of incommunicability and an analysis of their causes. If the preceding sentences give the impression that I am projecting medical terminology onto Locke's efforts to rigidly separate language from science, hold on to your hat. I argue later that this entanglement is deeply embedded in the way he invented—for want of a better term—language and fashioned communicability into a foundation for science and medicine.

Toward a Nosology of Incommunicability

In Locke's world, "language" had a bad reputation. Francis Bacon (1860, 101) denounced language—"the juggleries and charms of words"—as an intrinsically unreliable instrument that only distorted, not contributed to, knowledge. Accordingly, in constructing language and communication as a separate province of knowledge with its own ontology and foundational practices, Locke saved them from their condemnation as threatening the emerging infrastructures of modernity. However, the cost for this act of salvation was twofold: the project required a total commitment to transform communication and language into pure communicability; simultaneously, Locke wove incommunicability deep within their soul, creating a nosology of incommunicability that served—much like haranguing sermons warning that Christians were constantly on the verge of eternal damnation—to recruit his readers to a never-ending project of disembodiment and purification.[3]

A crucial dimension of Locke's work that would have profound implications for the place of communicability in ideologies of language, the body, science, and medicine for centuries to come is what C. B. Macpherson (1962, 231) refers to as "possessive individualism": "The core of Locke's individualism is the assertion that every man is naturally the sole proprietor of his own person and capacities—the absolute proprietor in the sense that he owes nothing to society for them". Communicability was accordingly possessed by individuals, even as each individual's moral worth and value to society could be evaluated by his—in Locke's androcentric lexicon—performance of communicability. More specifically, Locke incarcerated language and understanding in the individual mind. The project of modernity required the growth and exchange of ideas. However, they could not be directly shared with others: "Man, therefore, had by nature his organs so fashioned, as to be fit to frame articulate sounds, which we call words" (Locke [1690] 1959, III.1). In suggesting that making sound "was not enough to produce language," Locke created a multispecies ontology that differentiates humans from parrots and other species over which they have "dominion." He simultaneously subordinated form, the material properties of signs, to "ideas." He warned repeatedly that a focus on the sensuous dimensions of sound undermines the communicable labor of language: conveying ideas. Using the acoustic materiality of languages as more than a vehicle for conveying ideas thereby traps "men" in the realm of pleasure and incommunicability, reducing them to the status of parrots. Setting up the privileging of signifieds over signifiers, which Jacques Derrida ([1967] 1976) viewed as the heart of logocentrism right through Saussure and Claude Lévi-Strauss, Locke decreed that language requires having an idea in the mind first, which can then be paired with sounds. Herein lies the basis in Locke's foundational communicative ideology for one of the major limitations of how communication is conceptualized, enacted, and evaluated in medicine and public health: the isolated individual as its ontological locus. Here we can similarly locate an intellectual infrastructure for the personalist dimensions of white language ideologies that Jane Hill (2008) analyzed as obscuring the effects of linguistic racism.

Locke's nosology of incommunicable pathology is rooted in his origin story of language. Simple ideas are seemingly relatively immune to incommunicability, given that they emerge directly "from the existence of things" via the senses (Locke [1690] 1959, III.v.2). Incommunicability slips in right away, however, because economy of expression requires that words move, in pragmatic terms, from tokens to types, from particulars to classes of similar entities. This practice of decontextualization involves "separating from them the circumstances of time and place" (III.iii.4). From then on, the threat of incommunicability is always present as simple ideas get combined in "mixed modes," which involves making connections in the mind that do not correspond directly to "the existence of things." Given that complex modes pick out only some common characteristics of simple ideas and overlook others, the incommunicable threat expands as individuals include and exclude different features as they pursue this classification-and-combination process. Things get worse as people unthinkingly reproduce words they acquire through "education, custom, and the constant din of their party" (II.xxxiii.18). Locke extends the personalist locus of language in suggesting that communicability depends on recognizing that "words, in their primary or immediate signifi-cation, stand for nothing but the ideas in the mind of him that uses them" (III.xx.1). Tying words to "the ideas supposed to be in other men's minds" or in "the reality of things" (III.xx.4) is a recipe for incommunicability.[4]

The eighth circle of incommunicable hell comes, however, in the form of "the cheat and abuse of words," the "willful" disruption of fixed sound-idea relations. Here we find phatic uses of language (Jakobson 1960), where refer-ence is either absent or irrelevant, using words to signify ideas with which they are not reliably associated, and using obscure terms to dazzle or con-fuse hearers ("affected obscurity," in Locke's [(1690) 1959, III.x.3] terms). The worst incommunicable sin of all is rhetoric, by which Locke means uses of language for aesthetic effects or to persuade rather than to aid disinterested, rational reflection on the world. As Renato Barilli (1989) carefully traces, Locke participated here in a centuries-long effort to reduce the semantic and cultural scope of the concept of rhetoric to conscious attempts to use the seductive properties of form (or poetics, to return to Jakobson) to overpower the rational faculties of listeners and prompt them to do the speaker's bid-ding. Rejecting the possibility of connecting words with meanings in other "men's" minds helps close off the power of rhetoric that fosters interactional connections between self and other, positioning Locke as the opposite num-ber of Jacques Lacan's ([1966] 1977) view of language.

For Locke, incommunicability required a constant labor of imposing per-fect communicability, disciplining one's language. Worst of all, engaging in "the cheat and abuse of language" prompted becoming "the *slave* of vain-glory, ambition, or a party" ([1690] 1959, III.xi.7, emphasis added). Here we might want to reposition Hortense Spillers's connection between incommunicability and the total violence of slavery to look at how racialized violence and com-municability get connected. Locke invested in a corporation that transported enslaved people from the Gold Coast for sale in the West Indies and drew up a contract for and helped administer the "Council of Trade and Plantations" (Woolhouse 2007, 111) that regulated slave labor on New World plantations. Did this engagement with the violence inflicted on enslaved bodies in Africa and the American colonies afford him a privileged position to reflect on how slavery might enter into mis/understandings of language? Locke was thus invested, literally, in turning Black bodies into property. He also connected property to race, as Audra Simpson (2014, 101) points out, by suggesting that nature is turned into private property when mixed with forms of labor as-sociated with European and colonial forms of expropriation.

Characterizations of Asia and the Americas are common in the *Essay and Treatises*, reflecting Locke's status as "an enthusiastic though critical reader of travellers' accounts" (Gascoigne 2009, 541). Locke's colonial imaginary was informed by discussions in the Royal Society, of which he was a member, that exploited what its *Philosophical Transactions* called "'the advantage, which England injoyes of making Voyages into all parts of the World'" (quoted in Gascoigne 2009, 547) by training travelers to provide accounts of peoples they encountered that would be "appropriate for the stuff of natural history." The Americas, in particular, formed a site of nature untouched by reason: "The Woods and Forests, where irrational untaught Inhabitants keep right by following Nature" (Locke [1690] 1960, I.vi.58). Lumping together "merchants and lovers, cooks and tailors" (III.xi.10), "the day labourer in a country village" ([1706] 1966, 39), women, children, and the people of Asia and the Americas as unable to reflect rationally on language, this exclusionary logic positioned white, elite, European men as embodiments of communicability. Locke's map of communicability was thus built on a framework of colonial knowledge, power, and racial violence. Communicability was thus connected with the commodification of nonwhite bodies and nature as two tracks available to European, white, elite men to demonstrate rationality and agency and constitute themselves as political subjects. The point is not just that Locke profited from the slave trade but that communicability became a key foundation for slavery and colonialism as ontoepistemological, political, and economic projects and for the forms of white supremacy and racism that constitute their ongoing bitter fruit.

Incommunicability was as scalar as it was pernicious. Even as individuals could be "perpetually entangled" in the "endless labyrinth" of rhetoric (Locke [1690] 1959, III.x.9), incommunicability—particularly as promulgated by philosophers—"hath invaded the great concernments of human life and society; obscured and perplexed the material truths of law and divinity; brought confusion, disorder, and uncertainty into the affairs of mankind; and if not destroyed, yet in a great measure rendered useless, these two great rules, religion and justice" (III.x.12). These references reflect the book's emergence in tremendously chaotic times. Locke observed the violence of the English Civil Wars, both through periods in which he enjoyed high position and those in which he was faced with royal censure due to decades of work as Shaftesbury's philosopher and scribe (Woolhouse 2007). Locke positioned himself as able to diagnose the pathology that formed the roots of violence—incommunicability—and to assess its potential for social and political disruption.

Why all the medical metaphors? Having asserted that blurring the borders of the "provinces of knowledge" is a cardinal sin of incommunicability, we could accuse Locke of bad faith—or, at least, of a lack of full disclosure. In one of the vignettes that ground the philosophical framework of the *Essay*, Locke reports that he "was once in a meeting of very learned and ingenious physicians" in which he settled a heated debate by showing that it arose because the participants each defined a crucial term in different ways ([1690] 1959, III. ix.16). How might Locke have gained entrance into this conversation? Never does he mention in the *Essay* his training as a physician, receiving a bachelor of medicine and a license to practice, serving as Lord Shaftesbury's physician, treating patients (if somewhat infrequently), or drafting two (unpublished) books on anatomy and medicine (Anstey 2011; A. N. Williams 2005; Woolhouse 2007).

Locke studied at Christ Church, Oxford, from 1652 to 1667. Milton (2001, 224) suggests that, having rejected legal and religious careers, Locke turned to medicine as an occupation. He worked with noted physicians and participated in a group of natural philosophy experimentalists that included Hooke, Boyle, and Richard Lower (309), who introduced Locke to medicine (Cranston 1957, 40). Locke appears to have begun seeing patients only once he moved to London and sought out Syndenham, one of his "master-builders." Michel Foucault ([1963] 1973, 22) calls Syndenham "the initiator of classificatory thought," having "defined what might be a historical and geographical consciousness of disease." Georges Canguilhem credits Sydenham with delimiting diseases and finding their natural order. For Sydenham, "There are disease species just as there are animal or plant species" (Canguilhem [1966] 1978, 42). Particularly interested in plague and smallpox epidemics, Syndenham published *Methodus curandi febres, propriis observationibus suprastructura* in 1666. Locke accompanied Syndenham in his visits to patients, particularly those recovering from smallpox, having devised a new treatment. Beyond his departure from medical protocol, Syndenham's practice was controversial due to his reliance on the natural history of the illness of individual patients (Dewhurst 1963, 35), as the book's subtitle suggests. This collaboration, in biographer Roger Woolhouse's (2007, 80–81) words, "completely transformed [Locke's] thinking not only about medicine but about our knowledge of the natural world in general." His friends called him "Dr. Locke" (320).

This influence was not unidirectional. The first edition of Syndenham's *Methodus* relied on speculative reasoning that Locke, influenced by mechanical philosophy, rejected. In later editions, Locke's philosophical orientation moved

Syndenham toward a skeptical, observational framework. They collaborated on two unpublished works, "Anatomia" and "De Arte Medica," which elaborated the observational, natural history of disease approach. Their collaboration was so close that historians debate whether Locke wrote these works or served as Syndenham's scribe.

Patrick Romanell discusses a fragmentary note, intended for a preface to Syndenham's work on smallpox, that Locke wrote in 1670, some two years into their collaboration and a year before writing the *Essay*'s first draft. Romanell identifies an idea central to Locke's approach to medicine that, Romanell argues, becomes the *Essay*'s core principle: "Man cannot attain certainty with respect to hypotheses about questions of fact, because the human mind is too limited in capacity to know 'the essence of things'" (Romanell 1958, 198). In short, the world, like Clifford Geertz's (1973, 28–29) turtles, is incommunicability all the way down. Rather than a direct methodological and epistemological transfer from medicine to work on language and knowledge, as Romanell seemingly suggests, I see the relationship as dynamic and dialogic, viewing Locke's promotion of communicability as shaping his approach to medicine just as his medical engagement deeply informed his theory of language. I would also leave room for the influence of "master-builders" Boyle and Newton and other experimental natural philosophers. My assessment is less celebratory than that of many historians of science and medicine. Rather than lauding Locke and Syndenham for helping shape medicine in ways that presaged contemporary biomedicine, I am interested in how the language/medicine synergy rooted white supremacy, colonialism, and ableism within dominant understandings of knowledge, language, and medicine.

Syndenham's practice was driven by the principle that "'whatever is useful is good'" (Romanell 1958, 310), shaping Locke's proto-utilitarianism. Medicine, Locke similarly suggested, must be practical, directed toward curing diseases and extending human well-being. Poetry, rhetoric, and other uses of language for pleasure were useless, at best, because they did not advance the ends of language: "recording our own thoughts for the help of our own memories" and serving as "the easiest and shortest way of communicating our notions" ([1690] 1959, III.ix.108). The use of language in writing a book, the task in which he was engaged, is similarly justifiable only when "it may be useful to others." Locke (13) warned in the "Epistle" that "it savours more of vanity or insolence to publish a book for any other end." Sara Ahmed (2019, 8) calls attention to Locke's emphasis on use in *Two Treatises of Government* ([1690] 1960), emphasizing proper, industrious uses of land, as in converting it into property and wealth, thus shaping "how the category of 'unused' was used to justify the colonial appropriation of land." I would argue that notions of use and usefulness were equally crucial in constructing knowledge and medicine.

Locke was interested in finding ways to communicate his ideas to his readers, but his approach created several difficulties. Under the guise of functionalism, it enabled him to slip a very narrow view of language and communication under the door, positioning his brand of communicability as the only route to achieving understanding. As I have argued, a great deal of the *Essay* is devoted to discrediting other perspectives on language and modes of structuring communicative practices; branded as linguistic pathologies, they required constant surgical intervention. Constructing opposing modes of knowing, communicating, and embodying as markers of incommunicability, Locke brought into being categories of defective subjects who were ineligible for participation in modern projects until projects of surveillance and instruction had run their far-from-inevitable course. Finally, communicative functionalism enabled him to fashion communicability from the racialized odds and ends of colonialism, making it a key embodiment of whiteness that was exquisitely useful in constructing and naturalizing colonial projects. This chapter has, I hope, helped establish that tracing relations among race, communicability, and incommunicability is far more than a US preoccupation. These connections have deep and broad consequences, even if they hardly achieved the status of universals.

This issue brings me to a major point I raise in this book. I examine multiple ways that biocommunicability produces incommunicability, re/producing hierarchies that undermine efforts by people who are not professionals to contribute to the production of health knowledge. Health professionals do not necessarily have an intrinsic love of biocommunicability, given that it can interfere with efforts to provide care in as speedy a manner as possible and can afford spaces in which challenges to medical authority emerge. Some health professionals similarly struggle to counter the violence of biocommunicability in inscribing images of incommunicability on patients' bodies and thereby reproducing health inequities. So how did biocommunicability become such an essential part of biomedical infrastructures? Biocommunicability is generally justified on utilitarian grounds as promoting better patient outcomes, as necessary to make biomedical interventions successful. Biocommunicability, moreover, becomes imperative to the extent that it is deemed necessary to extirpate the very incommunicability that it creates. Given that medical profiling produces incommunicability in "encounters" with racialized patients and patient populations, racialization increases the power of logics of necessity and utility exponentially, a point that gains importance in discussing Frantz Fanon's contributions in chapter 3.

A remarkable difference—and hidden similarity—between Locke's medical perspective and language philosophy lies in issues of the body. The human body was a central focus in Locke's medical writing and practice. At the same time, Locke performs a disappearing act on the body in the *Essay*. Despite his concentration on the mind and sensation, he disavows any interest in physical considerations or bodily dimensions ([1695] 1714, 1). Demanding that speech be disembodied, severed of any connection to particular bodies, he excludes agricultural workers ("Where the Hand is used to the Plough and the Spade" [II:540]), laborers (as preoccupied with the struggle for survival), and women (as focused on reproduction). Whom does this leave out? The subject who can undertake a Lockean process of purifying language is male, elite, European, and adult. Moreover, the body, for Locke, is an ableist body. In suggesting that understanding is like "the eye," which "takes no notice of itself," he seems to foreclose the possibilities that eyes might confront disabling conditions. Communicability requires unimpeded sensory engagement with phenomena to have a firm idea of them, thus ensuring the reliability of language's Lockean semiotic foundation: simple ideas. Disabilities present disqualifications that result in incommunicability: words "are not intelligible at all" when "another has not organs or faculties to attain; as the names of colours to a blind man, or sounds to a deaf man" (III.ix.106).

Nevertheless, Locke's own body thrusts itself foundationally into making the *Essay*. Here I come back to the words in the first sentence of the "Epistle" that gave me pause: why were the hours he spent writing the *Essay* "idle and heavy"? He later elaborates that the book's completion required "a retirement where an attendance on my health gave me leisure." Locke had a chronic disability. As the physician and historian A. N. Williams (2005, 85) reports, "Throughout his life, Locke's health was blighted by asthma, which often incapacitated him for long periods." Much as he was drawn to London's scientific, medical, and philosophical circles, Locke was periodically forced to leave the city due to the coughing and respiratory insufficiency that resulted from its highly polluted air. This condition became so acute at times that Locke believed that he was dying (Woolhouse 2007, 105). Locke also faced problems with his legs, which sometimes kept him bedridden (429). Ironically, a disabled philosopher-physician provides a foundational ableist argument for the centrality of communicability that relies on tying the looming specter of incommunicability to disability.

Language has never fully recovered from Locke's banishment of poetics, rhetoric, context, indexicality, and embodiment—that is, of everything but communicability and reference. Ah, but what about incommunicability? It became the antithesis of modernity, the source of confusion, disorder, and violence. Threatening to appear at every turn, incommunicability was forever condemned to a teleological, never-ending game of whack-a-mole, constantly in need of being squashed in favor of communicability. Locke ([1690] 1959, IV.xxi.4) vociferously tried to expel the body and medicine from the province of "the right use of signs in order to knowledge," and he ardently demanded that we patrol the borders of the provinces of language, science, and politics and discipline trespassers. These fetishistic exclusionary efforts positioned communicability as the only authorized, rational way to think about language and communication. They simultaneously gave rise to proliferating forms of incommunicability that constantly threatened white, male, elite, European, ableist control over language and the body. Getting framed as referential, instrumental, teleological, and in constant need of policing and intervention turned medical discourse into the secret twin of communicability. The remaining chapters of this book analyze such efforts to diagnose and extirpate incommunicability and how this fixation thwarts scholarship and practice.

Before we get there, let's think about what might happen if we returned to the primordial moment of Locke's "meeting at my chamber" and decided to stay in the space of incommunicability. A first step would be to open up the meeting to bodies that are not male, white, elite, and European. We need to go further in asking for assistance in disarming the communicability-incommunicability binary itself. Who might help us deepen analytics that can enable us to stay within the incommunicable—and sometimes uncomfortable—space that Savannah Shange opened up in dialogue with her student interlocutors and that Simpson found in Mohawk practices of refusal? If Locke's legacy haunts us at every turn, we will need to draw insights from interlocutors who can help us keep from simply reproducing implicit links between white supremacy and communicability. Advancing this project requires listening to people forced to speak from within spheres of incommunicability, which I do in the remaining chapters of part I.

2

W. E. B. DU BOIS

Incommunicability and/as the Veil

How can we exorcise John Locke's curse of communicability and simultaneously turn his frightened and frightening attunement to the pervasiveness
of incommunicability into new ways to challenge and inhabit the perceived
chasm between language and communication, medicine and the body? Just
over two centuries later, William Edward Burghardt Du Bois's *The Souls of
Black Folk* provided a hymn to incommunicability whose tones still resonate
more than a century after its publication. Du Bois was born to a family of poor
agriculturalists in Great Barrington, Massachusetts, in 1868. He graduated
from Fisk University in 1888 and Harvard in 1890; with his 1895 dissertation
on the slave trade, he became the first Black person to earn a doctorate from
Harvard. Teaching at Atlanta University, Du Bois enlisted the social sciences in
attacking notions of racial inferiority. Lee Baker (1998, 139–40) valuably places
Du Bois within a broad context, writing, "In most cases, African American
social scientists were motivated by activism and the need to develop strategies
to solve social problems. In addition, they followed their artistic counterparts
and ignored discipline-specific boundaries by blurring the lines that delineated

them. In this respect, the scholars who emerged during the New Negro Movement foreshadowed multidisciplinary approaches to research."

As Booker T. Washington's industrial education program threatened support for Black higher education, Du Bois left for New York to become the founding editor of the National Association for the Advancement of Colored People's magazine *Crisis*. He traveled to Russia and China, defended socialism, and participated actively in peace conferences that challenged US Cold War politics. Du Bois was indicted in 1951 as a foreign agent and acquitted; he became a member of the Communist Party of the USA in 1961. Although much of his writing focused on the United States, Du Bois (1940, 132) challenged "provincial attitudes" toward race relations. Developing a cosmopolitan, global view of race relations, imperialism, and capitalism (see Briggs 2005b; Edwards 2003; Gilroy 1993; Posnock 1998), he stressed that US civil-rights struggles needed to connect with antiracist efforts in other countries.

Writing at the turn of the twentieth century, Du Bois illuminated how incommunicability structures the experience of Blackness in the United States and relations between Black and white people. Two of his most famous analytics—the Veil and double-consciousness—pinpoint how racism engenders incommunicabilities and produces their profound, pervasive impact:

> The Negro is a sort of seventh son, born with a veil, and gifted with second-sight in this American world,—a world which yields him no true self-consciousness, but only lets him see himself through the revelation of the other world. It is a peculiar sensation, this double-consciousness, this sense of always looking at one's self- through the eyes of others, of measuring one's soul by the tape of a world that looks on in amused contempt and pity. One ever feels his two-ness,—an American, a Negro; two souls, two thoughts, two unreconciled strivings; two warring ideals in one dark body, whose dogged strength alone keeps it from being torn asunder. (Du Bois [1903] 1990, 8–9)

In joining the many efforts to interpret this famous passage, I hope to make a modest contribution by focusing on how it—and other passages in *Souls*—provides us with a productive approach for developing analytics of incommunicability. Du Bois's picture of double-consciousness is far from contemporary celebratory understandings that depict individuals with open access to multiple intellectual, cultural, and textual worlds. These "double thoughts, ... double words and double ideals" instead constitute a "painful self-consciousness" that "is fatal to self-confidence" and "must produce a peculiar wrenching of the soul" (146). Contra Locke's attempt to decontextualize understanding and communication from bodies, double-consciousness inflicts forms of psychic and bodily violence on bodies racialized as Black. To be sure, double-consciousness is not the cause of this suffering, but it is one of the symptoms of the violence of racism and injustice. Moreover, despite its painful effects, I suggest, double-consciousness provided a means of turning incommunicability into a critical and productive locus of reflection and action.[1]

Du Bois maps double-consciousness in interactional and developmental terms. He painfully narrates his first experience of the shadow of the Veil—a complex notion that springs from anti-Black racism—when a girl marked him as "different from the others" by refusing to accept his gift in the course of an exchange of cards between classmates. Finding that he was shut out of the white world "by a vast veil, I had thereafter no desire to tear down that veil, to creep through" ([1903] 1990, 8). Du Bois argues that "despite much physical contact and daily intermingling" of Black and white people, the Veil structures social interaction between them in such a way that it precludes communicability: "There is almost no community of intellectual life or point of transference where the thoughts and feelings of one race can come into direct contact and sympathy with the thoughts and feelings of the other" (132–33). Du Bois notes that media sources enable incommunicability to jump scale: "The daily paper chronicles the doings of the black world from afar with no great regard for accuracy" (133). It is worth building on this insight. For white readers, such stories reproduce a reassuring one-sided sense of communicability: journalists can render Black alien worlds transparent for white people, even as they project Black people as incapable of grasping the seemingly rational world that white people believe themselves to inhabit. For Black readers, such reporting reconfirmed a double incommunicability: white people are ignorant of Black perspectives, content with reproducing shallow images, unable to assimilate evidence that would cast these stereotypes into doubt, and content with uncritically assimilating banalities and falsehoods about Black people as truth. Stories about Black people in the white-dominated press thus provided roadmaps for double-consciousness, mediatized confirmations of anti-Black stereotypes that Black people confronted in their daily interactions with white people. Ultimately, according to Du Bois, due to pervasive racialized incommunicability, "the white man, as well as the Negro, is bound and barred by the color-line" in such a way that even "the very representatives of the two races . . . are so far strangers that one side thinks all whites are narrow and prejudiced, and the other thinks educated Negroes dangerous and insolent" (133). Nahum Chandler (2014, 121) argues that Du Bois's formulation "confounds the ultimate premise of racial distinction, a categorical or oppositional logic of distinction or identification." Thus, the Veil does not divide the world into two separate and opposing communicabilities—one inhabited by Black people and one by white people—as liberal multiculturalism might project. The doubling, which Chandler emphasizes, simultaneously multiplies communicabilities and places Black Americans into uncomfortable, shifting spaces of racialized incommunicability.

The effects of the Veil and double-consciousness are not confined to social interaction and mediatization. "This sense of always looking at one's self through the eyes of others" also reaches inside, fracturing, according to Du Bois, identities and senses of self. The Veil affords "a painful self-consciousness, an almost morbid sense of personality and a moral hesitancy which is fatal to self-confidence" and that "must produce a peculiar wrenching of the soul, a peculiar sense of doubt and bewilderment" (Du Bois [1903] 1990, 146). Just as the power of racialized incommunicabilities is felt within lives, Du Bois does not see communicability as shaping connections "within the Veil"—that is, relations among Black people. Vividly recounting two summers teaching at a country school in rural Tennessee, he suggests that common experiences of poverty and racism and sharing the affective relations associated with births, weddings, and funerals engendered "a half-awakened common consciousness," leading him to "have called my tiny community a world." Nevertheless, although these connections "caused us to think some thoughts together; but these, when ripe for speech, were spoken in various languages" (54).

It is worth pausing here to return to Savannah Shange and Audra Simpson. Unlike Du Bois, they refuse to posit an originary ontological, ethical, and political ideal of communicability and then trace how pervasively racism produces incommunicability. Shange (2019, 120) merges what I would see as distinct notions of "Du Boisian/Fanonian and later Coulthardian double consciousness" by turning "noncommunicability" and ethnographic refusal into an analytical starting point. She suggests that Simpson "theorizes proliferating consciousnesses that refuse the recognition of an external gaze, producing 'endless play,' along the lines of 'I am me, I am what you think I am, and I am who this person to the right of me thinks I am, and you are all full of shit, and then maybe I will tell you to your face'" (Simpson 2014, 107, quoted in Shange 2019, 120–21). Simpson and Shange would push us, perhaps uncomfortably, to see how Du Bois's powerful analytic is also, in part, a product of communicability that positions incommunicability as a pathology produced by racism. Their formulation opens up more space for agency within incommunicability, as based on a politics of refusal—a refusal to be interpellated and incarcerated by white supremacy.

Du Bois does not simply map incommunicability as an object of research, as an entity that can be viewed from a distance by writer and reader alike, that can be made to disappear through dispassionate analysis. The experimental nature of *The Souls of Black Folk* enabled Du Bois to perform an incommunicable dance with his readers. He addresses the projected whiteness of his readers in the book's opening lines, offering to raise the Veil so "that you may view faintly its deeper recesses" ([1903] 1990, 3). Du Bois thus warned white readers that they inhabit spaces of incommunicability vis-à-vis Black worlds. Frequently alluding to the paltry interest and crude stereotypes that shape white claims to understand Black lives, Du Bois frequently warned white readers that the incommunicable barrier of the Veil would limit and structure their understanding of his words.

Du Bois advised readers that each chapter would begin with verses and music from a Sorrow Song, a message "naturally veiled and half articulate" in which "the slave spoke to the world" (185). In a detailed reading of ten Sorrow Songs, Du Bois suggested that "through all the sorrow of the Sorrow Songs there breathes a hope—a faith in the ultimate justice of things." Chapter 1 begins with these lines:

O water, voice of my heart, crying in the sand,
All night long crying with a mournful cry,
As I lie and listen, and cannot understand
   The voice of my heart in my side or the voice of the sea,
O water, crying for rest, is it I, is it I?
   All night long the water is crying to me.
(Arthur Symons, quoted in Du Bois [1903] 1990, 7)

Highly evocative, the song's powerful "I" is not readily identifiable, bounded, or stable. Rejecting Locke's call for monophony, Du Bois creates heteroglossic texts, to use Mikhail Bakhtin's (1981) term, in which the shifting tones of the songs and the changing contours of poetic and affective movement and degrees of complexity penetrate the text. As Du Bois ([1903] 1990, 12) writes about the anguish of seeing oneself "darkly as through a veil," ever fragmented by the doubling of consciousness, words, thoughts, and ideals, he uses the Sorrow Song quoted earlier to juxtapose the sounds of water and the "voice of my heart" as mournful cry. The songs go beyond increasing the heteroglossic quality of Du Bois's writing to demand multiple, complex, shifting forms of listening, demanding that white and other readers go beyond the referential to become attuned to the effects of violence inflicted on Black flesh.

Locke reduced language to pure referentiality and sought to ban poetics and, indeed, any attention to the formal properties of language. Communicability demanded individual, bounded, and stable subjects that were self-made prior to selecting signs to convey their thoughts. Du Bois challenged Locke's referentialist and personalist ideology of language by demonstrating how musicality and poetics enable subjects to constantly make, unmake, and transform in complex, multiple, shifting ways. I argued recently (Briggs 2021) that entextualization (Bauman and Briggs 1990)—the structuring of the formal features of utterances through recurrent generic and stylistic as well as emergent forms of patterning—goes beyond imbuing discourse with sensuous and aesthetic dimensions. It also opens up a process by which subjects hear, literally, their own processes of subject formation and, as entextualization anticipates its reception, reaches out in trying to establish affective relations with interlocutors or readers. *Souls* reaches beyond representation to invite readers to surrender fixed, self-confident senses of self to a challenging process in which both the carefully crafted poetics of the text and his powerful analysis of the effects of racism on Black and white people open up spaces of pain, uncertainty, and potential transformation. In *Mules and Men* and other work, Zora Neale Hurston ([1935] 1978) would later turn Black poetics into a site for ethnographic exploration, a mode of structuring her own heteroglossic, polyphonic text and a complex analytics of race.

For this reader, Du Bois most deeply plumbs the limits, terror, and potential productivity of incommunicability in a chapter that moves generically toward a lament, a Sorrow Song of his own, as he mourns the death of his eighteen-month-old son, Burghardt, on 24 May 1899 ([1968] 2007, 284). Du Bois ([1903] 1990, 151) begins with a gendered account of in/communicability, contrasting his initial sense of perplexity and his inability to feel love for his newborn as opposed to the mother's transformation into the only voice who could "coax him off to Dreamland, and she and he together spoke some soft and unknown tongue and in it held communion." Du Bois traces the affective transformation that occurred as he saw in Burghardt the "unbowed pride of a hunted race" (151) and "heard in his baby voice the voice of the Prophet that was to rise within the Veil" (152). The affective transformation evident in this period of emergent connection with the child was signaled by a chilling "till," marking seasonal temporalities in shifts from fall to winter and "the long Southern spring" into Atlanta's hot summer. The temporal, rhetorical, and affective rupture is signaled by a single sentence: "And then one night the little feet pattered wearily to the wee white bed, and the tiny hands trembled; and a warm flushed face tossed on the pillow, and we knew baby was sick" (152).

Du Bois's description draws readers into the anguish and fear of ten days of illness, followed by witnessing Burghardt's death.

The parents' contrastive forms of grieving plumb the limits of in/communicability, life, and embodiment. With a tone of gendered reductionism, Du Bois frames the mother's grief as reflecting "simple clearness of vision" as she (reportedly) said, "He will be happy There; he ever loved beautiful things." Du Bois locates himself in multiple layers of incommunicability: "And I, far more ignorant, and blind by the web of mine own weaving, sit alone winding words and muttering, 'If still he be, and he be There, and there be a There, let him be happy, O Fate!'"[2] Here Du Bois's reflection on his immersion in an even deeper world of incommunicability challenged the claims to transparency and linearity that constitute central features of communicability. Du Bois fractures linearity as he moves among the Sorrow Song, the present of the forms of racism he documented, the future racist violence that awaited Burghardt in life, and a world beyond the Veil. Du Bois thus musters musicality to help him keep going when representation and knowledge have failed him. He writes, "I might have known that yonder deep unworldly look that ever and anon floated past his eyes was peering far beyond this narrow Now" ([1903] 1990, 154). In reflecting on this passage, Chandler (2014, 125) comments, "Du Bois invokes the possibility of a temporality that extends both before and after the time of American slavery." Even as he captures the depth of anguish that it can engender, particularly as it is attached to and detached from racialized bodies, Du Bois still leaves room for the power of incommunicability to shatter Lockean illusions of the transparency and linearity of knowledge, and he opens up new temporalities and imagined spaces of justice.

In his powerful description of his child's final hours, Du Bois ([1903] 1990, 152) writes: "I hear now that Voice at midnight calling me from dull and dreamless trance,—crying, 'The Shadow of Death! The Shadow of Death!' Out into the starlight I crept, to rouse the gray physician,—the Shadow of Death! The Shadow of Death!" After this brief reference, the physician disappears from the scene, leaving the two parents to witness the child's passing. The doctor's brief role does not seem to be shaped explicitly by the Veil's pervasive effects. As much as the Veil structures Du Bois's biography of his son's short life and how he, as a father, experienced these events, he does not seem to entertain the possibility that racial inequalities might have helped turn a childhood infection into a death sentence. Why, we might wonder, was the child treated only after ten days of illness? Why would his critical condition warrant only a single, brief house call rather than hospitalization? Du Bois's biographers Charisse Burden-Stelly and Gerald Horne (2019, 32) write that the illness was diphtheria, and the visit by "the gray physician" followed Du Bois's frantic search to obtain help from one of the few Black doctors in segregated Atlanta, because no white doctor would treat the child. Despite Du Bois's sense that Burghardt might have survived if Atlanta's Black population had adequate access to medical facilities and services, racialized health inequities do not become part of his wide-reaching critique of structures of racism in *The Souls of Black Folk*.

Du Bois was certainly cognizant of racialized health inequities. In *The Philadelphia Negro* (1899), published four years before *Souls*, he devotes a chapter to "The Health of Negroes." Based on statistics and ethnographic observation, Du Bois analyzes factors that affect the health of Black populations, from slavery to the higher death rates of Philadelphia's Black residents. He attributes these figures primarily to "infantile mortality and consumption," the latter referring to tuberculosis (152). Du Bois identifies a range of structural factors related mainly to the "bad sanitary surroundings" in areas, such as the Fifth Ward, where low-income Black residents were concentrated (150). Suggesting that the statistics he compiled "would seem to adduce considerable proof that the Negro death rate is largely a matter of condition of living" (156), he deftly tied health inequities to those of housing, employment, and segregation. In the Seventh Ward, only 14 percent of dwellings had "water closets and baths," many of which were in poor condition, and many lacked private outhouses (161). At the same time, structural logics are closely entwined with the sorts of culturalist formulations that Hortense Spillers so pointedly criticized in "Mama's Baby, Daddy's Maybe." The "neglect of infants" is one factor Du Bois deems responsible for death rates (150). He suggests that "Negroes live in unsanitary dwellings, partly by their own fault, partly on account of the difficulty of securing decent house by reason of race prejudice." He adds, with respect to high mortality rates, "Primarily it is because the Negroes are as a mass ignorant of the laws of health" (160). Embracing a communicable logic that followed from his diagnosis that "in habits of personal cleanliness and taking proper food and exercise, the colored people are woefully deficient," he suggests that "a gospel of soap and water needs now to be preached" (161). Du Bois faults Black patients: "When in poor health the neglect to take proper medical advice, or to follow it when given, leads to much harm." His reproach also includes failing to return for follow-up care. He nevertheless goes on to attribute "a superstitious fear of hospitals prevalent among the lower classes of all peoples, but especially among Negroes" to, at least in part, "the roughness or brusqueness of manner prevalent in many hospitals, and the lack of a tender spirit of sympathy with the unfortunate patients" (162).

As Baker (1998) argues, Du Bois did not fundamentally embrace culturalist logics. In *Dusk of Dawn*, Du Bois (1940, 117) wrote with respect to African heritage that "the physical bond is least and the badge of color relatively unimportant save as a badge; the real essence of this kinship is its social heritage of slavery; the discrimination and insult; and this heritage binds together not simply the children of Africa, but extend through yellow Asia and into the South Seas." In wrapping up the chapter on health in *The Philadelphia Negro*, Du Bois (1899, 163) suggested that "the most difficult social problem in the matter of Negro health" is a genocidal attitude on the part of "the nation," which looks with "peculiar indifference" on racialized "human suffering" and seems "delighted" when bogus census statistics seem to suggest that "the Negroes were dying off rapidly, and the country would soon be well rid of them." As Natalia Molina (2006) and other researchers have shown, mortality statistics—particularly for infant and child mortality—provide key sites for producing stereotypes and justifying racist policies. Health inequities thus constitute one of those places in Du Bois's work where his remarkable ability to use a poetics and politics of incommunicability to challenge racism and call out its structural underpinnings became entangled with the sorts of communicable logics that keep hierarchies of race, class, gender, sexuality, and disability in place.

To be sure, as has been often critiqued, Du Bois was limited by class and gender ideologies, an arboreal projection of elites as leading ignorant masses to forms of enlightenment. He wrote that "to seek to make the blacksmith a scholar is almost as silly as the more modern scheme of making the scholar a blacksmith" (Du Bois [1903] 1990, 65). Here we might draw on Walter Benjamin (1968) and new materialities theory to suggest that blacksmiths can be remarkably prescient philosophers and storytellers. Echoing Locke's elevation of communicability as a pedagogical and civilizational program, Du Bois's notion of the "Talented Tenth" called on university-educated members of the Black middle class to develop "higher individualism" and "a freedom for expansion and self-development" ([1903] 1990, 81). He conferred on them the task of illuminating "an untaught people" (81) and overcoming its "narrowness of life" (106). The "primitive peoples of Africa and the world" need, in addition to land and home rule, "training through modern methods of educating children" (1995, 649). Du Bois celebrated knowledge and reason as the only "cure for war" (759), and he asserted that "the culture of the University" has been the source of the "broadest and deepest knowledge" that can promote a "catholicity of taste and culture" ([1903] 1990, 64, 69). Du Bois was harshly criticized for elitism by a subsequent generation of Black intellectuals (see Holloway 2002).

Nevertheless, Du Bois has much to teach us about in/communicability. Departing from the universalizing, decorporealizing, and scale-jumping tendencies we found in Locke, Du Bois presents us with a characterization of incommunicability that is vested not only in bodies racialized as Black and white but also in the specificities of class, geography, history, and political economy. He simultaneously globalized the contours of race, racialization, and racism by suggesting that "the problem of the twentieth century is the problem of the color-line,—the relation of the darker to the lighter races of men in Asia and Africa, in America and the islands of the sea" ([1903] 1990, 16). His analysis of ways that white claims to communicable superiority masked anti-Blackness helps extend our understanding of how communicability was tied to slavery, as signaled by Spillers's reading of Equiano's autobiography and our reflection on Locke's investments in slave companies and oversight of plantation economies.

Even as Du Bois sometimes characterized communicability as primordial and necessary, the depth at which he inhabited painful and productive dimensions of incommunicability helped disrupt the centuries-long hegemony of Lockean communicability. Denise Ferreira da Silva's discussion of Du Bois provides a crucial insight. In dialogue with Chandler (2014), Ferreira da Silva (2022) draws our attention to the first sentence of the first chapter of *The Souls of Black Folk*: "Between me and the other world there is ever an unasked question" (Du Bois [1903] 1990, 7). "The real question" that the "other world" wants to ask him, Du Bois notes, is, "How does it feel to be a problem?" Chandler (2014, 3) insightfully suggests that the space between "me" and "the other world" is not a simple binary, given how Du Bois calls attention to the otherness of a white, racialist world even as the unasked question situates his "me" along the "colorline." Chandler argues that Du Bois's provocation calls the foundations of Western metaphysics into question. Ferreira da Silva suggests that the sentence opens up a space in between that is not exhausted by either the "me" or "the other world," revealing possibilities for creating past and future worlds, possible worlds, or a world that is not a world at all. Du Bois's unasked question and the impossibility of responding ("I answer seldom a word") call into question the subject that is interpellated by communicability, demands an answer, and renders any response inadequate. The strategic assemblage that unfolds in *Souls*—calling out white incommunicability vis-à-vis Black social worlds, the concepts of double-consciousness and the Veil, and his multilayered, multigenre, heteroglossic experimental writing—issued a fundamental challenge issue to white claims to possess a singular, rational, enlightened consciousness.[3] The space of profound, multisided, incarcerated incommunicability that he opens up radically questions the very project of communicability and enables us to imagine worlds beyond communicability and incommunicability.

In *The Souls of Black Folk, Dawn of Dusk*, and other writings, Du Bois provides an archaeology of communicability's roots in white supremacy by analyzing the myriad ways that racism, colonialism, and imperialism produce incommunicabilities and turn liberal promises of communicability into daily acts of racist denigration. Du Bois challenged how communicability's claims of transparency and disembodiment infused education, journalism, and social-science research with forms of white supremacy. He suggested that any approach to language, communication, and the body must attend to issues of poetics and genre and be attentive to the racialized relations of voice among authors, readers, and the populations they analyze. Perhaps most significantly, Du Bois partially freed incommunicability from its subordination to communicability. Even as he offered ways of challenging instrumentalist, teleological demands for intervention, he sometimes succumbed to their power. Here is a point on which we have much to learn from Fanon in the next chapter.

3

FRANTZ FANON
Doctors, Tarzan, and the Colonial
Inscription of Incommunicability

In the preceding chapter, we followed W. E. B. Du Bois's remarkable ability to reveal scalar dimensions of how "the Veil" crushes lives and collective aspirations. The violence of health inequities and the racializing work of biocommunicability entered only obliquely, such as through his account of the death of his son, Burghardt, and his analysis of racial differences of mortality in Philadelphia. In turning to Frantz Fanon, we come face to face with how racism can turn biocommunicability into one of the most effective sites for constructing racial hierarchies and inscribing them on white and nonwhite subjects and bodies.

In moving from Du Bois to Fanon, we shift from a pivotal turn-of-the-twentieth-century figure in the United States to one of the twentieth century's most poignant critics of colonialism. It is hard to miss some striking similarities. Both classics, *The Souls of Black Folk* and *Black Skin, White Masks*, are early works, written while their authors were, respectively, in their midthirties and late twenties. Both are textually experimental. Fanon moved among prose, poetry, and dialogue as he commented on topics that included medicine, psychiatry, psychoanalysis, philosophy, literature, language, and more.

Both authors ranged across multiple registers and disciplinary perspectives, and they challenged the boundaries of genre even as they pushed readers intellectually, affectively, and politically. Du Bois and Fanon trenchantly analyzed the role of race and racism in constructing in/communicabilities and situating them historically, geographically, culturally, and politically. Both drew attention to how models of communicability encode whiteness, even as they provided systematic cartographies of the violent effects of incommunicabilities on Black lives and Black-white relations. Du Bois and Fanon examined how the imposition of racialized incommunicabilities constructs stereotypes of Black and Native American bodies and minds in ways that naturalize the violent effects of inequities. They traced how white people constantly fashion Black populations in biological terms as animals (Fanon) or as "somewhere between men and cattle" (Du Bois [1903] 1990, 68). Both warned white readers that their understanding would fall short of fully grasping the book's meaning, and both invited readers into spaces designed to unsettle their understandings of self and other. Finally, there are vast critical literatures on both figures; as was the case with Du Bois, I focus here on creating a dialogue with Fanon that explores the profound implications of his work for issues of in/communicability, bringing in other authors sparingly.

Fanon's role as a physician and psychiatrist offers crucial perspectives for my argument. Having trained and practiced in France, practiced in colonized Algeria, and renounced his hospital post to join a revolutionary movement that sought to liberate minds as much as bodies, Fanon analyzed how the colonial production of incommmunicability structured biomedical practice in ways that turned clinics and hospitals into key sites of colonial subjection and violence. Anticipating current forms of progressive medical practice, Fanon positioned diagnosis and treatment as political practices, using the details of individual cases in diagnosing the effects of racism on the minds and bodies of colonizers as much as on colonial subjects. He sought to turn the ward of an Algerian psychiatric hospital he directed into a site for transforming society. Patrick Ehlen (2000) reports that he integrated wards formerly segregated into "Europeans" and "Muslims." Fanon deemed efforts by himself and his staff to create "a fruitful experiment" in developing social therapy that would overcome incommunicability failed—with Algerian staff members as well as patients—in ways that led him to reflect on how these innovative practices had exacerbated incommunicability ([2015] 2018).

It might surprise some linguistic and medical anthropologists that Fanon began the first chapter of *Black Skin, White Masks* by declaring: "We attach a fundamental importance to the phenomenon of language" ([1952] 2008, 1). His biographer David Macey pointed to how Fanon's interest in language carried over into his own writing (see also Cherki 2000). When challenged by the editor of *Black Skins, White Masks* to explain an obscure passage, Fanon reportedly replied: "I cannot explain this sentence. When I write things like that, I am trying to touch my reader affectively, or in other words irrationally, almost sensually. For me, words have a charge. I find myself incapable of escaping the bite of a word, the vertigo of a question mark" (quoted in Macey 2000, 159). Resonating with Lacan, Fanon ([1952] 2008, 1) continued: "To speak is to exist absolutely for the other." He suggested that "a man who possesses a language possesses as an indirect consequence the world expressed and implied by this language" (2). He was quick to note, however, that racialization shapes the sorts of rights to and over language that people can claim. Fanon observed that being Black and Martiniquais, "I must watch my diction because that's how they'll judge me. He can't even speak French properly, they'll say with the utmost contempt" (4). This statement would, at first glance, seem to echo John Locke's demand for constant self-surveillance of one's speech. His point, however, was that demonstrating mastery of the language of the colonizers—including through the sort of bodily hexis so powerfully analyzed by Pierre Bourdieu ([1972] 1977)—subjected the colonized to heightened surveillance and deep distrust on the part of colonizers and colonized alike, constituting "evidence of a shift and a split" (Fanon [1952] 2008, 9). Nelson Maldonado-Torres and his colleagues (2021, 232) suggest that Fanon wrote about language not as an abstract universal but as it is "experienced in the lives of Black subjects in a fundamentally colonial and antiblack world."

Ever attentive to ideologies and pragmatics of linguistic differentiation, Fanon moved from dialect to French and Creole code-switching in the Francophone Caribbean to what he termed "pidgin."[1] His interest was in what scholars have discussed under such names as "motherese" and "foreigner talk" (Ferguson 1975; Snow and Ferguson 1977), how designing speech to match the perceived communicative features of designated recipients projects failures of knowledge, rationality, agency, and communicative competence. Fanon grasped that the process of faux recipient design encodes speakers' projections of the cognitive and linguistic status of the person they are addressing. These special linguistic registers are used mainly with those believed to possess linguistic or cognitive deficits, including children, the elderly, the sick, foreigners, and—the case in point—colonized subjects. The pidgin (*petit-négre*) that Fanon discusses also bears a strong racializing and racist dimension.

Even as he noted that other agents of colonialism—priests, policemen, and employers—also address colonized subjects in pidgin, Fanon devoted special attention to how physicians performed this form of linguistic violence:

> Consulting physicians know this. Twenty European patients come and go: "Please have a seat. Now what's the trouble? What can I do for you today?"
>
> In comes a black man or an Arab: "Sit down, old fellow. Not feeling well? Where's it hurting?" When it's not: "You not good?" ([1952] 2008, 15)[2]

Note that this statement overlooks ways that medical encounters in which racial difference is not present can generate incommunicability. In a statement regarding white people's modes of speaking with Black people in general, Fanon nailed the infantilization that drives pidgin: "A white man talking to a person of color behaves exactly like a grown-up with a kid" (14). Pidgin thus constitutes a racist poetics, where entextualization saturates lexical, grammatical, and intonational features with signs of the projected incommunicability of the addressee. Here we can return to the "white listening subject" (Rosa and Flores 2020) I raised in the introduction. Pidgin embodies colonial physicians' claims to have overheard their colonized patients' speech and to be able to reproduce it. Fanon suggests that pidgin, like Miyako Inoue's (2003) category of Japanese schoolgirl speech, is a denigrating linguistic imaginary, a "native" language no one speaks. Racist physicians, ironically, become the primary speakers of this language variety, constituting themselves as subjects through their self-proclaimed ability to x-ray the mind of the colonized. The biocommunicable frame surrounding this ventriloquism marks the doctor's relation to privileged registers—standard French and biomedical discourse—and the superiority invested in the purported need to use pidgin to care for people with cognitive, linguistic, and medical deficits. Fanon argues that by responding to physicians in pidgin, patients show that they have grasped doctors' modes of self-deception, constituting what Chela Sandoval (2000, 85) refers in a discussion of *Black Skin, White Masks* to as a "semiotic technology of the oppressed." Eduardo Menéndez (2002, 40, my translation) reads Fanon as suggesting that the work of physicians (specifically, psychiatrists) was so filtered by ideologies and the diagnostic categories of biomedicine that "their descriptions referred not to the true identity of the subjects they treated . . . , but to the reality that native subjects and groups 'allowed' professionals 'to see.'"[3]

White readers are thus in for a wild ride. For Fanon, pidgin is exhibit A of ways that, in Sandoval's (2000, 87) words, "subjugated peoples of color were reading Western cultural forms very differently than were white Westerners themselves." If colonizers read their subjects so abysmally and fail to recognize signs of their own self-deception, "Fanon's charge implies that dominant reality itself might be also a similar construction" (85). Fanon's insights were later echoed in work on raciolinguistics and linguistic racisms. In grasping how "linguistic and racial forms are jointly constructed as sets and rendered mutually recognizable as named language varieties and racial categories" (Rosa and Flores 2020, 95), linguistic anthropologists might fruitfully pursue Fanon's call to document the central role of biocommunicability and clinical communicative practices.

Fanon ([1952] 2008, 15) ironically voiced the raciolinguistic ideologies used to justify this mode of address: "Speaking to black people in this way is an attempt to reach down to them, to make them feel at ease, to make oneself understood and reassure them." The rationale thus reproduced the fundamental Lockean politics of language in assuming the primordial and paramount value of communicability, the need to diagnose perceived communicable obstacles, and the utilitarian obligation to enact interventions aimed at restoring communicability. Invoking the complex process of ironic voicing of racist speech that we also saw in Du Bois's writing, Fanon simulated a colonial participation framework (Goffman 1981) in which he pretended to defend the practice. He thus deployed, like colonized patients in speaking with doctors, what Homi Bhabha (1994) refers to as "colonial mimicry," in which performing features of the discourse and manners of colonizers encodes undercurrents of mockery and menace. Fanon often wove colonial mimicry into the poetics of his texts. Fanon's voice thus surrounded and split apart the voices of colonial physicians: "To speak gobbledygook to a black man is insulting, for it means he is the gook. Yet, we'll be told, there is no intention to willfully give offense. OK, but it is precisely this absence of will—this offhand manner; this casualness; and the ease with which they classify him, imprison him at an uncivilized and primitive level—that is insulting" ([1952] 2008, 15).

Taking us into the realm of what scholars would later term *doctor-patient interaction*, the subject of chapter 5, Fanon x-rayed the centrality of the clinic as a site for performatively constructing pervasive relations of inequality and pathologies of colonialism.[4] He developed these observations in three locations: his experience in the Antilles (including a short period in which he practiced medicine); the treatment of North African patients in France; and the medical system he encountered after accepting a post in Algeria in 1953, a year before the war of independence began in earnest. In the essay "The 'North African Syndrome'" (1952), later published in *Toward the African Revolution*,

Fanon extensively used colonial mimicry in re-voicing French physicians' stereotypes of North African patients they encountered in French hospitals. The chapter's title signals a critique of what psychiatrists identified as a "syndrome" in which North African patients presented with a wide range of complaints that seem to correspond to no identifiable pathology. Fanon reported exchanges in which physicians elicited only vague responses, leaving them frustrated. Afterward, patients returned before their treatments had run their course or sought help from multiple doctors. In clinical encounters, patients spoke "volubly" about their pain, "and after fifteen minutes of gestured explanations the interpreter (appropriately baffling) translates for us: he says he has a belly-ache" (Fanon [1964] 1967, 5). Here Fanon not only pinpoints how patients are forced into a space of incommunicability but how they assume the mantle of communicability in pressing for adequate treatment in the face of racist clinical inequities. When the patient returns before a treatment has taken its course, "he is made to understand this, or more precisely, he is told. But our patient has not heard what we said. He *is* pain and he refuses to understanding any language, and it is not far from this to the conclusion: It is because I am Arab that they don't treat me like others" (5). In these encounters, Fanon wrote, the patient's persistence in seeking treatment only confirms the stereotype of North African patients as incommunicable, which is grounded "not experimentally, but on the basis of an oral tradition" (10). This racist misrecognition not only defeated the instrumentalist logic that rationalized physicians' use of pidgin but achieved its opposite: it left colonized patients at *dis*-ease (see Perez Hattori 2004) and put them on guard.

Fanon ([1964] 1967, 9) described at length how French doctors mistreat North Africans: "Speaking to an Arab, the student or the doctor is inclined to use the second person singular. It's a nice thing to do, we are told . . . to put them at ease."[5] The incommunicable stereotype produces pervasive health/communicative inequities: "'I can't help it,' an intern once told me, 'I can't talk to them in the same way that I talk to other patients.'" Fanon continued mimicking the voice of medical profiling: "But anyway, you can't say it's our fault." Moving by steps to reclaiming his own voice, first of a medical practitioner and then, it would seem, of a colonized subject, Fanon replied:

—But that's just it, it *is* our fault.
It so happens that the fault is YOUR fault. (14)

Fanon's analysis of medical racism enabled him to identify two broader structural problems: the isolated, exploited, and ignominious position of North African men in France, living as workers with no family life, and the colonial oppression that left Francophone North Africa poor, oppressed, and lacking in infrastructure and resources. If no specific pathology can be located, the physician never concludes that "medical thinking was at fault; . . . He will find the patient at fault—an indocile, undisciplined patient, who doesn't know the rules of the game" (8). Projecting health/communicative inequities onto North African patients thus confirms the stereotype: "When you come down to it, the North African is a simulator, a liar, a malingerer, a sluggard, a thief" (7). Fanon used this discussion to question a basic tenet of medical semiology: if a specific pathology, as codified in nosological modes of classification, cannot be pinpointed, the cause is identified as incommunicability, and the blame is placed on the patient. This incommunicable failure was framed not only as a moral failing but, jumping scales, as condemning entire populations to incommunicability and thereby naturalizing health inequities and the violence of colonialism.

Fanon's criticism of French medicine in Algeria was particularly biting. In the chapter "Medicine and Colonialism" in *A Dying Colonialism* ([1959] 1967, 121), he identified the roots of incommunicability in the advent of colonialism: "Introduced into Algeria at the same time as racialism and humiliation, Western medical science, being part of the oppressive system, has always provoked in the native an ambivalent attitude." The medical historian Richard Keller (2007, 840) notes that Fanon saw French physicians in Algeria as creating a humanitarian façade for colonial domination and surveillance to diminish support for the National Liberation Front (FLN). Having already pointed to pidgin as the underlying structure that guides how white physicians addressed colonized patients in *Black Skins, White Masks*, Fanon ([1952] 2008, 126) elaborated there on Algerian patients' demeanor in clinical settings: "The colonized person who goes to see the doctor is always diffident. He answers in monosyllables, gives little in the way of explanation, and soon arouses the doctor's impatience."

In contrast to what he characterized as the stigmatized volubility of North African patients in France, here Fanon documents the place of what Roman Jakobson ([1939] 1971) calls the sign zero, communicative uses of silence in spaces where a linguistic form is expected, as a means of confronting colonial medical discourse. Fanon thus documents in various works a wide range of ways that colonized patients responded to racism and power in clinical settings: ventriloquizing physicians' denigrating uses of "pidgin," voluble and repeated attempts by North African patients in France to convey their symptoms to physicians, and Algerian patients' use of "monosyllables." Although these observations did not emerge from broad surveys of doctor-patient interaction in all of the sites in which Fanon practiced, it seems clear that he was attuned to the specificities of the effects of linguistic racism in different colonial settings and diverse ways that colonized subjects navigated relations among race, colonialism, clinical practices, and communicability.

Fanon ([1959] 1967, 131) argued that French physicians' words and actions were viewed by their Algerian patients not as evidence of a humanistic desire to lessen suffering but as "a link in the colonialist network, as a spokesman for the occupying power." For patients, clinical encounters are "always an ordeal," and diagnosis and treatment recommendations "are but sequels of the ordeal." Physicians' utterances were demedicalized by patients as reflecting "the lie of the colonial situation" (128). In short, they rejected a basic premise of biocommunicability that posits the clinic as a neutral contextual ground for producing and interpreting exchanges between providers and patients. Colonized patients instead positioned clinical discourse as tokens of broader, power-laden exchanges between colonizers and the colonized. Fanon analyzed accusations of noncompliance with treatment recommendations and failure to appear for follow-up visits as expressing reluctance to prolong the "ordeal." Anticipating later research on divergences between physicians' and patients' perceptions of clinical encounters, he concluded: "The doctors say: 'Those people are rough and unmannerly.' The patients say: 'I don't trust them'" (128). For Fanon, the colonial production of incommunicable patients constituted "this enormous wound."

Translation provided a point at which Fanon judged his efforts to analyze and transform the structure of colonial medicine in Algeria as having fallen short. In his clinical practice in Algeria, Fanon sought to diagnose and treat the pathologies not just of patients but of clinical institutions, as David Marriott (2018) emphasizes. In the ward he directed at the Blida-Joinville Hospital, Fanon attempted to build on his previous experience in radical psychiatry working under François Tosquelles at Saint-Alban in France, who remained an important influence on him. He sought to level hierarchical relations among physicians, patients, and nurses and to give patients the power to make collective decisions about some aspects of life in the asylum. Nevertheless, Fanon did not speak Arabic, despite his modest efforts to learn it. As a result, he relied on translators to communicate with many patients: "At best a nurse or orderly; at worst, another patient had to be pressed into service" (Macey 2000, 228). A major problem here is that, in colonial Algeria, translation was associated with colonial oppression, with contexts in which Algerians faced colonial administrators or were forced to appear in court. Disclosing to a physician through an interpreter thus could feel more like being forced to make a confession than asking for help from a therapist (232). At times in his writing, Fanon took a reductionist stance on the politics of translating.[6]

Fanon coauthored an article with his Algerian intern, Jacques Azoulay, whose dissertation Fanon supervised, based on a section of Azoulay's dissertation. The authors recount "a fruitful experiment" in social therapy that began shortly after Fanon took charge of a ward with a mixed "Muslim" and "European" population. Forms of "ergotherapy" that involved handicrafts, movies, ward meetings, bimonthly celebrations, and newspaper production inspired intense participation among European women. Fanon and Azoulay ([1954] 2018, 357) assess these attempts, however, as a "total failure" with "Muslim men." They invoke a perspective of "cultural relativism" to suggest that these activities were based on European logics and practices that collided with those of their Algerian Muslim patients.[7] They accordingly conducted "a functional analysis" (364) of the "cultural existence" of poor Algerian patients, going beyond atemporal reifications to gauge the effects of colonialism on landholding, labor, demographics, and poverty, nevertheless suggesting that these factors "by and large explain their state of ignorance, their traditional primitivism" (365).

Their assessment of the shortcomings of their therapeutic efforts is quite relevant for my discussion: "Now we can understand the reasons for our failure. We said that the ward meetings had turned out not to be productive. This is essentially because we did not speak Arabic and had to make use of two interpreters (for Kabylian and Arabic). This need to have an interpreter fundamentally vitiated doctor-patient relations" (Fanon and Azoulay [2015] 2018, 367). They note that "the image of the interpreter" was associated with colonial administrators and the penal system; when transferred to the hospital, "the same need for an interpreter spontaneously triggers a distrust that makes all 'communication' difficult." (The quotation marks around "communication" seem to point to Fanon's ongoing concern with the politics of in/communicability.) The authors then present insights that move in the direction of an ethnography of the failure of medical translation. When a patient's trust "had been won" and "his speech was filled with enthusiasm," it was directed to the psychiatrist directly, erasing the presence of the interpreter (367). The authors grasp the importance of multimodal dimensions of provider-patient communication, including "gestural and verbal components" (367–68), in shaping how "the doctor, especially the psychiatrist, makes his diagnostic through language" (367). When translation was necessary, however, the patient's facial expressions and "profuse" gestures were lost as the psychiatrist "had to wait until the patient has stopped talking in order to grasp the meaning. At which point, the interpreter sums up in two words what the patient has related in detail for ten minutes" (368). Overlooking the pragmatics and politics of highly power-laden speech "when it comes to explaining something simple or transmitting an order," they suggest that reliance on translators "is perhaps valid" in such cases (368). In clinical encounters, however, "when it is necessary to begin a dialogue, a dialectical exchange of questions and replies, alone able to overcome reticence and bring to light abnormal, pathological behavior," translation undermines the therapeutic process. Noting that this essay reflects the active participation of Algerian psychiatrist Jacques Azoulay, Fanon's analysis positions him as the prophet-in-waiting of critical perspectives not only on doctor-patient communication but also on medical translation as well.

Fanon's revolutionary perspective blossomed in Algeria. He reported that "every doctor has his vineyards . . . , and is likewise the owner of mills, wine cellars, or orange groves, and he coyly speaks of his medicine as simply a supplementary source of income." Indeed, the broad features of the colonial economy of racism—"the colonialist arrogance, the contempt for the client, and the hateful brutality toward the indigent"—were woven into the fabric of medical practice ([1959] 1967, 134). Fanon was appalled at the greed and lack of professionalism of the French doctors he encountered there. Macey (2000, 216–17) reported that French colonial physicians in Algeria commonly defrauded patients by using bogus practices of diagnosis and treatment to increase their incomes.

In a powerful letter addressed to a colleague returning to France during the war, Fanon went on to analyze how silence also shaped physicians' responses to illness in Algeria, albeit in ways different from the silence of their patients. He chided the physician for practicing for eight years in Algeria without ever associating with "Arabs" or taking note of "this enormous wound" that characterizes the situation of the population ([1964] 1967, 48). He placed the silence of his physician addressee as reflecting the utter self-imposed incommunicability of French physicians concerning Algerian suffering, both within and outside the clinic: "the collective silence of 800,000 Frenchmen, this ignorant silence, this innocent silence" (49). As Carolyn Ureña (2019, 1646) points out in an insightful commentary on these texts, French doctors during the Algerian War were required by law to report any injuries that might indicate that the patient was engaged in the armed struggle, thereby turning medicine even more directly into a tool for colonial surveillance and military violence. Fanon recounted in *The Wretched of the Earth* that he treated both French military torturers and the Algerians they tortured in the ward he directed of the Blida-Joinville Hospital. In speaking of Fanon's positioning of the revolution as opening up a space of uncertainty, a new beginning that "signifies both experience and dissolution," Marriott (2018, 37) puts it succinctly: "It is in the context of his clinic that Fanon first apprehends this poetics of dissolution—its grammar, tenses, and modes."

Fanon perceptively pointed to how clinical interactions with Black patients also racialized physicians. White colonial physicians simply assumed their biocommunicable success without assessing whether or not they were actually helping patients understand—or really had a clue about the worlds of communication and health in which all parties were entwined. Indeed, producing incommunicability confirmed the white physicians' power and superiority. In *Black Skin, White Masks*, Fanon ([1952] 2008, 15) suggested that "if the person who speaks to a man of color or an Arab in pidgin does not see that there is a flaw or a defect in his behavior, then he has never paused to reflect." This lack of self-awareness was tied to the role of racialized clinical incommunicabilities in re/producing communicative/health inequities—and, thus, power relations—between physicians and patients and between colonizers and the colonized in general. Fanon argued that Black people can never become doctors per se; they can become only "the Negro physician." A constant monitoring ensues: "As long as everything was going smoothly, he was praised to the heavens; but watch out—there was no room whatsoever for any mistake. The black physician will never know how close he is to being discredited" (97). Fanon observes how the stigma arising from a single error would jump scale: "I knew for instance that if the physician made one false move, it was over for him and for all those who came after him. What, in fact, could one expect from a Negro physician?" (97). Black patients' recognition and rejection of how the racializing character of white physicians' treatment of Black patients produced incommunicability did not vaccinate them or Black physicians against its violent effects.

Contra a strong current in the contemporary doctor-patient interaction literature, Fanon, like Algerian patients, refused to draw an analytic boundary around clinics vis-à-vis other colonial contexts. Reading pidgin as a Rorschach test that can help us understand "the psychology of colonialism" ([1952] 2008, 16), Fanon summarized the incommunicable bottom line of this supposedly communicable, humanistic gesture: "It is already safe to say that to speak pidgin means: 'You, stay where you are'" (17). Anticipating work on linguistic racisms, Fanon went on to analyze how Black minds and bodies are preconfigured in such a way that racist speech effects its violence even when it is detached from white mouths: "Speaking pidgin means imprisoning the black man and perpetuating a conflictual situation where the white man infects the black man with extremely toxic foreign bodies" (18–19).

Fanon's criticism was not directed exclusively at white colonial physicians. In a crucial passage, it was self-directed: "At a personal level, during certain consultations, I have felt myself lapsing," he wrote. "In the company of this seventy-three-year-old peasant afflicted with senile dementia I suddenly feel I am losing my touch. The very fact of adopting a language suitable for dementia and the mentally retarded, the fact of 'leaning over' to address this poor seventy-three-year-old woman, the fact of my reaching down to her for a diagnosis are the signs of a weakening in my relations with other people" ([1952] 2008, 15–16).

We can learn a great deal from this remarkable passage. Here Fanon alludes to what he projected as his personal model of clinical communicability: a reciprocal, respectful, and laterally organized exchange that proscribed the use of derogatory registers and the production of incommunicability. In this instance, however, class, age, and ableism intersected in such a way that "suddenly" he slipped into a form of denigrating address, a hierarchizing, stigmatizing practice of producing incommunicability that was instrumentally rationalized ("the fact of my reaching down to her for a diagnosis"). Having confessed to this slip, Fanon quickly goes on to defend himself by suggesting: "I always make a point of speaking to the 'towelheads' in correct French and I have always been understood. . . . I refuse to indulge in any form of paternalism" ([1952] 2008, 16). This statement elevates "correct French," a speech variety that he had placed within the contours of colonial linguistic racisms, to the status of a neutral, seemingly politically solidarity medium, and it seemingly "always" prevented incommunicability. Fanon wrote this statement while practicing in France; the complexities of multilingualism were, perhaps, easier to overlook there than in colonial Algeria. Again, linguistic anthropologists and other scholars who have so deftly engaged the politics of multilingualism, language ideologies, and racialization would have much to add in analyzing these issues.

Fanon restricted his trenchant analysis of doctor-patient interaction to colonial medicine, whether practiced in Algeria or the Antilles or with North African patients in France: "In a non-colonial society, the attitude of a sick man in the presence of a medical practitioner is one of confidence. The patient trusts the doctor; he puts himself in his hands. He yields his body to him. . . . At no time, in a non-colonial society, does the patient mistrust his doctor" ([1959] 1967, 123). In "Medicine and Colonialism," Fanon contrasts the monosyllabic responses of Algerian patients "with the kind of inhibiting fear that patients usually feel in the doctor's presence" (126). Bringing up the possibility that incommunicability might be commonly produced by clinical interactions outside of what he identifies as colonial contexts, Fanon seems to place the cause inside the patient—precisely the opposite of his assessment of patients' reticence in French-Algerian colonial medicine. He goes on to suggest: "We often hear it said that a certain doctor has a good bedside manner, that he puts his patients at ease" (126). Although the use of reported speech potentially distances Fanon from this assessment, it seems to indicate that a physician's communicable skill can extract this affective relation from patients' interiors and restore communicative efficacy. As I argue in chapter 5, the imperative to foster communicability and the role of communicability and clinical practices in producing incommunicabilities are important issues for clinical medicine in general. It is thus unfortunate that Fanon stopped short of expanding his brilliant insights to open up the broader implications of incommunicability in clinical medicine.

Fanon seemingly embraced a fundamental concern of psychoanalysis by beginning the chapter titled "The Black Man and Psychopathology" focusing on the family. He immediately turned the tables on white psychoanalysts, however, by critiquing how they deprovincialized (Chakrabarty 2000) white European constructions of "the family" as putative universals. Even as Fanon agreed that families constitute a key site in which psychopathologies are preconfigured, he moved the analytical ground from individual psychosexual relations with parents to a structural process of socialization that takes place around age ten to twelve, at the onset of puberty. He argued that at this age, children are exposed to a critical mechanism of "*collective catharsis*" (Fanon [1952] 2008, 124) for releasing aggression in the form of illustrated magazines, such as comic books, Mickey Mouse, and Tarzan. "Written by white men for white children," these texts locate images of violence in the racialized Other, particularly images of African savagery and cannibalism and violence at the hands of Native Americans (124). Through a process that Sigmund Freud ([1900] 1965) referred to as symbolic condensation, here pushed beyond individual pathologies, the image of "the Negro as savage and cannibal" (Fanon [1952] 2008, 184) becomes the quintessential embodiment of sin, evil, violence, and sexuality.

Fanon positioned these symbolic repertories as central to race relations and forms of psychopathology experienced by Black and white people, albeit in different ways. According to Fanon, "the Negro as savage and cannibal" becomes an internalized figure of fear and attraction for white women and, for white men, an image of unattainable mythic hypersexuality. When "these same magazines are devoured by the local youth" in the Antilles ([1952] 2008, 124), the Black child "always identifies with the good guys. Accordingly, "the little black child, just like the little white child becomes an explorer, an adventurer, and a missionary" (125), thereby forming unconscious identities as white people. Black children thus experience a profound sense of rupture when, "at the first white gaze, he feels the weight of his melanin" (128), thus becoming iconically associated with the very figure that they had learned to fear and despise. This traumatic discovery follows from racialized contacts with white people and "through books, newspapers, school texts, advertisements, movies, and radio" (131). Here again, Fanon anticipated work by Jane Hill (2008), Barbra Meek (2006, 2013), and others on the role of media in constructing linguistic racisms and making them pervasive in daily life. These condensed symbols of racist stereotypes become internalized as "a host of information and a series of propositions slowly and stealthily work their way into an individual . . . and shape his community's vision of the world" (Fanon [1952] 2008, 131), creating wounds in sites that have been preconfigured for trauma. Stefania Pandolfo (2010, 27) beautifully points to the dynamics of this process: "Fanon pronounces his phenomenological diagnosis of the annihilation of being in the form of a psychodynamics of 'intrusion.' . . . He describes the raced/colonized subject as constituted by the violent intrusion of the other, the colonizer, in the psychic space of the self, an intrusion that evacuates the self, and replaces it with the poisonous object of the other's fantasy, an object with which the self will coincide." Fanon's stress on the power of the trope of cannibalism as the distant and indelible past of Black populations provides an analytic for rereading Locke's recurrent and gratuitous references to cannibalism as marking the zone of maximum distance from rational, elite, white Europeans. In an ominous return of the figure of prohibited musicality, the imaginary sound of "tom-toms" haunts white psyches.

Fanon provided a crucial perspective on racism as structure and event, on how individual acts of racism—such as physicians' use of pidgin—can engender such pervasive incommunicability for racialized subjects that even communicating with oneself can seem impossible. His chapter "The Lived Experience of the Black Man" provided perhaps the most poignant, and undoubtedly the most famous, treatment of the sudden eruption of these performative racist acts and, in John Austin's (1962) terms, their perlocutionary effects. Fanon reproduced a primordial act of racialization in the opening lines of the chapter and returned to it often, creating a poetic structure that alternated between bald, disturbing presentations of a racist act, recollection of his reactions, and analysis:

"Look! A Negro!" It was a passing sting. I attempted a smile.

"Look! A Negro!" Absolutely. I was beginning to enjoy myself.

"Look! A Negro!" The circle was gradually getting smaller. I was really enjoying myself.

"*Maman*, look a Negro! I'm scared!" ([1952] 2008, 91)

Rather than prefacing these words with the unfolding of a narrative or a sense of "the context," Fanon prepared readers by discussing how encounters with white people fractured his desire "to uncover the meaning of things" and "to be at the origin of the world" (89). I need not remind readers of Du Bois's account of the first profoundly racializing and racist act he experienced as a child. Attempting to follow Du Bois and Fanon, I would suggest that racist performatives create ruptures for Black subjects through the imposition of definitions of Blackness "by the Other, the white man, who had woven me out of a thousand details, anecdotes, and stories" (91). Like Du Bois, Fanon thrusts readers into the middle of the unfolding of a performance of linguistic racism and its radical disruption of affective relations and a sense of identity; only after beginning to trace his reactions does Fanon reveal that the racializing event unfolded while sitting opposite a white boy and his mother on a train.

Fanon poignantly traced how such acts of racialization produce highly situated and broad, enduring forms of incommunicability through dimensions of objectification and embodiment. He articulated how the speech act turned him into "an object among other objects" ([1952] 2008, 89), an observation that takes us back to Hortense Spillers's trenchant observations on the status of Black flesh in the wake of slavery. A "feeling of not existing" (118) emerged as "the eviscerated silence surged toward me with paralyzed wings" (119). This rupture in the possibility of communication and the sense that the white man "had no scruples about imprisoning me" in incommunicability deprived him of the status of fellow human being (92). Jumping scale, Fanon concluded that "the white world, the only decent one, was preventing me from participating" (94). He reported that he reproduced internally this drive for anonymity, invisibility, and silence, trying to escape incommunicable imprisonment: "I transported myself on that particular day far, very far, from my self, and gave myself up as an object" (92).

Glen Coulthard (2007) suggests that Fanon reads Hegel in such a way as to theorize a move to turn away from white oppressors or, in Audra Simpson's (2014, 24) terms, "to avert one's gaze and refuse the recognition itself." Reversing Locke's depiction of performativity as a "cheat and abuse of language," Austin (1962) famously identified "felicity conditions," the "conventions" regulating the social, institutional, and material "conventions" and psychological dispositions required for successful performance of speech acts. Nevertheless, Fanon's account suggests how Austin's seemingly deracialized performative acts are shaped by racial hierarchies. The racial injury that Fanon so poignantly reveals shows how performativity is tied fundamentally to racialization and racial violence, operating differently when performed by subjects racialized as nonwhite and white.

Fanon's chapter could not be more forceful in positioning the experience of racist incommunicability in the body. The racist act burst him apart, only to have "the fragments put together by another me" ([1952] 2008, 89). Deprived of the constructions of subjectivity and agency seemingly produced by communicability, "the image of one's body is solely negating. It's an image in the third person" (90). In the classic line, Fanon reported: "My body was returned to me spread-eagled, disjointed, redone, draped in mourning on this white winter's day" (93), a mourning required by the social death that resulted in banishment from white projections of communicability. He was permanently relegated to a Blackness of incommunicability and an incommunicability of Blackness, "deafened by cannibalism, backwardness, fetishism, racial stigmas, slave traders, and above all, yes, above all, the grinning *Y a bon Banania*" (92).[8] The iteration of racist performatives in the text induces a bodily semiotic in which white gazes, even silent ones, led to his "body schema, attacked in several places, collapsed, giving way to an epidermal racial schema" (92). A fascinating scientific metaphor captured how "the Other fixes me with his gaze, his gestures and attitude," locking him in incommunicable disembodiment "the same way you fix a preparation with a dye" (89). In commenting on this passage, Pandolfo (2010, 27) describes the assault as "an occupation understood in spatial, almost military terms, as a shrinking of vital space, which snatches the self and pulverizes its corporeal schema, halting the work of the imagination and producing in its place a somatic hallucination."

Returning to Savannah Shange's (2019) provocation, we might ask where incommunicability becomes productive for Fanon, helping us explore a politics of ethnographic refusal. At first glance, Fanon's analysis seems to leave little room for Black subjects to challenge the violent, imprisoning effects of the imposition of racist incommunicability. Echoing Du Bois, Fanon bitterly decries how mastering French, attaining education, and gaining professional credentials only shifted racist comments from denigration to patronization, anticipating raciolinguistic analyses of how racialized "compliments" reproduce white supremacy (Alim and Smitherman 2020). As he pinpointed how as a "black physician" he was walled in by white people's efforts to find a way to discredit him and prove the inferiority of Black professionals, he concluded: "Neither my refined manners nor my literary knowledge nor my understanding of the quantum theory could find favor" ([1952] 2008, 97). As he continued to develop the train scene, Fanon suggested that displaying anger freed him from his "rumination" and that he "realized two things at once: I had identified the enemy and created a scandal. Overjoyed. We could now have some fun" (94). In both *Black Skin, White Masks* and *The Wretched of the Earth*, Fanon often paired laughter, sarcasm, and violence as strategies of decolonial incommunicability. The forms of colonial mimicry that Fanon wove into the poetics of his texts suggested ways that mimicking pidgin and other colonial stereotypes provided modes of exposing and challenging their denigrating effects. Given that racist acts are structural as well as situated, Fanon's complex poetics challenged both racism and its philosophical, medical, and scientific underpinnings as he wove together complex shifts of voices, a nonlinear style of argumentation, forms of indirection, and forceful analyses in reproducing, parodying, and challenging the racialized imposition of incommunicability.

In the end, Fanon projected speech acts emerging within spaces of incommunicability as critical sites for sparking revolutionary transformation. Detailing settlers' use of zoological terms to dehumanize colonial subjects, Fanon suggests: "The native knows all this, and laughs to himself every time he spots an allusion to the animal world in the other's words. For he knows that he is not an animal; and it is precisely at the moment he realizes his humanity that he begins to sharpen the weapons with which he will secure its victory" ([1961] 1963, 430). Commenting on how exhortations on Western values produce a bodily reaction, "a sort of stiffening or muscular lockjaw," he adds: "When the native hears a speech about Western culture he pulls out his knife—or at least he makes sure it is within reach" (43). In *The Wretched of the Earth*, Fanon traced the forms of interrogation, torture, and rape used by French security forces—including some of his white patients—to overpower efforts by Algerian militants and their family members to use silence as a tool for transforming incommunicability into a means of preventing disclosure of revolutionary identities and strategies. Fanon's clinical studies pointed to the complex effects of both communicabilities and incommunicabilities in the contexts of war and colonialism on Algerian and French patients alike. Adopting the familiar form of the case study, Fanon engaged in sociodiagnosis, analyzing the forms of colonial violence that gave rise to psychic disorders. Rather than focusing on individual patients, he argued that it was colonial society that was sick and generated a range of pathologies. In the end, the cure for colonial communicability was revolution, a commitment to use "absolute violence" in overturning the foundational violence of colonialism.

Toward the end of the "Medicine and Colonialism" essay, Fanon undercut the power of his positioning—political and clinical—of incommunicability as a starting point for struggles to overturn racism, colonialism, and their effects on communication, health, and human relations. Noting how liberation was turning "'the' doctor" into "'our' doctor, 'our' technician," Fanon ([1959] 1967, 142) suggested that medicine, hygiene, and ideas about disease transmission were being readily accepted as "the people wanted to get well, wanted to care for themselves and were anxious to understand the explanations proffered by fellow doctors or nurses." Simultaneously, witchcraft and belief in the *djinn*, "all these things that seemed to be part of the very being of the Algerian, were swept away." Fanon continued: "Even instructions difficult for highly technological societies to accept were assimilated by the Algerian" (143). In short, the revolution had allowed the world of perfect communicability falsely promised by colonial medicine finally to appear. Fanon had argued that a key goal of colonial violence is to undermine the colonized population's belief in its own cultural traditions (McCullouch 1983), and he had conducted research with Islamic healers to learn about Algerian theories of and treatments for sexual dysfunction (Fanon [2015] 2018, 385–93). In celebrating what he deemed to be the transformative effects of the revolution for medicine, however, he applauded as "old superstitions began to crumble" (Fanon [1959]1967, 143).

I have argued that Fanon has much to offer us in taking up Shange's challenge to decolonize incommunicability as a point of departure and embrace it as a crucial analytic. He points, in both his writing and his clinical practice, to possibilities for displacing racialized, denigrating incommunicabilities and stripping communicabilities, including biomedical ones, of their roots in white supremacy, racism, classism, and colonial violence. For Fanon, in short, incommunicability becomes a revolutionary force. Nevertheless, even Fanon was not vaccinated against communicable hegemony, against the sense that communicability—and biocommunicability, at that—is the teleological horizon we all must embrace.

4

GEORGES CANGUILHEM AND THE CLINICAL
PRODUCTION OF INCOMMUNICABILITY

Even as Frantz Fanon points us in the direction of grappling with ways that
producing incommunicability is a constitutive feature of clinical medicine, this
topic is a central desideratum for our third philosopher-physician, Georges
Canguilhem, and his book *The Normal and the Pathological*. Canguilhem is particularly important for our inquiry, because he focuses on how the body itself
enters centrally into affording an individual's passage into states of communicability and, particularly, of incommunicability. Similarly, the clinical production of incommunicability constitutes, for him, not a special case but a
common result of clinical practice, at least in the case of chronic disease.

Canguilhem began his career studying philosophy under the neo-Kantian
Émile Chartier, known as Alain. A close disciple of Alain's, Canguilhem
embraced his Cartesianism, with its separation of mind and body, and his
pacifist position. Starting in 1936, thirty-one-year-old Canguilhem took two
decisive moves, joining the French Resistance and beginning medical studies. Why study medicine? Giuseppe Bianco (2012, 247) reports that the main
difficulty in answering this question is "Canguilhem's absolute silence: he
never talked explicitly about his medical training, and he only very rarely

mentioned his intellectual itinerary before the publication of his medical doctoral dissertation, *The Normal and the Pathological.* In the introduction to the 1966 edition, Canguilhem noted:

Having taken up medical studies some years after the end of our philosophical studies, and parallel to teaching philosophy, we owe some explanation of our intentions. It is not necessarily in order to be better acquainted with mental illnesses that a professor of philosophy can become interested in medicine. Nor is it necessarily in order to exercise a scientific discipline. We expected medicine to provide precisely an introduction to concrete human problems. . . . The present work is thus an effort to integrate some of the methods and attainments of medicine into philosophical speculation. ([1966] 1978, 33–34)

The result was genuinely transdisciplinary, not simply working between disciplines but moving beyond fixed disciplinary boundaries to rethink basic disciplinary presuppositions. Canguilhem's approach to the philosophy of science focused on key concepts, which he saw not as transcendental categories fixed in universal grids but as historically contingent notions inherited from the past and periodically reshaped. In David Peña-Guzmán's (2018, 29) characterization of Canguilhem's work, concepts provide "schemas of perception, discourse, and thought that affect how and what scientists *see, say,* and *think.*" Canguilhem traced how concepts are historically mutable, appearing in multiple theories and often attempting to erase their histories to gain a sense of power and correspondence to reality. In Roman Jakobson's ([1957] 1971) terms, they are shifters, conveying different meanings in different contexts. A historical analysis of concepts gave him a crucial means of working between philosophy and medicine. Nevertheless, Canguilhem's historical orientation placed him at odds with many professional philosophers of science, given that his "aim was not to attack science but to show it in action in its specificity and plurality" (Rabinow 1994, 13). His deep engagement with philosophical concepts sometimes alienated scientific and medical practitioners, and his close attention to scientific ideologies and practices seemed marginal for many historians. Peña-Guzmán (2018, 29) thus suggests that, "for most of his life, Canguilhem found himself trapped in the negative space between these disciplines: too historical for the philosophers, too philosophical for the scientists, and too scientistic for the historians."

Digging deeply into European histories of medicine, Canguilhem traced a growing emphasis on disease rather than health. Here he converged with a fundamental tenet of Latin American social medicine and critical epidemiology

(Breilh 2003; Menéndez 2009), which have critically engaged this shift in orientation. A crucial point of departure for *The Normal and the Pathological* is rejecting the notion, advanced by the positivist physician Victor Broussais and the philosopher Auguste Comte, that the difference between normal and pathological states is a matter of degree, a quantitative difference, rather than of kind. Canguilhem instead looked to René Leriche, who, as Kevin Gotkin (2016) notes, "takes seriously the testimony of a sick person." Paul Rabinow (1994, 15) suggests that "this work signaled a major reversal in thinking about health." Rather than following Comte in viewing knowledge of the normal as preceding understanding of the pathological, Canguilhem followed Leriche in reversing this relation, quoting his assertion that "the sick man can thus advance knowledge about the normal man" (quoted in Canguilhem [1966] 1978, 100). Viewing life as "not statis, a fixed set of natural laws" but as "action mobility and pathos" (Rabinow 1994, 17), Canguilhem went on to examine the lifeworld occupied by a patient with a serious chronic disease, suggesting that she cannot understand it in terms of her previous, "normal" bodily experience. He brilliantly traced the transformations experienced by patients on entering into a prolonged illness. Shifting frames of reference away from the absence of the prior, "normal" state, he suggested that "the pathological state . . . must be understood as one type of normal, as the abnormal is not what is normal but what constitutes another normal" ([1966] 1978, 203).

Canguilhem's essay "The Living and Its Milieu" ([1965] 2008) can help us grasp how his argument unfolds. He rejects the characterization of living beings as surrounded by and acted on by the objective forces of the environment. Beings instead engage relationally and dynamically with a "milieu." The living being structures, as the essay's title suggests, its milieu through forms of perception and pragmatic experiences as beings pick out objects and position them in relation to one another and to the being in question (118). Relations are determinative in both directions, with the being "both dominating the milieu and accommodating itself to it." (113). As Todd Meyers (2019) observes, "'The living' resides on one side of the conjunction in the title, the living and *its* milieu—not a general milieu concept, not a generic environment, but a milieu proper to *that* organism, to the living." There are interesting resonances between Canguilhem's notion of the milieu and work in linguistic anthropology of several decades ago on "contextualization," which sought to replace reified, static notions of "the context" with dynamic, ongoing processes that both structure elements of surrounds and are continually affected by them (Gumperz 1982). With the advent of a serious chronic illness, a person transforms even what might seem to be the same environment into a different milieu. Canguilhem ([1965] 2008, 113) added that unlike "a healthy life," "the pathological state" transforms this relationship into "a struggle, . . . an opposition."

The relationship to language here is crucial. In Canguilhem's formulation, life provides the patient with expressions tied to what is perceived as "the normal," how healthy bodies and minds function. This "normal" state is no longer cognitively and affectively accessible as the pathological state becomes the only normal available to the patient. Accordingly, words and speech acts that depend on "the normal" are incapable of capturing the patient's experience. Canguilhem referred to "cases of insanity where the patients seem incomprehensible to others as well as to themselves" ([1966] 1978, 115). To his credit, he did not rigidly separate physical and mental health as opposing spheres but saw this process as applying to both. Reflecting his training in medicine and philosophy at each turn, Canguilhem emphasized how this rupture produces an impasse in clinical exchanges. Starting again from reference to particular "cases of insanity," he noted that "it is impossible for the physician, starting from the accounts of sick men, to understand the experience lived by the sick man, for what sick men express in ordinary concepts is not directly their experience but their interpretation of an experience for which they have been deprived of adequate concepts" (115).

In his medical historiography, Canguilhem traced a movement from anatomy to physiology to pathology that cast pathology as "a natural extension of physiology," thereby conditioning how physicians address "the relations between the normal and the pathological" ([1966] 1978, 42). Replicating stages in the training of physicians from dissections that provide a sensuous relationship to anatomy to rounds that provide experience with a broad range of nosologically defined pathologies, physicians' relationship to pathologies would seem to reproduce the ontological priority of the normal. Even as the pathological is defined vis-à-vis its transformation from the presupposed physiological "normal," the instrumentalist, curative goal of medicine is to restore "the normal." Like Fanon's critique of instrumentalist logics in medicine and science, Canguilhem commented on the work of the sociologist Auguste Comte and the natural scientist Claude Bernard in pinpointing "the fundamental positivist idea" that casts technologies and interventions as "the application of a science" that constructs the function of knowledge teleologically as grounds for intervention: "to know in order to act" (99). Herein lies another way that Canguilhem is important for my argument.

Canguilhem helps us think about experiential and communicable problems confronting patients in two ways. First, Canguilhem stressed that for patients, the abnormal is a land of no return: "The fundamental biological fact that life does not recognize reversibility" ([1966] 1978, 196) means that "no cure is a return to biological innocence. To be cured is to be given new norms of life" (228). Thus, demanding that patients acknowledge a lost "normal," use it in articulating their present experience, and express a desire to return to a "normal" state of being—all fundamental features of biocommunicability—produces a profound state of incommunicability. He argued that this attempt to normalize pathological states thwarts both patients' ability to communicate with their physicians and patients' efforts to develop new modes of perception and articulation. Think about the common use of numerical rating scales for pain. When patients report that they are in pain, physicians ask them to rate their pain on a scale of zero, meaning no pain, to ten, designating the worst possible pain. When asked this question during moments of intense pain, I remember my confusion. "What," I silently asked myself, "did it feel like to be without pain?" Living at that moment only in a world of pain, I found the comparative task both impossible and frustrating. Such encounters thus push patients whose prior relationships among experience, language, environments, and body have suddenly collapsed further into incommunicability, even as they promise a return to biocommunicability. Rather than discovering the new milieu that their patients inhabit and helping support their efforts to explore ways that incommunicabilities associated with emerging pathologies can become productive of novel ways of thinking, feeling, and being, the normalizing functions of clinical communicability unwittingly edge patients further into potentially despondent and debilitating positions of incommunicability.

I want to use these insights in rethinking in/communicability. Canguilhem emphasized that the normal is not simply the patient's experience of health but the result of a constant process of normal*izing*, of imposing medical and scientific normativities. "The norm, by devaluing everything that the reference to it prohibits from being considered normal" ([1966] 1978, 240) renders "the sick man" abnormal "because of his incapacity to be normative" (186). Clinical encounters impose a normalizing process on and through the ideological work of communicability. I focus in chapter 5 on the dominant models of clinical interaction that physicians and other practitioners acquire during their professional training and how patients learn to respond to the cues that providers offer. Rather than coproducing pragmatic features of a specific interaction, physicians' imposition of biocommunicability—as justified by an instrumental, teleological logic that makes good "patient outcomes" seem contingent on good doctor-patient communication—is a normativizing force that continually regiments each party's conduct in terms of general, unstated biocommunicable norms. Even as both providers and patients must self-monitor in each clinical encounter to ensure that they are displaying bio-communicable competence, physicians are extensively evaluated in medical school for their ability to produce signs that they are engaged with patients; this process of assessment is also lodged in patients' comments, now elicited through surveys. Evaluations of patients' biocommunicable competence, on the other hand, emerge continually through providers' verbal and nonverbal reactions, as well as much more subtly and consequentially through decisions regarding the bestowal of more or less desirable forms of treatment (or none at all), and, more rarely, being dropped as a patient. Despite being adopted as a part of patient-centered medicine, biocommunicable demands push patients into new spaces of incommunicability that engender senses of confusion and discomfort, exacerbated by the feeling (often reflected in the provider's face and intonational features of their voice) that they have failed communicatively. If good health requires good communication and if you are judged to have failed communicatively, patients are made to feel responsible for their illness and problems arising in treatment and recovery. Thus, thinking with Canguilhem can help us see how the instrumental and normative dimensions of this demand for biocommunicability can undermine the clinical process.

Canguilhem's work can deepen our understanding of the transformative potentialities that lie in ways that people inhabit spaces of incommunicability. Physicians generally pathologize incommunicability as a failure and a threat to biomedical efficacy that must—if possible—be eliminated. Communicable regimes thus foreclose the possibility of gaining insight into ways that voices emerging from within incommunicable spaces, like the "stand" that drove Locke to create his communicable nosology, could yield new understandings not just of a particular patient but of medicine and experiences of health and disease in general. In suggesting the value of Canguilhem's work for disability studies, Gotkin (2016) draws attention to a passage in which Canguilhem cites Leriche: "'At every moment there lie within us many more physiological possibilities than physiology would tell us about. But it takes disease to reveal them to us'" (quoted in Canguilhem [1966] 1989, 100). Canguilhem thus concludes: "Diseases are new ways of life" (100).

Although Canguilhem thus has much to offer in coming to understand communicability and incommunicability, his insights would come at a considerable cost if we were to leave Fanon's critique of race, racism, and clinical practice behind. Interestingly, it appears that Canguilhem and Fanon spent time (one summer and two years, respectively) in the same center of radical psychiatry, Saint-Alban, although at different times. It seems that Fanon came across Canguilhem's *The Normal and the Pathological* due to this connection (Macey 2000, 143). Fanon attended to issues of multilingualism and language variation; speech styles (including racist ones); and the importance of performativity, poetics, and genre, including in his own writing. Canguilhem's view of language, by contrast, was primarily limited to the lexical and referential, to how physicians' understanding of illness is limited by requiring patients to "express in ordinary concepts" experiences "for which they have been deprived of adequate concepts" ([1966] 1978, 115). Here Canguilhem missed the communicative power of silence and such nonreferential features as intonation and sound symbols, from groans and slight variations in voice timbre, loudness, and pitch to the corporeal semiotics of gesture, gaze, head movement, bodily movement and orientation, and the like, a topic to which I return in later chapters.

Finally, Canguilhem individualized the boundary between the normal and the pathological, suggesting that its analysis can only become "perfectly precise for one and the same individual considered successively" (182). Carlo Caduff (2019) suggests that "he starts from the premise that there is an individual who constitutes her milieu. This is perhaps the most important limit in Canguilhem's approach." Canguilhem did not focus on how differences of race, class, and nation shape perceptions of normality, pathology, diagnosis, and treatment, thereby deprovincializing European constructions of physicians and patients and elevating seemingly deracialized minds and bodies to the status of universals. We have learned to be more critical about invocations of "the body," given its universalizing and abstracting power. As Hortense Spillers (1987) powerfully suggests, the flesh of enslaved people—particularly women—was seen more as property than as human bodies. Canguilhem's formulation needs to undergo substantial revision in coming to grips with Fanon's ([1952] 2008, 92) description of how his "body schema, attached in several places, collapsed, giving way to an epidermal racial schema" in the face of racist acts. Fanon's powerful analysis of how white physicians performed the incommunicability of their colonized patients challenges Canguilhem's projection of the "normal" and of physicians' practices of normalization. Recall Carolyn Rouse's (2009) ethnography of how doctors normalized requests by Black sickle cell patients for pain medications as reflecting a racialized norm of baseless requests for drugs. When daily life is structured by profound inequities in education, housing, employment, political rights, access to health care, land expropriation, and the sorts of everyday acts of racist denigration analyzed by W. E. B. Du Bois and Fanon, does life become abnormal only when pathogens or chronic diseases have been diagnosed? Du Bois's ([1903]

1990, 154) powerful lament clearly positioned his son, Burghardt, as born in the shadow of the Veil, destined less to experience a normal life than to have "this little soul . . . grow choked and deformed within the Veil."

In short, Canguilhem provided us with fundamental insights into how medical perspectives and practices systematically produce incommunicability, and he opened up possibilities for thinking about how incommunicabilities can give rise to new ways of being, understanding, communicating, and healing. He analyzed how imposing biocommunicability on patients with chronic or serious illnesses thwarts the goals of physicians and patients alike. Building on his insights will, however, require displacing the same sorts of normative projections of white, socially and economically privileged Euro-American subjects that haunted Locke's view of language and knowledge.

PART II

*How Incommunicability Shapes
Entanglements of Language and Medicine*

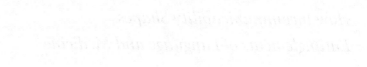

5

BIOCOMMUNICABLE LABOR AND THE
PRODUCTION OF INCOMMUNICABILITY
IN "DOCTOR-PATIENT INTERACTION"

In the introduction and chapter 1, I devoted considerable attention to examining the ideological labor that has attempted to separate language and communication from medicine and the body. Subsequently, dialogues with W. E. B. Du Bois, Frantz Fanon, and Georges Canguilhem helped me trace how ideologies of communicability and incommunicability; discursive practices relating to medicine, colonialism, and psychiatry; forms of linguistic racism; and everyday acts of racism reveal how language and medicine are continually coproduced. These chapters also suggested how incommunicabilities can be inhabited in ways that radically question communicability and the forms of white supremacy on which it rests.

In part II, I explore two research areas in which health-communication connections have, however, long been apparent: doctor-patient interaction and health communication. Each of these is tied to massive domains—one might almost say industries—of practice. They are crucial in configuring health care and health outcomes, particularly for racialized and other disadvantaged populations, but they also have much broader implications in shaping racial and other hierarchies. I argue that the tense tangos they dance between making communication and medicine seem ideologically autonomous and revealing their imbrications generally result not in challenging the production of incommunicabilities but in deepening their negative consequences and making them seem like natural effects—if not causes—of health and other inequities. The stakes for challenging how dominant communicabilities thwart the goals of health professionals and patients and constrain the emergence of radically new approaches are thus high.

Given how communication between doctors and patients emerged in our discussions of Du Bois, Fanon, and Canguilhem, I begin with this subject. I surmise that it may be the arena in which intersections of health and communication have perhaps gained their greatest visibility, as much in scholarly research as in clinical practice. Known variously as doctor-patient, physician-patient, and provider-patient interaction or communication, this research trajectory has drawn scholars from various disciplines. It is a remarkable example in which academic research has been taken to heart by physicians, nurses, and the faculties that train them. Advertisements for healthcare systems and clinical facilities—from billboards to television and digital advertisements—project smiling, concerned physicians. They are designed to attract patients by using visual images that project doctors and nurses as engaged, caring listeners. Both providers and the patients who seem to return their warm smiles and attentive forms of engagement provide models, literally, of biocommunicability in health care.

This body of research is analytically centered primarily in conversation analysis (CA), which was initiated mainly by sociologists. Harvey Sacks (1984) and other scholars laid out several key CA methodological tenets. First, research centers on "actual occurrences" of social interaction. John Heritage and Maxwell Atkinson (1984, 2) commented that "within conversation analysis there is an insistence on the use of materials collected from *naturally occurring* occasions of everyday interaction by means of audio- and video-recording equipment or film." According to Emanuel Schegloff (1992, 106), CA "departs from, and can always be referred to and grounded in, the details of actual occurrences of conduct in interaction." Charles Goodwin and Alessandro Duranti (1992, 22) similarly stated that "face-to-face interaction provides the primordial locus for the production of talk." Second, published texts present segments of these recordings in the form of transcripts that center on the format presented by Gail Jefferson in her appendix to the paper by Sacks and his colleagues (1974). Researchers have isolated different interactional phases of clinical visits: Opening, Presenting Complaint, Examination, Diagnosis, Treatment, and Closing (Heritage and Maynard 2006a, 14).

The central role of communicability in informing research in this area and its extension into medical practice emerged in the opening lines of an influential review by two leaders in the field, the sociologists John Heritage and Douglas Maynard (2006b, 351):

> In the 1970s, two major studies established doctor-patient interaction as a viable research domain. The first, conducted by Korsch & Negrete (1972) at the Children's Hospital of Los Angeles, was based on observations of 800 pediatric acute care visits and used a modified version of Bales's (1950) Interaction Process Analysis (IPA) to code the data. The results were striking. Nearly one fifth of the parents left the clinic without a clear statement of what was wrong with their child, and nearly half were left wondering what had caused their child's illness. A quarter of the parents reported that they had not mentioned their greatest concern because of lack of opportunity or encouragement. The study uncovered a strong relationship between these and other communication failures and nonadherence with medical recommendations, showing that 56 % of parents who felt that the physicians had not met their expectations were "grossly noncompliant."

This statement is strikingly similar to John Locke's account of the meeting with friends in his chamber (see chapter 1). Locke reported that he identified a disorder (the emergence of confusion and disagreement), began a diagnostic process, pinpointed incommunicability as the cause, and proposed a solution: a new regime of communicability. Heritage and Maynard provided an origin story that similarly positioned a "striking" crisis of incommunicability as catalyzing this line of research. Presupposing the expectation that physicians should produce knowledge and patients should receive it—that is, the dominant, unilinear, hierarchically ordered model of biocommunicability—their summary suggests that a quarter of parents missed the opportunity to elicit the advice and intervention that physicians should provide; others either did not receive or grasp the content that physicians provided. This communicable failure is granted causal status, producing "nonadherence with medical recommendations" and the labeling of communicably deficient parents as "'grossly noncompliant.'" Heritage and Maynard's argument followed biomedical logics. Correct diagnosis of the causal agent—incommunicability—required a specific, bounded treatment: the transformation of doctor-patient interactions to make them maximally communicable.

This growing emphasis on doctor-patient interaction in medical education and practice is not isolated. Rather, it forms part of a shift that stresses not just medical knowledge but competence (DelVecchio Good 1995), "more emphasis on what physicians could *do* rather than what they *know*" (Hodges and McNaughton 2009, 282). Janelle Taylor (2011) details the associated rise in the use of "standardized patients" who are trained to play patients with particular pathologies in simulated medical interactions. In addition to their role in training sessions, standardized patients participate in examinations, enabling educators and examiners to evaluate candidates through quantitative scores provided by the standardized patients and through observers watching from behind one-way mirrors. These exercises have had high stakes for physicians since the National Board of Medical Examiners stipulated in 2004 that US physicians demonstrate "Clinical Skills" in national licensing examinations before they can practice. As Taylor notes, the use of standardized patients went hand in hand with diminishing emphasis on bedside teaching medical faculty, thus relying on low-paid nonmedical personnel (standardized patients) more than more highly paid professors. Crucially, using pretend rather than real patients fostered the standardization and quantification of biocommunicable competence, thus forming part of the shift toward "evidence-based medicine" (EBM) that emphasizes standardized clinical guidelines based on systematic reviews of randomized controlled trials (RCTs) over clinical judgment (Mykhalovskiy and Weir 2004; Nichter 2013; Ødemark and Engebretsen 2022; Sackett et al. 2000; Solomon 2015; Timmermans and Kolker 2004; Timmermans and Berg 2003). Evidence-based medicine forms part of broader processes that make claims for biomedical knowledge and authority in the face of challenges to "expert" authority and the dominance of neoliberal demands for efficiency and effectiveness (Lambert 2006). Physician-patient communication protocols thus allow the qualitative, experienced-based "art" of clinical practice to be reconfigured in terms provided by the growing emphasis on seemingly objective, quantitatively based guidelines.

My goal here is not to underestimate the value of a highly visible research trajectory and a prominent feature of clinical training. Rather, given the dominance of doctor-patient communication guidelines, particularly in the United States, I am interested in how particular types of biocommunicability become markers of successful medical practice and how incommunicabilities are created by this foundational move. I explore how ideological and pragmatic forms of labor associated with projecting biocommunicability as natural and necessary can exacerbate and naturalize communicative/health inequities.

Not all physicians embrace EBM, and some are highly critical of efforts to standardize and regiment how they relate to individual patients. Similarly, critical voices among researchers have pushed back on these issues for decades. Elliot Mishler (1984) points to how this focus directs attention away from more significant contextual problems toward technical biomedical frames and leads researchers to augment biomedical authority by adopting doctors' perspectives in analyzing medical encounters. Sue Fisher and Stephen Groce (1990, 226) similarly suggest that, by focusing on physicians' roles in medical encounters, "researchers in this tradition have unintentionally obscured the patient's point of view." In an influential critique, the physician-sociologist Howard Waitzkin (1991, 19) argues that communication protocols enable "doctor-patient interactions [to] convey ideologic messages under the rubric of scientific medicine." He analyzes how clinical encounters not only reproduce broader social inequalities, including the effects of racism, but help produce and naturalize them. Conversation analysis methodology focuses exclusively on what is audible and visible in recordings; everything outside this frame becomes invisible, augmenting the decontextualizing effects of the dominant biocommunicable model in reifying the clinical scene. Jennifer Guzmán (2020) provides an excellent example of what gets left out of recordings made in the clinic. She details how Mapuche families' cartographies of health/communicative labor include the long journeys and huge expenditures required to transport patients, but physicians' time-space calculations and definitions of care include only what transpires after they enter the clinic's door. In other words, as Eduardo Menéndez (2009) stresses, doctors render most of what transpires outside the spatiotemporal parameters of the clinic incommunicable. (I return to this point later.)

Heritage and Maynard (2006b, 362) suggest that "CA begins from the presumption that physician and patient, with various levels of mutual understanding, conflict, cooperation, authority, and subordination, jointly construct the medical visit." Researchers have revealed how speech in clinical encounters follows gross power asymmetries that enable what Mishler (1984) calls the "voice of medicine" to dominate. Nancy Ainsworth-Vaughn (1992, 1998) looked in detail at a number of features of doctor-patient interaction, including topic transitions and such features as questions, responses, and interruptions. Although she suggests that all participants are continually involved in constructing power through interaction, physicians and male patients exercise more control. Fisher and Groce (1990, 227) suggest that "accounting practices," ways that physicians and patients account for their actions, "function strategically" in shaping "a moment-by-moment battle in which patients struggle to get heard, simultaneously displaying yet another manifestation of the asymmetry in the medical relationship." Although physicians thereby display "the dominance of the medical role" (229), patients are not entirely passive.

Rather, they "manipulate the architecture of a conversation enabling patients to tell their stories, to provide information, and to display their competence," thereby exploding "the myth that patients are incompetent and have little to say that is relevant to their health care" (241). Framing these issues as a binary and zero-sum calculations of power between only two, seemingly homogeneous classes of actors fosters generalizations about "physicians" in such a way to overlook the tremendous heterogeneity among the ranks of doctors and their ways of interacting with patients. Such efforts to measure or challenge the standardizing power of communications protocols, particularly when articulated through a narrow scripting of medical discourse as doctor-patient dyads, overlook the role of the institutions (including healthcare corporations and state agencies) that employ physicians and the insurance companies and governmental bodies that impose diagnostic and treatment guidelines. Indeed, many doctors have turned away from clinical practice in response to the limitation and sidelining of their clinical judgment. Capturing these relations requires going beyond analyzing isolated recordings of doctor-patient interactions to include the sort of fieldwork conducted by Aaron Cicourel (1992) in which he traced how initial encounters were progressively recontextualized in subsequent face-to-face, recorded, and written contexts. One of the goals of this book is to provide doctors and patients with a framework that can help them extend their critiques and aid them in forging new perspectives and practices.

As long as linear, hierarchically ordered biocommunicability informs models of interaction, concepts of negotiation and mutual understanding introduce contradictions that apply with particular force in the face of racialized inequities. The role of biocommunicability here is direct and consequential. Assessments of patients as health communicators enter into the clinical judgments that, according to the Institute of Medicine, result in poorer care for African Americans and Latinx patients (Smedley, Stith, and Nelson 2003). Michelle Van Ryn and Jane Burke (2000) found that physicians assumed African Americans abused drugs and alcohol more frequently, were less educated and intelligent, were less attentive to medical guidance, and were less likely to follow treatment guidance than white patients. The ideal patient—whose seemingly deracialized features align with identifying whiteness as the "normal" baseline—is thus largely a biocommunicable construct.[1] Carolyn Rouse's (2009) careful study of sickle cell suggests that racialized stereotypes of incommunicability lead Black patients' statements about the excruciating pain associated with the disease to undergo a transformation of speech act classification—to be interpreted as illegitimate requests for drugs.

Indexical Landscapes of Care: Positioning Other Forms of Labor in the Work of Care

I drew on Canguilhem's insights in analyzing how clinicians can exacerbate incommunicability by asking patients to express their symptoms with reference to their prior, "normal" states, rendering "the sick role" (in Talcott Parsons's [1951] terms) even more incommunicable. Nevertheless, Canguilhem reproduces the analytical and empirical blinders of much doctor-patient interaction research by limiting his analysis to encounters between physicians and patients in the clinic. This constraint can limit physicians' ability to learn about dimensions of patients' lives outside these spaces.

The geographer Carl Sauer (1925) drew attention to the status of landscapes as palimpsests, where new cultural features were continually mapped onto spaces inhabited by previous inscriptions (Anschuetz, Wilshusen, and Scheick 2001).[2] The linguistic anthropologist Keith Basso (1996) wrote influentially about the power of narrative to create landscapes, spaces that are shaped by the words and actions of humans and nonhumans. Visiting them, either physically or narratively, then opens up narrators and audiences to the effects and affects that linger within them. Putting Sauer and Basso together, we could see clinical settings as potentially operating as palimpsests, spaces that are potentially continually transformed as patients imaginatively construct the landscapes they view as most deeply affecting their health and well-being, such as homes and (un)houses, worksites, schools, prisons, and social-service agencies. Patients can, again potentially, collaborate with providers in projecting clinical concerns back into them, thereby transforming their features. We need to ask, however, about the extent to which communicable constraints enable this process to unfold.

The following example comes from Waitzkin's classic *The Politics of Medical Encounters*. Compiling audio recordings of a random sample of 336 doctor-patient encounters, Waitzkin (1991, 64) and his team took transcription seriously, guided by work in CA and sociolinguistics. In the following transcript, a white doctor (D) speaks with "a 41-year-old man who works as an assistant food operations manager in a hotel. He is Catholic, black, divorced, a high school graduate, and the father of three children" (84). "Leading into a series of questions about the patient's neck and back pain," the physician links the primary diagnosis of "'acute muscle spasm'" to the patient's employment:

D: All right. And you're working somewhere?
P: At the _____ . . . (words)

D: What is your job there?

P: I'm the assistant food and beverage manager.

D: All right. Are you a healthy man basically?

P: I am.

D: Any chronic diseases?

P: I have, uhm, they call it, um, mature diabetes.

D: Do you take medicine for that?

P: No. I control my weight.

D: Good. (84)

Waitzkin's work provides fascinating analyses of how class and race inequities are produced, embodied, and made to seem natural. In this example, which he characterized as "routine and prosaic," Waitzkin focuses not on race but on how the doctor discusses issues of work (84).

To capture how clinical interactions could superimpose landscapes in such a way as to pinpoint the structural factors that shape health and disease, I would like to build on Michael Silverstein's notion of indexical order. Silverstein suggests that potentially relevant contexts are ordered, starting from the immediate spatiotemporal dimensions of the interaction. Nevertheless, indexical orders do not spring directly from contextual features. Instead, they emerge from how those features get reconfigured. "First-order indexicality" construes the interactional context in particular ways, a process that Silverstein (2003, 193) refers to as "schematization."[3] Contexts are thus transformed into semiotic constructions that shape subsequent discourse. (Note here the similarity to Canguilhem's notion of "the living and its milieu.") Things then get complicated as first-order indexical orders become the basis for further acts of schematization, a process that can create multiple, superimposed layers. Let us take a hypothetical example of a conversation among three individuals while taking a walk. Person A draws attention to "a pretty flowering tree" (first-order indexicality). Person B responds: "The species in question is not 'a pretty tree' but a white flowering dogwood or *Cornus florida*," thereby building second-order indexicality on A's schematization of this feature of the context. Person C then accuses B of always acting combative and competitive, creating a third-order indexicality that schematizes the first and second orders.

Even as the concept of indexical orders can help us rethink doctor-patient interaction, analyzing this case through the lens of in/communicability can point to limitations of Silverstein's valuable framework. He would identify first-order indexicality with features of the context, then examine how additional orders unfold across time and scale. Doctor-patient interaction research fixes us even more solidly on interactions that emerge in the space of the clinic as "the context." Even as Waitzkin challenged the doctor-patient interaction literature in other ways, he similarly identified "the context" with the patient and physician and the clinical space they occupy, thereby drawing attention away, for example, from the role of nurses and receptionists. Waitzkin accordingly encodes participant frameworks in his transcripts as "D" and "P."[4]

Enabling the patient to join the physician in jointly constructing a "schematization" that would calibrate work and clinical contexts would have helped figure out how the job site entered into producing the injury; it could become an essential locus for care. As Ainsworth-Vaughn (1992, 419) suggests, physicians often use "all right" at the beginning of a speech turn to acknowledge reception of the patient's previous utterance and mark the transition to a new topic. After asking for a job title, the physician closes the exchange about work and shifts to eliciting the patient's medical history. The doctor thus has allowed "working" to enter into clinical communicability only minimally and referentially. Instead of permitting the worksite to transform "the context" of the clinic and increase its communicable power and breadth, a later job-related discussion heads in the opposite direction: the doctor urges the patient to take time off from work and take breaks by lying down on a heating pad. By expressing "difficulties in staying home or even cutting back on job-related physical activity" (Waitzkin 1991, 85), a further attempt to lay out the contours of the worksite landscape, the patient signals that the treatment plan is unrealistic. Rather than picking up on how he has produced incommunicability, the physician offers to prescribe a narcotic.

My goal is hardly to second-guess the doctor, a task that I am neither inclined nor qualified to undertake. I instead wish to show that by controlling and restricting the unfolding of indexical orders, the physician misses a vital opportunity to pinpoint the causes of his patient's condition and collaborate in devising a plan to ameliorate them. Here I need to introduce a couple of terms from linguistic anthropology. In discussing communicability, I have been discussing the *ideological labor* that goes into constructing notions of health professionals, patients, knowledge, and communication in particular ways. Analyzing indexical orders also requires thinking about *pragmatics*, which involves the detailed way signs are used in actual examples. In a conversation, how people take turns, build on one another's words, shift topics, display attentiveness, and the like are issues of pragmatics. Finally, co-conversationalists also comment on what is being said; frame particular utterances as authoritative, hesitant, or humorous; and register their agreement or disagreement with what the other has said (stance taking). *Metapragmatic* elements are thus communication about communication. "Hold on. Could you repeat that, please?" is a metapragmatic sign that seeks to stop the flow of conversation, mark a particular stretch as not having been heard or understood, and requests a particular type of response. Doctor-patient protocols teach physicians to provide standardized metapragmatic signals that they are attentive to patients' concerns and needs. Metapragmatic cues also structure and control clinical interactions. In the earlier example, the physician's "All right. And you're working somewhere?" was a metapragmatic sign that signaled a shift of topic and the selection of work as the next focus of discussion. The second "all right" was a metapragmatic sign that closed off the work discussion. Pragmatics and metapragmatics dance a sort of tango, with metapragmatics attempting to control pragmatics in such a way as to shape how discourse proceeds and is interpreted—but without ever fully succeeding.[5]

The ideological basis that shapes the doctor's attempt to metapragmatically regiment or control the exchange revolves around narrow biomedical definitions of pathology, diagnosis, and treatment, which Menéndez (2009) refers to as the hegemonic medical model (*modelo médico hegemónico*). Projecting an individual patient and clinical visit as the indexical horizon, the physician places other structural inequities beyond the scope of clinical communicability. Many jobs—including agricultural labor, factory work, and the ever-growing demand for rapid package delivery—involve constant pressure on muscles and joints, stress, and exposure to toxins that commonly leave workers with disabling injuries at relatively young ages. By avoiding moving indexically beyond the context of the visit, the physician never learns whether his patient has faced unreasonable physical demands or whether occupational safety regulations might have provided guidelines for bringing them under control. By incarcerating the exchange within a narrow sphere of biocommunicability, the physician leaves no space for extending the indexical order to include ways that racialized inequities might be contributing to the patient's situation, from pay inequities and unequal access to promotions to the sorts of microaggressions—brief, often subtle nonverbal or verbal forms of bias and denigration that target members of racialized populations—that have been linked to health problems (Gómez 2015). In short, the doctor fails to transform the encounter into an opportunity to seek greater justice, both in the clinic and at the patient's worksite. The physician in question is hardly alone here. Fisher and Groce (1990, 242) suggest that physicians' accounting practices "function strategically to limit the scope of the discussion to medical topics and to legitimate the authority of the medical role," while patients' accounts "function strategically to expand the scope of the discussion to include social topics and to legitimate themselves as competent."[6]

Let us take a step back from this example. The production of incommunicability in clinical settings is particularly acute when health inequities intersect with health/communicative inequities (Briggs 2017). Research on the role of translation in health care provides a particularly clear window on this issue. Professional translators are paid to sustain communicability in the face of what are projected as potential sources of incommunicability: language differences between providers and patients. Generally more aligned with practitioners' perspectives than those of patients, translators often collaborate in hiding ways that patients resist professional ideological and metapragmatic control (Davidson 2001). Such erasures (Gal and Irvine 2019, 21) can withhold evidence that patients are displaying signs of active engagement and attempting to contribute communicatively to diagnosis and treatment, thereby jeopardizing their classification as good, cooperative patients and increasing the likelihood they will be deemed incommunicable.[7]

Commonsense understandings of medical translation reduce complex processes of moving back and forth between multiple ways of speaking (including technical, medical varieties), experiences of health and illness, and ways of being in the world to a simple matter of finding words in one language that seem to match those in another. Emily Yates-Doerr (2019, 299) argues that "translation, when treated as a process of making differences equivalent, functions to make nondominant languages and practices disappear." When translation becomes a means of imposing dominant communicabilities across terrains of communicative and medical difference, it can help project patient populations as incommunicable and silence their possible contributions to forging perspectives and practices that could enhance providers' and patients' goals. Indeed, the need for medical translation can itself be a symptom of race and class hierarchies that limit the recruitment of physicians with similar race, class, sexual, and other features of patient populations. As I noted in chapter 3, the problematic status of translation as a key element of colonial control was a limiting factor in Fanon's remarkable analysis of medicine and colonialism and his clinical practice.

The demographics of nurses and patient populations are often more closely matched, but biomedical orientations of training programs and nursing protocols can diminish the potential advantages that this concordance offers for bringing diverse communicabilities into dialogue. In a sensitive study of how nursing pedagogy in Papua New Guinea "transforms 'receivers'" of biomedical knowledge "into 'translators and disseminators,'" Barbara

Andersen (2017, 759) analyzes how nurses shift between Tok Pisin and vernacular languages and among medicalized registers, taboo terms for sex, and forms of metaphor and indirection. These choices, accompanied by extensive metapragmatic discourse, are not simple reflections of EBM protocols or the need to promote comprehension. They instead perform "a kind of ethical metapragmatics" (759) that constitutes "an indigenized 'confessional technology'" (764) used "to extract 'hidden' truths" (760), promote Christian values, increase adherence to treatment and prevention protocols, and manage the purportedly uneducated affective repertoires of patients. In other words, even as they incorporate Christian logics and vernacular speech practices into dominant communicabilities, their imposition reinforces the perception that Papua New Guinea populations are irremediably incommunicable.

In Delta Amacuro, Spanish-speaking physicians rely on Warao-speaking nurses as translators. Given that patients are often their neighbors and sometimes relatives, nurses could provide crucial details to aid physicians in diagnosis, particularly in complex cases. The physicians, who define the role of translation as moving referential content between two bounded, opposing linguistic codes, recruit nurses to help imprison discourse within the narrow biomedical frames they provide, maintaining their metapragmatic control over the indexical orders that emerge. When nurses occasionally display their ability to link diverse communicabilities in bridging communicative and medical practices, such departures from their assigned role are generally read as affronts to physicians' authority. Conversations in Warao outside the clinic often enable nurses to break through the Veil of incommunicability and learn a great deal more about the issues that patients are facing. Few of the Spanish-speaking physicians I have interviewed and observed were interested in the insights that emerged from exchanges they did not control—even when a mysterious disease that had gone undiagnosed for a year killed scores of people (Briggs and Mantini-Briggs 2016).

Anthropological research on the role of bilingual children as translators is striking (Urciuoli 1996). Interpreting between parents and health professionals confronts children with unfamiliar medical registers and institutional procedures "while managing a synchronous, multiparty interaction" (Reynolds and Orellana 2009, 215). Beyond uncomfortably participating in discussions of parents' sensitive health and other issues, child translators face difficult decisions about whether to acknowledge metapragmatic signs of communicative and medical profiling and patient resistance to biocommunicability. Despite the immensity and precarity of the task, they often face both parents' and providers' "critiques of their linguistic, cognitive, social, and behavioral competencies" (221). Such biocommunicable contradictions can entwine providers, patients, and families in practices that undermine the achievement of health/communicative justice, even as they all attempt to provide care.[8]

What I would call communicable racial profiling thus dances a complex tango in which perceived social characteristics are tied to micro-monitoring of each utterance in the clinic, even as patients' words and actions are sometimes interpreted and assessed through the filter of incommunicable stereotypes. Problems evident in follow-up visits and lab results are often interpreted retrospectively as empirical evidence of in/communicability, often labeled "noncompliance." Herein lies a major contradiction. Social-science studies of provider-patient interaction and how doctors are trained to communicate more effectively with patients certainly spring from a genuine interest in improving care. A focus on clinical translation similarly emerges from concern with how perceived linguistic divides can jeopardize clinical outcomes. Nevertheless, we seem to return to Locke's foundational diagnosis: identifying incommunicability as a pathology and threat that requires remediation. The treatment protocol is remarkably similar: creating a standardized regime of biocommunicability that seeks to identify and extirpate dimensions of incommunicability. As for Locke, the cure is mainly responsible for the disease: imposing biocommunicability itself constitutes a major force for creating incommunicability and turning it into a stigmatizing force that can thwart the goals of providers and patients. To return to the discussion of Sara Ahmed (2019) on use: rather than examining how doctor-patient protocols can affect the experience and well-being of patients, their use is rationalized by their projected usefulness in improving care. Rather than helping physicians grasp the broader contexts and social forces that shape their patients' health, this communicable order helps seal the clinic off from much of the rest of the world that surrounds it.

Narratives in Clinical Spaces: Encounters on Borders of Incommunicability

One of the areas in which the communicative versus medical binary has been most fruitfully bridged is in work on narrative. I focus here on a book that provides a celebrated point of reference: Arthur Kleinman's *The Illness Narratives* (1988). In the prologue, Kleinman recounts a moment during his medical training when his role is to support a seven-year-old girl whose severe burns require a daily whirlpool bath in which physicians remove her burned flesh. Kleinman is tasked with holding her uninjured hand and reducing her resistance to the excruciating treatment; his initial efforts reflect a communicable model that projects narrative disembodiment: getting the girl to talk about "her home, her family, her school" might prompt less of a focus on the procedure and her pain, thereby easing her agony and increasing compliance (xi). He thus initially tries, in classic Lockean fashion, to separate the communicative task with which he has been charged from the medical procedures being performed and, following Canguilhem, to suggest that she describe her previous, "normal" life in order to draw attention away from an agonizing pathological state. A sense of failure prompts Kleinman to ask the girl to tell him about the experience of being so terribly burned and the painful treatment. By joining the girl in her descent into incommunicability, the two are able to coproduce a distinct communicable model that gives rise to novel subject positions and relationships to knowledge, embodiment, and medicine.

Kleinman describes a reciprocal transformation as the patient seems "noticeably better able to tolerate the debridement" and the physician-in-training learns "a grand lesson in patient care" (xii). Dell Hymes's (1981) narrative research can help us slow down the story and further appreciate what happened. Hymes distinguishes between narratives that are "interpretable," "reportable," and "repeatable" and those that mark a "breakthrough into performance." The first three produce distanced relationships between what Roman Jakobson ([1957] 1971) terms narrated events and events of narration; in them, storytellers point toward narratives whose enactment seems to unfold elsewhere, taking responsibility only for characterizing their meaning or reporting on or repeating an act of narration. With a "breakthrough into performance," narrators take responsibility for creating lifeworlds that unfold in narratives and ongoing, performative acts of bringing them into being. In his classic work on performance, Richard Bauman (1977) emphasizes the emergent quality of performance and how unique configurations of participants, circumstances, and desires shape the form and content of narratives. In performances, narrative processes are as much on display as narrated events. Bauman stresses the active role of audiences, analyzing how even brief responses ("Wow!"), gestures, and facial expressions constitute forms of co-narration.

Kleinman's move here is innovative in two ways. First, he opens up a form of communicability that centers on the coproduction of knowledge about illness and medical forms of treatment by patient and provider. Second, the patient—a seven-year-old child—is interpellated not in the subordinate role as a recipient of the understandings produced by health professionals but as a partner in generating and articulating them. This breakthrough into performance enables subject positions, subjectivities, and social relations to become more open to scrutiny and transformation. I surmise that holding the girl's hand similarly shifts from an enactment of biomedical authority to an embodied register of co-narration. Rather than attempting to normalize her experience, Kleinman avoids the trap that Canguilhem identified by joining the patient in cocreating a form of communicability that helps her articulate the world of pathology and incommunicability that she inhabits.

For Kleinman (1988, xiii), this vignette articulates a different vision of medicine: eliciting patients' narratives of their experience of illness and their "explanatory models" becomes "a core task in the work of doctoring." As the voice of a badly burned seven-year-old is transformed from cries of resistance into sources of insight, a challenge emerges to linear, hierarchically organized biocommunicable models, unlocking potential breakthroughs in confronting health/communicative inequities. Menéndez (2009) suggests that much labor on which biomedicine depends is *autoatención*, or care enacted by laypeople outside clinical settings as they monitor their bodies and those of family members, friends, and coworkers; make decisions regarding possible interventions; allocate resources and provide transportation; respond to diagnostic questions; and support treatment regimes. Nevertheless, this labor generally becomes invisible or is denigrated when patients and their relatives enter clinics; it is turned into evidence of ignorance, misinformation, resistance, or noncompliance—in short, of incommunicability. In the preceding example, Kleinman focuses on care provided by health professionals in the clinic. Nevertheless, eliciting patients' narratives can open up spaces for making lay forms of labor—including care and much more—visible and acknowledged. I would urge the expansion of illness narratives to include patients' accounts of how they have been treated as incommunicable and their efforts to articulate how they struggle to render communicability less narrow, constraining, and hierarchal. In this way, illness narratives could help transform incommunicability into productive spheres that yield not stigma but new possibilities for caring and living.

Rethinking Kleinman's contribution through the lenses of in/communicabilities and health/communicative inequities suggests ways to deepen this challenge to dominant modalities. He notes that narratives emerge through "clinical and research interviews" (1988, xv) as practitioners engage in "the sensitive solicitation of the patient's and the family's stories of the illness" (10). Interviews impose important restrictions if the goal is to challenge dominant biomedical communicabilities and to collaborate in devising alternatives. Interviewers and interviewees face unequal power relations: interviewers claim rights to decide what counts as knowledge, who will elicit it, and how it will be used (see Briggs 1986). When physicians serve as interviewers, two power asymmetries converge.[9] Interviews rest on communicable models that picture interactions as structured by interviewers' search for particular kinds of content, requiring interviewees to fit their unique experiences, perspectives, and semiotic practices into the discursive boxes provided.

In that health professionals are expected to extract information in responding to patients' health needs, interviews conducted in clinical settings are in some ways less artificial than those created by strangers (fieldworkers) to further projects that figure into researchers,' not respondents,' agendas. Clinical interviews are ideally oriented toward goals shared by both parties, although their understandings and agendas do not perfectly coincide. Coproducers of the form and content of what emerges, clinicians largely control the metapragmatics that structure interviews. As with research interviews, once the encounter ends, the clinician is invested with the power to interpret the exchange and decide what future lives it will lead, whether in charts, referrals, clinical presentations, or publications, even as their power here is shared—often reluctantly—with administrators, insurance companies, and state regulators. At the same time, interviews are generally treated as black boxes, such that the complex and collective process of knowledge production and the interviewer's positionality and goals fade into the background as results seemingly provide transparent windows on interviewees' lifeworlds. Members of racialized populations have decried for generations that interviews often produce incommunicability and stigma, especially when they are conducted by white, middle-class social scientists. More than four decades ago, Américo Paredes ([1978] 1993) analyzed cases in which Latinx respondents asked white researchers to join them in x-raying how researchers, journalists, and politicians produce incommunicability and stigma. Anthropologists nonetheless reproduced denigrating images of cultural difference and positioned themselves as embodiments of white communicability, "the *transparent I*" that, Denise Ferreira da Silva (2022, 13) argues, lies at the heart of white supremacy. Interviews and surveys are crucial technologies in positioning white, middle-class professionals in what Nadine Hubbs (2014, 2) refers to as the role of "the narrating class."[10]

As I argued in an ethnographic critique of the use of interviews in social-science research, my goal is to suggest not that interviews should be outlawed. It is to suggest that what comes out of them should be analyzed not as if they are transparent windows on interviewees' lifeworlds but complex, problematic, power-laden coperformances with interviewers, as well as to suggest the value of documenting interviewees' communicable models and knowledge-exchange practices (Briggs 1986). For one thing, interviews are not well suited for gaining insight into the social lives of stories, given that they generally render invisible practices patients use in producing, circulating, interpreting, and evaluating knowledge about health and disease outside of clinical settings. Linguistic anthropologists have long focused ethnographic attention on ecologies of narrative and how they form part of and help constitute daily life, social inequities, and, as Veena Das (2007) shows, catastrophic events and their deep historical residues. Cheryl Mattingly (1998) suggests that rather than reflecting on preexisting events, stories are performative acts that bring events and social worlds into being, adding that bodies themselves tell stories in clinical settings. The "multimodal" approach used by many linguistic anthropologists focuses on how bodies and objects are not accessories to words but are central to producing interaction and meaning. Interviews, especially after researchers reduce them to verbal transcripts that record only referential content, primarily present bodies—when they appear at all—as objects of representation, not agentive and performative forces. Linguistic anthropologists have extensively explored the formal or poetic features and patterns that imbue narratives with complexity and meaning, opening up different ways to explore their significance.[11]

I would anticipate that some medical anthropologists and health professionals might dismiss such issues as being of interest only to linguistic anthropologists, but such a view would be mistaken. Let us return to Menéndez's (2009) signature focus on *autoatención*, to the work of care that laypeople do outside of the clinic. I would add to his discussion that narratives and other discourse forms are crucial components. They provide archives of *autoatención* that capture knowledge about the health of individuals, families, and collectivities; illness events; and what has been done—by health professionals and laypeople alike—to address them. They render this knowledge accessible when facing new or worsening symptoms, decisions about available treatments, or attempts to seek additional help, offering potential caregivers insight into what has taken place. Rather than representations that exist apart from symptoms and acts of care, they are woven into their textures, as Mattingly suggests, and play a crucial role in shaping both what is and isn't done and how people perceive and react to what is taking place. To use an analogy, Walter Benjamin (1968) argues that craftsmen learn their trades and repertoires of stories simultaneously, such that voices, bodies, and hands are trained by both work and storytelling. Further connecting materiality and narration, he richly suggests that "traces of the storyteller cling to the story the way the hand-prints of the potter cling to the clay vessel" (92). To extend his analogy, traces of stories cling to bodies and acts of care, even long after an illness has ended. After all, the aroma of chicken soup or of Vicks VapoRub (often pronounced *vaporu* in Spanish) can evoke embodied senses of (grand)parental caregiving. Beyond the content of the narratives embedded in *autoatención*, their poetic and embodied features—gestures, facial expressions, intonational changes, rhythmic repetitions, and the like—iconically produce understandings of embodied states and indexically attach them to times, places, people, and events. As Menéndez emphasizes, *autoatención* is relational, constantly shaped by ways that laypeople actively assimilate biomedical formulations and layer them with nonbiomedical forms of knowledge and practice. Thus, if our understanding of illness narratives is confined to those produced in clinical spaces through interviews and features of narrative performances are overlooked, researchers and practitioners will have lost most of the insights that they can engender.[12] Canguilhem (2012, 25) observes that "the doctor's ambition" is "to procure for the sick man, by efficacious interventions, an amelioration or a restitution that he would not know how to obtain by his own means." This foundational move projects lay perspectives and practices as incommunicable—it is only through their presupposition and erasure that clinical spaces and perspectives gain value.

Kleinman's brilliant book has affected medicine: learning to listen to patients' narratives has become a standard part of clinical practice. Unfortunately, temporal and fiscal pressures constrain the emergence of narratives and transform them into entries in electronic records and requests for reimbursement. Reducing care to standardized, monetized services limits the potential of Kleinman's call to use patients' narratives for producing critical perspectives on medicine. Linguistic and medical anthropological research on inequities can come together in productive ways if we look critically and ethnographically at who gets to tell their stories, to which audiences, who controls their poetics, who gets rights to retell them, and whose voices become more powerful in the process. Innovative reflexive practices of this sort could be used as much in academic research as clinical practice. In sum, although eliciting narratives can provide a crucial means of critiquing biocommunicability, it is crucial to maintain "presence of mind," in Benjamin's (1968) terms, to keep from losing sight of how their elicitation can produce incommunicability and project it as a ready explanation for the effects of health/communicative inequities.

Caregiver-Patient Interaction beyond Biomedical Spheres

Beyond marginalizing other health workers, such as nurses, technicians, and receptionists, the doctor-patient interaction focus elevates an ideological and institutional feature of biomedicine to the status of a universal feature of care. Anthropological work on other healing systems opens up possibilities for thinking more critically and comparatively about clinical participation structures, in Erving Goffman's (1981) terms. Ethnographic studies point to the ethnocentrism that underlies models of clinical communicability as starting with bounded individuals who fit neatly into D-P dyads. Paul Kockelman (2007) documents K'ichi' views of health and disease as distributed over several individuals rather than a single person (identified as "the patient"); this assemblage can then be classified as a single social person. T. S. Harvey (2008, 2013) argues that Mayan healing encounters often involve multiple patients who co-narrate illness narratives. In biomedical encounters, individuals who are receiving treatment may also be absent, their place taken by others. He cautions against depicting "'patienthood'" as a "universal," as an "intuitive way of being-in-the-world" (2008, 578). In her research on the participation of medical tourists in Mazatec healing, Paja Faudree (2020) not only widens understandings of participation frameworks to grant central roles to psychotropic plants but examines how the juxtaposition of contrastive communicable models can structure and destabilize healing interactions.

An extended ethnographic example can help us decolonize perspectives on in/communicability in biomedicine by looking beyond the referential bias of biomedical modalities. I focus on a respiratory illness presented by the six-year-old son of a close friend, Manuel Rivera, in June 1990. It occurred in a rainforest community near the Mariusa River, an area in which people did not practice agriculture but moved seasonally between the forest and the coast. The center of life in the former context was an annual ritual cycle focused on the moriche palm (*Mauritia flexuosa*). Residents erected a two-story structure with a huge palm-stem basket on the lower level and filled it with palm starch. Moriche palm starch was a crucial food source for humans in an area without stores or refrigeration and a gift to a class of invisible pathogens, *hebu*, deemed responsible for various diseases. Accompanied by sacred tobacco smoke, ritual dialogues enacted by healers through song chanting, and all-night dances, palm offerings constitute the community's efforts to induce the *hebu* to stay away during the coming year. Any misstep during the process could anger the *hebu*, inducing them to attack one or more humans, which is precisely what purportedly happened to the boy.[13]

The child developed a high fever and respiratory congestion. He slept little that night; since houses lack walls, we all slept poorly. By morning he lay weak and listless, his gaze unfocused. I supplied aspirin, but this proved to be small comfort. Manuel Torres is a *hoarotu*, a curer skilled in extracting and inflicting *hoa* spirits. While massaging the child's chest and abdomen, he was led to believe by the size and relative hardness of the perceived spiritual pathogens that other spirits, *hebu,* were to blame.[14] Everyone became concerned that the child might soon die. Visiting the Nabasanuka Clinic was nearly impossible, given that it would involve carrying the child through several kilometers of marshland and then a long ride through treacherous coastal waters in a dugout canoe. Thus, in the late afternoon, the family summoned José Medina, a specialist in controlling *hebu* spirits, upon his return from the forest. Medina already knew a lot about the case from listening to the child during the previous night and hearing talk circulating in the small group; conversations with Torres and other relatives provided additional diagnostically relevant details. Medina retrieved his rattle, which he had been using to engage with visiting *hebu* spirits, and arrived at Torres's house as darkness was falling. Laying the boy in a hammock, Medina alternated between sitting next to him on a stool and crouching or standing above him to press the rattle against his body. Torres and I sat just outside the small house.

On three occasions, Medina pressed the rattle firmly against the boy's abdomen; I had the impression that he was performing a sort of invisible surgery using a gourd decorated with parrot feathers. The performance was divided into seven songs, corresponding to the seven *hebu* spirits that he removed.[15] Once they had been extracted and sent away, the performance ended and the child went to bed. The fever had broken by morning, but the child remained relatively weak. He was up and playing by the afternoon. The child's grandfather commented that he would have been dead by morning if the cure had failed.[16]

The movement between incommunicability and communicable control enacted in the performance was complex. The patient, his relatives, and Medina started from a position of incommunicability. The boy could only say that he felt feverish and in pain, and no one could pinpoint the likely cause. The initial conversations and observations provided Medina with hypotheses, however, as to which *hebu* might be responsible, each of which he tested using a different song. Each began with a slow, circular motion of the rattle above the child's body, which activated the *kareko* stones inside the rattle. *Kareko* are seen as types of *hebu* and extensions of Medina's own "helping spirits." Each song included the name of the suspected *hebu*. Given that the *kareko* enabled Medina to feel changes in the *hebu's* activity within the patient, this phase allowed him to see whether his hypothesis was correct or whether he needed to name a different *hebu*. When he was on the right track, Medina shifted to the "spanking" phase by increasing the tempo and moving the rattle close to the child's body or, for some songs, pressing the rattle against it. When successful, the *hebu* loosened its grip and submitted to the *wisidatu's* control.

In the third section, which returned to the slow tempo, other partici-pants took control over Medina's voice. This began with a series of vocables, sounds that lack referential meaning and grammatical inflection. *Wisidatu* say that these sounds emerge as the helping spirits press their way out of Medina's larynx to engage the *hebu*. In the body of the song section, the *hebu* itself reported how and why it afflicted the boy and admitted its inten-tion to kill him. The final section, primarily spoken, consisted of a dialogue between Medina and the boy's father in which the healer relayed, translated, and elaborated on the *hebu*'s words. The *hebu* announced that it grew in-creasingly angered as it observed ritual infractions, including some commit-ted by Torres and the boy's grandfather, and the greed of some participants in taking and consuming palm starch before the *hebu* had ritually consumed it. A rivalry between Torres and another healer also formed part of the *hebu*'s story. In other words, there were broader social and political components to what seemed to be an individual case of respiratory illness.

When beginning to diagnose and treat a patient, healers start from a posi-tion of incommunicability, one induced not by humans but by *hebu* or other pathogens, who deliberately hide their identities, how they have sickened the patient, and their motives. Medina progressively asserted communicable con-trol through his voice and rattle, increasingly displaying his knowledge and power through a first-person pronoun: *ine sike* (I myself am the one). This air of communicable arrogance overlaid rather than erased the incommunicable sub-ordination to the unpredictable machinations of invisible pathogens. Indeed, not only did Medina surrender his vocal apparatus to the *hebu* to succeed, but he faced the possibility of failure—and thus the patient's death. This movement produced incommunicability for the patient and his father, who is not a healer. Much of the song is in "healer's language," consisting of lexical stems and com-plex nominal and verbal forms unintelligible to non-initiates. The rationale is that *hebu* and other invisible pathogens do not understand ordinary Warao, so they can be controlled and extracted only through this specialized code.

It would be possible to draw a parallel to biomedicine, suggesting that heal-ers produce incommunicability, thereby putting their own power and special-ized knowledge on display. Although tempting, I believe that this statement would be analytically shallow, particularly if it involved transposing the tele-ology of communicability. As each song progressed, Medina complemented healer's language with forms interpretable to the patient and his father. What we might refer to as a breakthrough into communicability, to adapt Hymes's (1981) expression, occurred during the dialogue between Medina and Rivera, which was held almost entirely in everyday language. To posit a problem of communicability would similarly involve a reductionist emphasis on referential language. Indeed, even in sections of the song where father and son have limited ability to decode lexical items referentially, the rattling, vocables, melodic structure, tempo, pitch, and voice quality enabled them to sense the shifting relations among healer, rattle, helping spirits, *hebu*, and the boy's body. The patient and his father felt the contours of invocation, confrontation, overpowering, and expulsion, the latter signaled by a single rapid thrust of the rattle in the direction of the *hebu*'s usual domain.

Anthropologists of all stripes are likely to recall the classic analysis by Claude Lévi-Strauss ([1949] 1963) of a healing song of the Kuna nation that lies off the coast of Panama. I am still impressed by his ability to explore the depth and complexity of the text and his efforts to analyze it on its own terms. Nevertheless, Lévi-Strauss makes precisely the move this chapter's argument has sought to resist in that he implicitly imports key features of biomedical conceptions of doctor-patient encounters. He focuses on the relationship among the healer, a woman experiencing obstructed childbirth, and assemblages of nonhuman beings who either helped or hindered the process.[17] This reduction eliminates the role of the midwives beside the mother, just as the doctor-patient interaction literature generally overlooks the role of nurses and receptionists. Lévi-Strauss presupposes a binary opposition between incommunicability and communicability, casting the intervention as moving the patient from the former to the latter, arguing that the chant "provides the woman with a *language*, by means of which unexpressed, and otherwise inexpressible, psychic states can be immediately expressed" (198). He adds, "Once the sick woman understands, . . . she gets well" (197). Setting aside the remarkable poetics and musicality of the chant, Lévi-Strauss focuses on its referential content. Macpherson Chapin (1976, 1983) asserts that Lévi-Strauss is off base in that the chant uses a "stick doll language" that is unintelligible to the patient. Building on a critique offered by Joel Sherzer (1983, 134), however, we could say that positing a rigid opposition between communicability and incommunicability would be misleading, given that patients are familiar with the "purpose and general structure" of curing chants and can understand part of what is sung and said. Embracing a biomedical orientation that would later be shared by the doctor-patient literature, Lévi-Strauss is—as the title of his article suggests—fundamentally concerned with questions of efficacy. Nonbiomedical healing thus become intelligible for his readers when similarly submitted to a utilitarian logic.

Here I want to make the opposite move. Instead of using dominant communicable models of doctor-patient communication for validating and rendering interpretable—for nonindigenous audiences—an example of nonbiomedical healing, I would like to attend to how the Mariusa example can suggest new perspectives. Rather than positing a binary between communicability and incommunicability, it would be more productive to characterize the positionalities of healer, patient, the rattle, *hebu*, relatives, and other Mariusa residents as lying along shifting borderlines of in/communicability. In the Mariusa case, artificially imposing a dyadic model of caregiver-patient communicability and fetishizing reference would draw our attention away from thinking more carefully about the bodies of healer, patient, and father; the rattle and its *kareko*; the invisible but felt engagement of nonhuman actors; acoustic features of the healer's multiple voices; and the broader social and political context.

Might we not think of biomedical encounters, too, as occupying shifting in/communicable borderlines rather than either embodying perfect communicability or problematically producing incommunicability? Might the bodies, hands, and faces of nurses, patients, doctors, and relatives and the more than referential properties of their voices be as crucial as routinized metapragmatic phrases for eliciting patients' concerns and explaining diagnosis and treatment? Think about the technology that plays a central role in clinical visits and even in creating the iconic image of the doctor: the stethoscope. When using it, doctors and nurses do not attend to patients' words, and patients cannot hear what nurses and doctors are hearing. Nevertheless, I (as a patient) have the sense that they are using special listening skills to hear what is happening inside me, attending to what I may feel but cannot hear. Finally, take the dominant logic of differential diagnosis, a process that consists less of naming one definitive cause than progressively ruling out other possibilities. Does it not embody a sense of communicable humility, albeit one that often gives way to assertions of biomedical authority in communicating diagnoses to patients?

Conclusion

The issues addressed in this chapter take me back to Fanon, given his trenchant critique of how colonial physicians spoke with colonized patients. His account seems far from current efforts to improve medicine through extensive training of clinicians in standard protocols for interacting with patients. It is crucial to remember, however, that Fanon ([1952] 2008, 15, 16) reports that "I have felt myself lapsing" during "certain consultations," in particular with an elderly woman with dementia. Is it possible that this self-critical observation points to how Fanon revealed a broader tendency within doctor-patient interaction? Might the danger lie in both biocommunicability and how it is rationalized? Fanon mimics the sort of instrumentalist rationalizations that physicians often use to justify ways of interacting with patients, suggesting that they constitute "an attempt . . . to make them feel at ease, to make oneself understood and reassure them" (15)—again, the seemingly transcendent power of utilitarian logics. Even as we bracket the gut-wrenching racism of Fanon's example, the similarity in instrumental reasoning that often motivates research and training in doctor-patient interaction remains.

Thinking with Canguilhem would suggest that feeling sick introduces a disconcerting element of incommunicability, given that illness renders frameworks into which physicians draw patients' speech to a greater or lesser extent out of reach. Given that each patient's subjective experience is different (and varies from moment to moment), both patients and physicians face a common starting point of incommunicability. Biocommunicable models for provider-patient interaction superimpose a normativizing force that constantly evaluates and regiments the words and actions of patients and physicians vis-à-vis a distant, presupposed standard that rests on hierarchically ranked roles and differential access to communicative power. Patients and providers are constantly faced with performing, to redeploy a term developed by Dell Hymes (1974), *communicable competence*. Even as communicable competence would seem to produce a sense of confidence and mutual understanding, it rather infects and inflects encounters with biocommunicable anxieties. Patients wonder, Did I ask enough questions? Too many? Did I successfully convey to the doctor or nurse practitioner what is wrong with me? Does the doctor think I understand her/him/them? Did the information I drew from the news, social, media, advertising, or a medical source threaten the physician's sense of authority? And on the physician's side: Did I understand what the patient told me? Did I give the patient a chance to convey what is really going on? Did I explain things clearly? Did the patient trust the diagnosis and treatment plan? In short, doctor-patient communication guidelines pathologize the forms of incommunicability experienced by both providers and patients, constantly demanding that they be replaced by biocommunicable transparency. Moreover, not only is the biocommunicable competence of some patients and—Fanon, would add, some physicians—more closely scrutinized than others, but racialized patients are sometimes deemed biocommunicable failures before they utter a word.

I would like to return here to Miyako Inoue's (2003) discussion of the listening subject. She draws attention to how dominant social roles can be defined vis-à-vis particular ways of listening to specific discursive forms, reversing how the process actually works: the stigmatized speech modalities are brought into being through acts of constituting listening subjects. I have traced here how the normativizing force of doctor-patient interaction guidelines teaches physicians to listen for incommunicabilities, for gaps in patient's assimilation of biocommunicability. The case of racialized biocommunicable profiling is particularly striking, given that providers hear communicable stereotypes that, like Inoue's example and Fanon's characterization of colonial clinical pidgin, may bear little or no relation to what patients actually say and do. There is a more general phenomenon here. Doctor-patient interaction guidelines choreograph exchanges in such a way that patients must insert their questions, responses, accounts, observations, and narratives into the discursive structure that, although largely controlled by the physician, is an external regimenting framework to which doctors must similarly submit. Although patients are not expected to be able to mirror physicians' perspectives, they are expected to calibrate their contributions vis-à-vis the biomedical perspectives that professionals control. We can build on Eeva Sointu's (2016) observations on how medical students are taught to classify patients as "good" or "bad": good patients align with physicians biocommunicable models and interaction protocols, whereas bad ones seemingly fail to grasp or even challenge them. Fisher and Groce (1990, 242) note that physicians are more likely to listen to patients, take their input seriously, and give them time to provide the information they deem important "if they do not upset the asymmetry in the medical relationship." To extend Du Bois's term, patients are expected to exhibit double-consciousness, reflexively viewing their own perceptions in anticipation of the ways that physicians are likely to evaluate their perspectives. A statement offered by a medical student that is quoted by Byron Good and Mary-Jo DelVecchio Good (2000, 56) perceptively captures the communicable contradiction that emerges from how doctor-patient interaction guidelines teach physicians to listen: "Clearly I'm being told my job is to control that interaction. . . . You ask an open-ended question, but you guide. You give the illusion of the patient controlling the situation when in fact you're controlling the situation."

Three crucial caveats are in order, lest these points be misunderstood. First, it would be both ethnographically incorrect and ethically problematic to paint all physicians—let alone all clinicians—with a single broad brush. Many practitioners push back on attempts to standardize how they can interact with patients and highly unequal power relations. Indeed, as I have noted, some have quit medicine rather than accept the regimenting dictates of corporate and state regulators. Second, I do not want to suggest—in classic anthropological fashion—that I can see what is hidden from others. Practitioners and patients have discerned, commented on, and complained about these issues for decades. Rather than claiming clairvoyance, my goal is to provide an analytical framework that can help advance such efforts. Third, I am not pretending to offer a form of knowledge translation, a smooth process in which a research finding can be mechanically converted into a formula for changing how medicine is practiced (Ødemark and Engebretsen 2022). I do not think that analyzing how doctor-patient interaction protocols can unintentionally produce incommunicability will magically transform how patients and providers interact. Such a belief would incarcerate me in the Lockean trap, the belief that diagnosing a communicative disorder can yield a treatment formula that will remedy the problem. This move would repeat the three-hundred-year-old fallacy that, when offered enlightenment, rational people will immediately change the ways they think, speak, and act. It would also mistakenly construe the sort of control that physicians and other providers have over their own labor. Health professionals face immense time constraints and pressure from administrators, insurance companies, and government agencies.[18]

I do not, however, believe that the preceding discussion is "only academic," that it cannot be used in rethinking and reconfiguring medical education and practice. The "structural competency" approach suggests how accepted approaches can change in ways that challenge the production of incommunicability. This approach, developed partly by physician-anthropologists, prompts clinicians to look beyond patient-specific parameters. Advocates for "structural competency" training urge medical students and practitioners to critically scrutinize stigmas "enacted" in clinical encounters "due to structural causes" (Metzl and Hansen 2014, 127). A structural approach requires widening the physician's vision "from an exclusive focus on the individual encounter to include the organization of institutions and policies, as well as of neighborhoods and cities" (126). Jonathan Metzl and Helena Hansen instructively argue that such training should not provide formulae for clinical implementation; instead, conversations within and beyond clinical settings should be "beginning points" (131).

An example in the prestigious *New England Journal of Medicine* points to a physician who challenges the biocommunicable status quo and collaborates with her patients in extending indexical orders beyond the space of the clinic. The doctor leaves the clinic to look for the factors responsible for a case of acute wrist tendinitis after noting that other agricultural workers picking blueberries as much as twelve hours a day presented with similar symptoms (Seymour et al. 2018). After asking to visit the fields, one of her patients invited the physician to observe. She pinpointed the source of the injuries: a blueberry rake that was not ergonomically designed. "Watching these movements in person, the physician understood clearly how weeks of this work could lead to overuse injuries" (2386). Rather than simply providing ibuprofen and a wrist brace, the physician worked with community health workers and farmworkers to learn more about the broader set of factors, including available tools and working hours and conditions. Securing funds from a community-based research network, the clinic invited her patient, other farmworkers, growers, community-health workers, and people skilled in metalworking and ergonomics to collaboratively conduct research and explore alternatives, leading to the creation of a two-handled rake that was acceptable to all parties and significantly reduced the incidence of this type of injury.

Although Cheryl Seymour and her colleagues' article is not explicit on this point, I suspect that the clinical visit began with biocommunicable routines in place. Following up on Waitzkin's example, the doctor refused, however, to reduce the patient's work environment to referential content that could be stuffed into the indexical order of the clinic. She realized that the clinic did not provide an adequate indexical ground for diagnosis and collaborated with her patients in bringing the indexical order of farm labor into the space of diagnosis and in extending the indexical order of the clinic into the fields by observing patients at work. Agricultural workers are not only forced to accept oppressive working and living conditions, but they are largely excluded from discussions that shape them and—due to the threat of job loss and often deportation—face obstacles to reporting abuses (Holmes 2013; Saxton 2021). Rather than thinking that the medical gaze would enable her to identify the structural roots of the injuries, she asked farmworkers and community health workers to teach her about the indexical orders and material conditions of the fields, which reached into those associated with the commodification of workers' bodies in the drive for agribusiness profits, immigration policies, nativist ideologies, and police and other enforcement actions. Rather than producing incommunicability, the physician and the group formed through the physician's initiative— but that she did not control—thus challenged communicative inequities in a small victory for health/communicative justice.

I would suggest that advocates for structural competency might build on this example to include health/communicative inequities centrally in the "structural differential" process of diagnosis and transformation they promote. This step would seem crucial to displaying "structural humility" (Metzl and Hansen 2014). Metzl and Hansen (128) suggest that "we train doctors to listen to individualized stories, not to structural ones." Might forms of training include not only listening to the content of patient narratives in different ways but also challenging doctor-patient interaction normativization itself? Might structural competency—if it is to transform clinical medicine—not also include learning to listen to different languages, genres, and contexts in which patients offer their insights into health and disease?

A key question is how to think, research, train, and interact differently. Writing shortly after Paul Farmer's unexpected death, I invoke his lifelong goal to redefine health not as profit, development, efficiency, or technological spectacle but as an issue of justice. If language and communication, health and care are woven so tightly together—like health and communicative inequities—then there will be no justice in health if there is not also health/communicative justice. If provider-patient interaction is a crucial site in which these seemingly disparate realms are inextricably connected, perhaps research, training, and practice programs might best come together not around instrumentalist and interventionist logics but collaborative attempts to promote justice.

6

HEALTH COMMUNICATION

How In/communicabilities Jump Scale

Knowledge is the enemy of disease.
—SIR MUIR GRAY, chief knowledge officer, UK National Health Service

Communicability never gets to steal the show entirely in provider-patient interaction. What gets labeled communication is always entangled with relationships among bodies, technologies, viruses and bacteria, insurance companies (in some countries), and the like. The corporeal dimension of biocommunicability—interventions aimed at halting the disruptive effects of pathogens in bodies—remains a vital part of the labor enacted. Practitioners who are judged to be the worst communicators and yet excellent diagnosticians project the seeming separability of medicine and communication—and the higher status of the former. The US television medical mystery series *House* provides a limit case for popular imaginaries: the misanthropic Dr. Gregory House commits acts of biocommunicable violence in a fictional teaching hospital in New Jersey with malicious glee, casting colleagues and patients alike into incommunicable hell, even as he provides the lifesaving diagnosis that eludes everyone else. When we come to health communication, by contrast, the dominant material artifacts are not CT scans, stethoscopes, or X-ray machines. Instead, they include spoken words, pamphlets, flip-up charts, Google searches, and digital newsletters. Health communication thus seems to place us squarely in a realm of "communication" in which biocommunicability is positioned as the tool invested with the power to produce better outcomes—and to judge the success or failure of laypeople in fostering their own well-being.

I have traced the linear teleology of dominant biocommunicabilities that project the mobility of biomedical knowledge from its production in laboratories, leading hospitals, and epidemiologists' offices to its seeming end point in the transformation of laypeople's understandings and "behavior." The very label "health communication" marks a projected boundary between the biomedical *knowledge* of researchers and clinicians and its transformation into forms of *communication*. This makeover requires armies of specialized workers: in addition to clinicians enacting "doctor-patient communication" with patients, it includes health communication and media specialists in public health offices, people hired by nongovernmental organizations (NGOS) to give workshops and training sessions, *promotoras* (community health workers) who visit households, people creating online courses and media content, and media workers, among others. Whether we begrudgingly include legions of well-paid workers charged with bringing health knowledge to vast audiences through advertisements for pharmaceuticals and medical devices might be controversial. Except for physicians, nurses, and physician assistants, people charged with health communication are defined both by their access to biomedical knowledge and their exclusion from the ranks of those designated as clinical professionals; they are, rather, characterized by their ability to translate health knowledge across borders of communicability and incommunicability.

And then, at the end of this linear imaginary, come laypeople, defined by exclusion from both domains. We confront a governmental obligation, in Michel Foucault's (1991) terms, to work on our selves in such a way as to responsibly assimilate the fragments of medical knowledge that have been translated for our benefit. Equally important is the construction of some populations, with apologies to George Orwell, as more incommunicable than others—as never deserving an individual, self-interested, agentive role or capable of playing their assigned communicable role of listening to, understanding, and corporeally reflecting the knowledge provided. I develop these issues later.

My discussion thus far might seem to position health communication as Doctor-Patient Interaction 2.0, meaning an extension of the dominant biocommunicabilities we explored in chapter 5. Nothing could be further from the truth. Research and training in doctor-patient interaction project in/communicability onto a tiny screen of individual bodies, minds, and examining rooms, then populate the world with these seemingly universal biomedical atoms. As Frantz Fanon warned us long ago, this illusion obscures how broader inequities of race and class shape what transpires in clinics and how the biocommunicable violence of clinical interactions reproduces colonial inequities and hides efforts to resist them. Here I want to go much further. The preceding chapter faced the scalar restraints imposed by the doctor-patient interaction frame, another of the boundaries that restrict our understanding of how in/communicabilities move in the world. Simply extending biocommunicable models from provider-patient interaction to health communication would thus leave intact the same sorts of conceptual restraints evident in Locke's projection of communicability as a self-help program to help individual elite, white, European men to perfect their language or Georges Canguilhem's interest in how individual patients conceptualize and communicate their new pathological worlds. If the ideological labor of biocommunicability enacted in clinical settings imposes communicable profiling on individual bodies, health communication models jump scale, interpellating entire populations as incommunicable.[1]

Racializing Health Communication

The movement from clinical knowledge to health communication takes on concrete spatial and temporal parameters when a clinical encounter produces both prevention and treatment recommendations and a referral to a health education program. Being diagnosed with a chronic disease—quintessentially, diabetes—is likely to afford not only pills, pamphlets, and technologies but classes, workshops, and other activities. Two observations seem pertinent here. One is that a referral to a specialist who is usually not a clinical professional does not displace the authority of the physician or physician assistant but, rather, confirms and extends it. The incommunicability that purportedly caused or, at least, exacerbated the pathology that afflicts you seemingly cannot be ameliorated by words uttered in the clinical space alone but requires a more sustained and complex intervention—one explicitly focused on "communication." Another is that this transition opens up possibilities for entangling communicative and medical profiling in new ways. Even as structural inequities enter profoundly into the clinic, transforming particular human beings into exemplars of racialized or other stereotypes, health communication provides a powerful force for scaling up health/communicative inequities, enabling them to help shape global maps of difference, inequity, and stigma.

Let us start with a couple of examples. They are features of what linguistic anthropologists often refer to as linguistic landscapes, markers in built environments that point to the semiotics of difference. Kevin Kenjar's (2020) elegant documentation of the contested multilingual and multiconfessional character of a single area of Sarajevo from the late Ottoman period exemplifies how linguistic landscapes map difference. By examining street signs, commemorative inscriptions, public notices, storefronts, and graffiti, he traces the succession of languages and scripts and how they constitute pasts, presents, and futures. This analysis enables him to analyze how new state formations and nationalisms emerge, claim legitimacy, and erase competing and past formations and inconvenient historical narratives.[2]

Health communication also projects space and social difference onto linguistic landscapes. A first example comes from billboards in the San Diego area and elsewhere in Southern California in the early 2000s, particularly in areas with sizable Latinx populations, which Ruby Tapia (2011) has beautifully analyzed. As Leo Chávez ([2008] 2013), Otto Santa Ana (2002), Natalia Molina (2006), and others have documented, a key trope in anti-immigrant and anti-Latinx discourse in California is projecting Latinx women as excessively fertile. The image of the pregnant Latinx teen generated sufficient moral panic among conservative white politicians and their constituencies that the California Department of Health Services placed public health communications on billboards and in magazines in the early 2000s featuring young women and men seemingly trapped by unwanted pregnancies—most seemingly Latinx. In one example, a young man pushes a baby stroller; exhibiting a look of consternation, he seems to be addressed by the billboard's text: "Are these the kind of wheels you had in mind?" The young man's aspirations, seemingly focused on driving a flashy car or truck—not higher education, professional success, or political office—are thwarted by uncontrolled sexuality: an unwanted pregnancy. These images ensnare other residents' imaginaries of young Latinx people by littering the Southern California landscape with stereotypes dressed up as state efforts to address a health "crisis." Being interpellated as a seemingly bounded, homogeneous population by a health communication campaign marks it as a projected source of health problems and social disorder, becoming a threat in a "tale of a general crisis of social and corporeal distinctions" (Reid 1997, 554).

The power of these billboards, posters, and other ways of inscribing health communication on the linguistic (or, better, semiotic) landscape is augmented by their projection as parts of communicable strategies that also emerge in magazines, mainstream journalism, and social media. Take a contemporaneous story by a Latinx journalist, Héctor Becerra, "Program Is Fighting Teenage Pregnancy," published in the *Los Angeles Times*.[3] Becerra suggests that "traditional Latino households" are so pervaded by sexual taboos and failures of communication among family members that information about sexuality and family planning cannot break in. He quotes the executive director of a program seeking to educate young Latino men about sex and contraception, saying, "Especially in the Latino community, we have so many secrets. 'You don't talk about this, you don't talk about that. God will punish you.'"

What impact do these images have on their supposed targets: Latinx teenagers and youth? Here we can fruitfully return to Fanon's analysis of the effects of colonial physicians' use of pidgin with their patients: they elicited not enhanced understanding or rapport but the sense that doctors are incapable of transcending their racist blinders to deliver adequate care. Rather than prompting viewers to police their sexuality, these billboards were more likely to convince Latinx viewers that state health authorities cannot see beyond stereotypes to perceive Latinx residents in their complexity and diversity. These magazine advertisements and billboards were unlikely to invite people who do not identify as Latinx to ask their Latinx neighbors about their lives and aspirations. They were more likely to prompt other residents to see Latinx youths as too incarcerated by excessive sexuality and fertility to escape the incommunicable barriers erected by images of immigrant invasions (Chávez [2008] 2013; Santa Ana 2002) and raciolinguistic profiling: "This is the United States: speak English!" (Zentella 2003). In a study of the semiotics of 1990s anti-tobacco advertisements in California, Roddey Reid (2005, 98) nicely captures a fundamental contradiction of how incommunicability unfolds in public health campaigns. Targeted public health "messages" cast populations as in need of hypodermic injections of biomedical knowledge, even as they project them as "outside the community of knowledgeable citizens"—that is, "as unsuccessful pedagogical subjects."

A more recent example emerged early in the COVID-19 pandemic. Ventura County Public Health distributed two posters illustrating the "social distance" needed to prevent COVID-19 transmission. One, sent to businesses, pictured a woman in business attire and a man wearing a white shirt and tie separated by two skis. The caption read, "6 FEET IS ABOUT THE LENGTH OF SKIS" (figure 6.1). A poster distributed for display on farms featured a man and woman in work clothes with three vegetable or fruit crates between them; the caption read, "6 FEET IS ABOUT THE LENGTH OF 3 PRODUCE CRATES" (figure 6.2). Most agricultural laborers in the county are Latinx, some drawn from Mexican and Central American indigenous populations. In addition to critiquing the contrastive objects used to measure distance, social media posts commented on the detailed hair, facial, and other features of the figures in the skis poster and the faceless silhouettes on the crates image. The graphic dimensions of these posters exemplify the everyday use of multimodal semiotic features as forms of recipient design—how discourse is patterned in such a way as to match the perceived cognitive and linguistic capacities of the person or people targeted. The implicit semiotic analysis in the media posts suggested that the depersonalized images invite distance and de-identification—that is, stereotyping.

A discussion with Gisselle Rosales, a Latinx resident of Ventura County and student at the University of California, Berkeley, who kindly brought this example to my attention, pointed to the significance of a state effort to mark spaces of business with signs of middle-class status versus attributes associated with Latinx agricultural laborers. The differential distribution of the skis posters to businesses and the crate signs to farms enacted a semiotic segregation effected by a government agency. Like the billboards example, these posters suggest that the linguistic marking of landscapes is tied to corporeal and material semiotics rather than formal markers of linguistic codes alone: both sets of posters appeared in Spanish and English. A study of signage in London during the COVID-19 pandemic pointed to a different sort of health/communicative inequity: fewer signs appeared in low-income areas, and the ones that did appear were less up to date on emerging guidelines and emphasized messages about helping keep public areas open. Signs displayed in higher-income areas, by contrast, emphasized staying at home and saving lives (Kalocsányiová, Essex, and Poulter 2023).[4]

In the billboards example, I pointed briefly to how health communication can use health/communicable profiling to interpellate multiple audiences simultaneously. Media accounts of health communication play important roles here. A column published in the *San Diego Union-Tribune* profiles a Medicare-funded "education program" in California designed to assist Latinx type 2 diabetes patients. The racialization of Latinx populations seemingly requires that health communication efforts inform them about health care and education. Why? The problem lies not with systemic inequities, including access to and quality of care, but with what are projected as the cultural contours of Latinx populations. The article quotes the perfect spokesperson: Ana Pérez, a nurse managing the program, seemingly ipso facto fluent in biocommunicable circuits about type 2 diabetes and what is portrayed as Latinx culture. Pérez reportedly characterizes the need to invite Latinx pop-

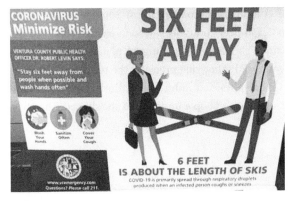

FIGURE 6.1. Ventura County poster illustrating social distancing using skis

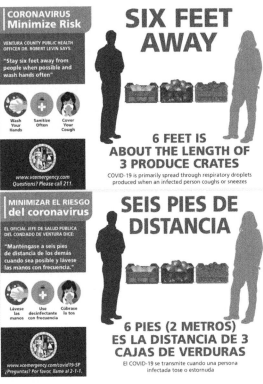

FIGURE 6.2. Ventura County poster illustrating social distancing using crates

ulations into clinical spaces as requiring intervention into cultural-religious incommunicability: "'Latinos go to doctors just when they feel sick; if they feel OK, they don't go,' says Perez. 'But sometimes with diabetes, there are no symptoms.'. . . And she says there's a tendency to define a disease as 'God's will, that there is nothing they can do.'"[5] The article then jumps scales in racializing diabetes type 2 incommunicability to include "Vietnamese, Filipinos and African Americans," embracing a broad swath of Southern California's population. The solution lies in peer counselors, who in eight weeks provide "self-management education classes and . . . bilingual materials on how to keep the disease under control." Embodying precisely the teleology provided us by our master philosopher-physician, John Locke, the article concludes with a quote from a doctor: "'Once people understand the disease, they become empowered.'"

Diving In, Ethnographically: Sitting with Fanon in Venezuelan Public Health Communication

My friend Fernando Coronil, whom I still dearly miss, defined Venezuelan modernity through the lens of oil, the country's "natural body" (Coronil 1997). Performing membership in Venezuela's social body and claiming citizenship rights included demanding a share of the wealth derived from fossil fuel extraction. Coronil pointed to the legacy of President Rómulo Betancourt in transforming Venezuela into a modern petro-state. I claim a different, equally ambivalent ancestor, Arnoldo Gabaldón, as a father figure of Venezuelan nationalism. Gabaldón was not an elected official or oligarch: he was a dedicated public health official. His job was to make Venezuela safe from the Anopheles mosquitos that transmitted malaria, which kept buzzing around the segregated oil camps where Texan and Oklahoman oil workers and their families enjoyed housing, clubs, and magazines that excluded all but a few professional Venezuelans.[6] Gabaldón mustered contacts with fellow practitioners of what would become international health to obtain access to DDT, the magical chemical afforded by US World War II industrial technology. A remarkable public health professional with access to extensive petroleum-funded resources, Gabaldón brought Anopheles mosquitos "under control" and rid the country of malaria (Gutiérrez 1998).

Unfortunately, decades later not only did the Anopheles and their parasite companion species return, but another type of mosquito—*Aedes aegypti*—brought dengue fever to Venezuela, like much of Central America and South America. Because of its toxic effects, DDT was banned, requiring the use of other insecticides. Unlike malaria, dengue was an urban as much as a rural pest, proliferating outdoors as rain collected in discarded containers and tires and inside houses through water in flower pots and uncovered storage containers. Fumigation alone did not solve the problem when dengue became a significant health problem in the 1980s. Health education was needed to teach people to drain, treat, or cover the water that enabled *Aedes aegypti* to breed.

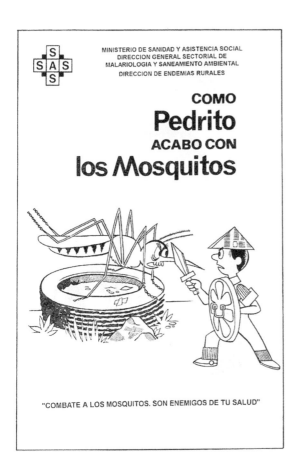

FIGURE 6.3. Pedrito
pamphlet, title page

In addition to television spots and posters, one of the most common vehicles for interpellating members of Venezuela's social body for participation in the "fight" against dengue was via pamphlets massively distributed
by ministry employees, including on the street; in shopping centers; at ministry clinics; and, when case numbers were particularly worrisome, door to
door. The Ministry of Health and Social Assistance unit that Gabaldón created, the General Sectorial Office of Malarial and Environmental Sanitation,
produced a classic example of this genre at the turn of the millennium. Its
cover features a boy, Pedrito (Little Pedro), pictured as an infantilized war-
rior hero with a paper hat and a garbage can for a shield, fighting a huge
Aedes aegypti with menacing eyes and teeth. Pedrito, according to the pamphlet's title, "finished off the mosquitos" (figure 6.3). Mosquitos, declared to
be "enemies of your health," are fitted with a proboscis that is as phallic as Pedrito's toy sword. As Alex Nading (2014) has detailed for Nicaragua's dengue

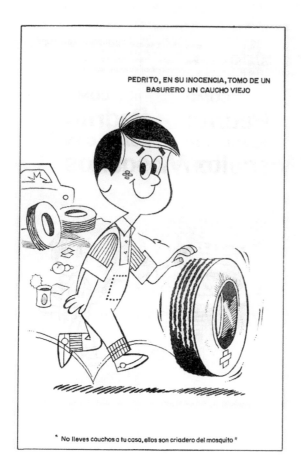

FIGURE 6.4. Pedrito pamphlet, child with old tire

prevention program, the representation of mosquitos in anthropomorphic—including gendered—terms can help shape how humans position themselves in relation to them, dengue, and eradication programs.

The origin of the old tire on the cover was revealed in the following image: a trash dump. It is Pedrito's "innocence" that led him to remove the tire as a plaything, seemingly representing lay incommunicability vis-à-vis the knowledge produced by Gabaldón's unit: tires "are breeding sites for the mosquito" (figure 6.4). The tire is a powerful symbol of Venezuelan modernity, part of the twentieth-century project of transforming a premodern patchwork of diverse regions primarily linked by river and sea into a major petroleum producer united by a strong national government, roads, and automobiles. Projecting old tires as bordering middle-class houses suggests fears that premodern, unsanitary, barbarous qualities still lurk within the country's claim to modernity (Coronil 1997).

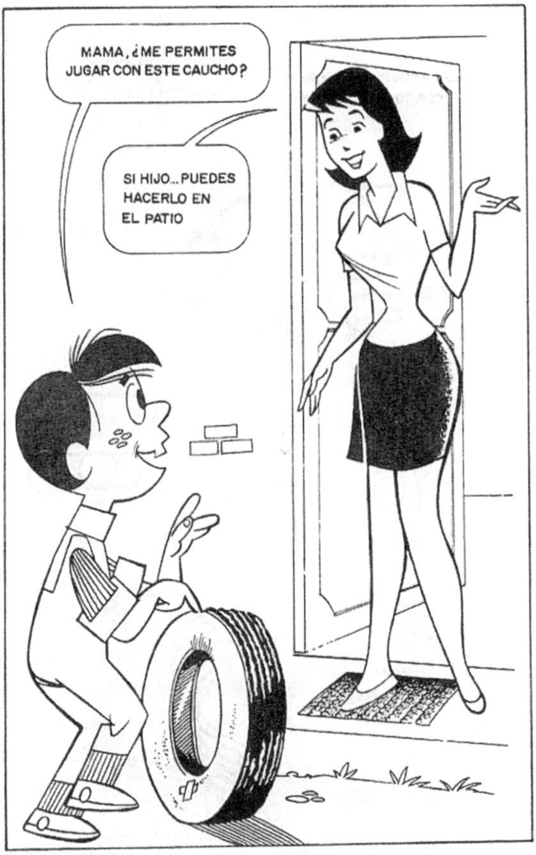

FIGURE 6.5. Pedrito pamphlet, child with mother

The pamphlet positions "the family" as "an important element in this campaign against the mosquito," exhorting that families "must participate actively in the elimination of breeding sites in their houses." The performative inscription of class, race, and gender features of this seemingly primordial social unit becomes strikingly apparent on the third page as Pedrito's mother appears (figure 6.5). She is not only as well dressed as Pedrito, marking "the family's" class status, but her body is sexualized. Her response, allowing Pedrito to play with the tire only on the patio behind the house, creates narrative tension: why would a woman who looks and speaks like this figure allow her son to play at a dump, pick up a tire, and bring it into the space of domesticity, even if she relegates it to the backstage area of the patio?

The next page creates a visual and linguistic rift as Gabaldón's successors, scientists associated with the General Sectorial Office of Malarial and Environmental Sanitation, seem to speak directly to readers rather than through

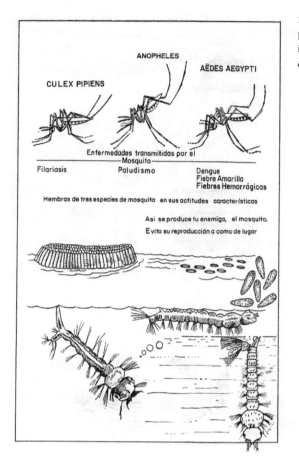

Pedrito and his mother (figure 6.6). Classic scientific illustrations replace infantilized cartoon drawings; Spanish is interrupted by Latin names for mosquito species; and a narrative gives way to scientific projections of cause and effect: eggs turn into larvae and then into mosquitos, and mosquitos become vectors for various diseases. The contents of Gabaldón's remarkable entomological museum in Maracay seem to spring onto the pages of the pamphlet. The story of a boy's and his mother's innocent entrapment by incommunicability gives way to inviting readers to enter the space of biocommunicability.

As the pamphlet returns to the narrative in figure 6.7, we see the "lamentable consequences" of incommunicability: Pedrito gets bitten. His previous affective positionality—the fighter who turns a defiant face to the mosquito and a happy, smiling countenance to mother and reader—have given way to an angry or painful relationship with the mosquito. In the image that follows (figure 6.8), Pedrito's countenance expresses febrile dependency. Interest-

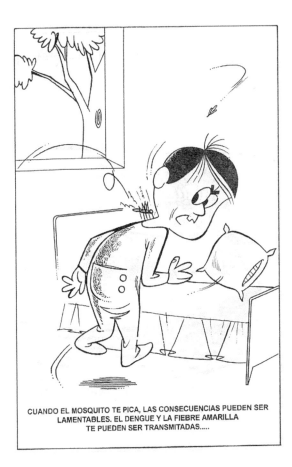

FIGURE 6.7. Pedrito
pamphlet, the bite

CUANDO EL MOSQUITO TE PICA, LAS CONSECUENCIAS PUEDEN SER
LAMENTABLES. EL DENGUE Y LA FIEBRE AMARILLA
TE PUEDEN SER TRANSMITADAS.....

ingly, the clinician in this public health pamphlet does not speak but only looks attentively at his patient, even as he wields an equally phallic needle and syringe. The mother's embracing smile and relaxed gestures (see figure 6.5) have given way to a "worried" relationship to her child.

The last drawings provide a happy ending to the story. Pedrito's mother demonstrates proper gardening techniques—placing plants in dirt or sand rather than in larvae-breeding water—and picking up vessels "that can accumulate water" and throwing them into a garbage can, against which the old tire has been positioned (figure 6.9). The state's benevolent role emerges as a neatly uniformed sanitation worker and garbage truck complete the task. The final drawing shows an infuriated mosquito, his proboscis bent, looking for a new home and Pedrito standing, sword and garbage can shield back in hand, next to his mother, their smiles gracing the poetic motto, "Health is the fountain of happiness." The last page of "BASIC NORMS FOR DENGUE PREVENTION"

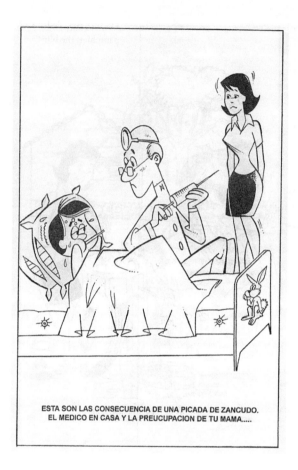

FIGURE 6.8. Pedrito pamphlet, boy, mother, and doctor

ESTA SON LAS CONSECUENCIA DE UNA PICADA DE ZANCUDO.
EL MEDICO EN CASA Y LA PREUCUPACION DE TU MAMA.....

makes explicit the principles that guide the mother's and child's transformation into model biocommunicable subjects of dengue discourse.

Pedrito and his mother seem to stand for the transformation of all Venezuelans from incommunicable subjects to model communicable and sanitary citizens.[7] Nevertheless, linguistic and, particularly, visual details performatively construct "the family" in ways that would have excluded most of the people who received the pamphlet. The depiction of the mother's body revealed the status of the pamphlet—and, thus, health communication—as part of the national project of constructing the idealized feminine body in Venezuela as hyperfeminine, hypersexualized, and anatomically distorted, as powerfully documented by Marcia Ochoa (2014). Mother and child become models of middle-class civility and familial relations through their mutually attentive gaze and polite two-part exchanges. The mother projects the home and its public façade as a symbol of modernity and class status by restricting Pedrito's

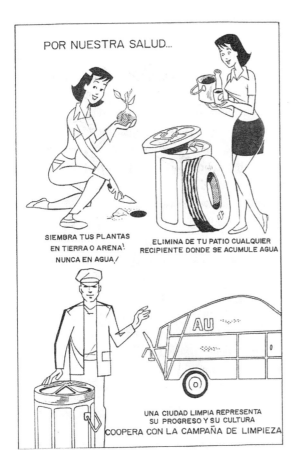

FIGURE 6.9. Pedrito pamphlet, the cleanup

POR NUESTRA SALUD...

SIEMBRA TUS PLANTAS
EN TIERRA O ARENA!
NUNCA EN AGUA/

ELIMINA DE TU PATIO CUALQUIER
RECIPIENTE DONDE SE ACUMULE AGUA

UNA CIUDAD LIMPIA REPRESENTA
SU PROGRESO Y SU CULTURA
COOPERA CON LA CAMPAÑA DE LIMPIEZA

unsightly toy to the back patio. Beyond the figures' neat clothing, the class narrative is extended as we see that Pedrito seems to have his own tidy small bed in, it would seem, his own room—symbols of a middle-class lifestyle that was inaccessible at the time for the vast majority of Venezuelan children.

The pamphlet constructs health care in ways that disguise the deterioration of Venezuela's previously substantial health allocations and public health facilities (Armada and Muntaner 2004; Jaén 2001). It projects the causes of health problems as "consequences" of laypeople's behavior produced by lapses into innocent incommunicability rather than as related to policies enacted by the World Bank, International Monetary Fund, and other multilateral agencies and the Venezuelan government. One element of this transformation that seems to emerge indirectly in the pamphlet is privatization, pushing patients out of free public facilities and into private clinics, many staffed by the same physicians. The economic privilege required to access fee-based health care is symbolized by a house call by a private physician, which was not accessible even to the middle-class subjects imagined in the drawings.[8]

In short, the Venezuelan state legacy of Gabaldonian modernity created its own version of Tarzan books and attempted to distribute them to all residents. This story of a happy transformation from incommunicability and disease into communicability and health would, however, have been unlikely to make all Venezuelans feel included. Those who could identify with its material and linguistic projections of modernity and middle-class status were more likely to live in homes with air conditioners and screened windows. In the pamphlet, the burden of communicability falls on women; adult males, except for the physician and the sanitary worker (who, unlike the mother, is paid to clean up), are nowhere visible. Middle-class mothers would be less inclined to identify with a woman who would allow her son to go, unsupervised, to a garbage dump and return with a dilapidated tire. For the roughly 60 percent of Venezuelans classified as living in poverty at the time, the pamphlet offered less an invitation to communicability than a life sentence of incommunicability: if becoming a communicable citizen depended on the material resources and forms of idealized age- and gender-defined embodiment pictured, the pamphlet projected salvation from dengue, yellow fever, and incommunicability as inaccessible. In short, as an in/communicable project, this health communication effort was designed to fail—but in ways that held the state guiltless and extended logics that blamed poor and racialized Venezuelans for global and national policies.[9]

A health communication "campaign" crafted when a cholera epidemic began in Peru in January 1991 enables us to follow the health communication pamphlet version of Tarzan books through various stages of articulation vis-à-vis health inequities. Before the first cases appeared in Venezuela in December 1991, public health officials worked closely with specialized health journalists for leading national newspapers and broadcast media through a consensus that they were partners in educating publics about cholera.[10] Latin American populations had no experience with cholera, given that the disease had been absent for nearly a century. The Ministry of Health and Social Assistance (MHSA) also produced videos for television broadcasts. A widely disseminated version featured a woman who embodied middle-class femininity by performing cholera prevention in a well-furnished kitchen. She demonstrated washing her hands with soap, rinsing fruit and vegetables, and boiling drinking water and storing it in a nearby freezer refrigerator. As with the dengue materials, the burden of preventing a massive epidemic fell on women's unpaid labor.

Although these television spots reached most Venezuelans, a vast portion of the population lived in homes that did not boast access to running water, refrigerator-freezers, or income to supply the props used in the performance. Moreover, health officials had already collaborated with journalists in constructing a narrative that depicted poor Venezuelans living in urban shantytowns (*barrios*), street vendors of food and drink, and indigenous people as the "at-high-risk groups" that would likely become cholera vectors—even before a single case had been reported. As a result, middle-class and elite viewers possessed the material resources and domestic spaces that enabled them to feel communicably interpellated as the sanitary citizens who could prevent cholera. Nevertheless, perceiving themselves as not being poor, indigenous, or informal workers, most thought that they did not need to worry about the disease. However, this communicable assemblage of health education materials and news stories communicated to members of the three "at-high-risk groups" that they were deemed incommunicable by fiat: they were cast so profoundly into the ranks of cholera vectors and so lacking in material resources required for cholera prevention that no efforts to perform their communicable engagement with prevention efforts could afford sanitary citizenship.

Photographs in newspaper articles aimed at middle-class audiences seemed to capture the filthy incommunicability of the three "at-high-risk groups." Articles focusing on cholera—published before any cholera cases appeared in Venezuela—frequently included images of poor, scantily clad children playing in unsanitary spaces in poor urban neighborhoods. An image of an indigenous mother with her infant, published several times in what was then the national reference newspaper, *El Nacional*, pictured an attentive health worker and a woman whose incommunicable status is embodied in how she seems to turn away from the offer of biocommunicability, simply staring off into space (figure 6.10).[11] A massive project of producing cholera communicability and modern, sanitary citizens cast the majority of the people in the country into a realm of incommunicability that depicted them as threats to the communicable body politic.

The version of the national anti-cholera campaign undertaken in Delta Amacuro State, where an indigenous-nonindigenous racial binary structures daily life and access to services and justice, provides a deeper sense of how health communication gets racialized. There, some five hundred people died in the Orinoco Delta after the first cases were reported in the state in August 1992. While cholera can kill an adult through dehydration in as little as ten hours, it can be treated by rehydration and antibiotic therapies. The number of deaths resulted not only from gross inadequacies in available biomedical services

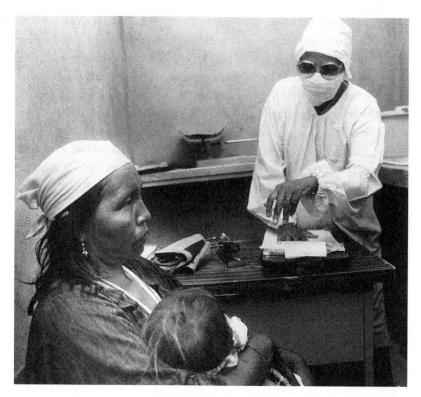

FIGURE 6.10. *El Nacional*, photograph of indigenous mother and child

but also from the failure of public health institutions to inform residents that cholera was likely to arrive and that patients had to seek treatment immediately. In some small communities (figure 6.11), as many as a third of the adults died in a single night. The epidemic thus compounded insecurity around issues of life and death in a region in which more than a third of the children died before reaching puberty and the incidence of tuberculosis was approximately 60 percent.[12]

The national publicity that focused on the epidemic threatened the legitimacy of public health institutions in Delta Amacuro State and the regional government's hold on power. The Regional Health Service peremptorily countered criticisms that its own failure to provide adequate sanitary infrastructures and health care for the rainforest area was responsible for the high morbidity and mortality by blaming rainforest residents. In collaboration with journalists, they devised a logic that targeted "indigenous culture"—specifically, beliefs that spirits cause illnesses and reliance on "shamans" rather than doctors—for unconscionable morbidity and mortality.[13]

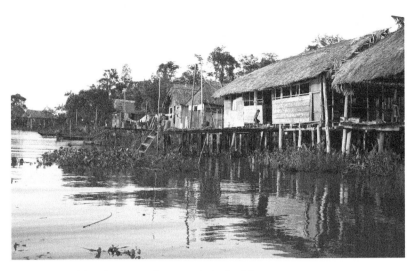

FIGURE 6.11. Hubasuhuru, a small community in the delta

Health communication materials produced during the outbreak reproduced the racial binary in biocommunicable terms. A pamphlet handed out
on the streets of Tucupita, Delta Amacuro State's capital, prominently features parents who lack any of the features used in racializing individuals as
indigenous (figure 6.12). In stark contrast to the seeming incommunicable
distraction of the indigenous mother pictured in figure 6.10, the couple focuses intently on the child and, it would seem, its health. It would be hard to
find a more striking difference, both visually and textually, between the main-
land version and a pamphlet created by the leading branch of the Venezuelan
military (the Guardia Nacional) for the rainforest area—geographically adjacent but projected as racially and culturally foreign. The first image contrasts
a military physician whose prominent mustache emphasizes his masculine
and nonindigenous identity (figure 6.13). His bespectacled eyes engage the
reader directly, and his stethoscope marks his professional position. Beside
him is a man whose dress (consisting only of a woven loincloth), armbands,
haircut, and anatomy place him as a quintessential exemplar of the national
imaginary of indigenous peoples. I have worked in the Orinoco Delta for
nearly four decades and have never seen anyone who resembles this figure.

The text is Warao, using a strange mixture of Spanish and International
Phonetic Alphabet orthographies. The content, expectedly, consists of basic
biomedical knowledge about cholera and prevention guidelines. In the first

FIGURE 6.12. Middle-class family in cholera pamphlet

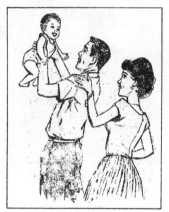

FIGURE 6.12. Middle-class family in cholera pamphlet

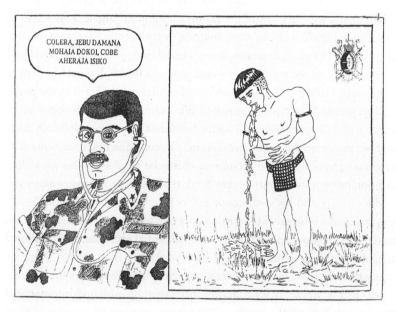

FIGURE 6.13. Guardia Nacional cholera pamphlet for delta, military doctor and vomiting patient

image, the physician speaks to a plural "you" (*yatu*), seemingly to all who are expected to understand the text and feel interpellated by the drawings. He warns of vomiting and stomach aches as cholera symptoms. The man seems to bring the doctor's warning to life, standing on open ground, looking down, vomiting, and grasping his stomach. The figure seems doubly locked in incommunicability: he not only exhibits an illness that seemingly results from failing to adopt the proffered norms, but he exhibits no signs of auditory or visual attention, let alone any attempt to pass along prevention advice. The image that follows (figure 6.14) presents an even more bizarre disjunction between communicability and incommunicability. The words grammatically, addressed to a plural "you," echo those of the physician, but they are attached to a naked figure with his back to the reader, buttocks exposed, defecating on open ground. This image could be read psychoanalytically as suggesting that cholera patients can speak only biocommunicably, well, through their anuses. The figure seems to take ventriloquism to an extreme as a denigratingly incommunicable figure sustains the flow of communicable advice.

Later pages picture people complying with cholera guidelines. As in the Pedrito series, the final images bring this communicable transformation to a happy conclusion as a mother walks with her ailing child toward the clinic. She bears the important message that people should obtain medicine in the clinic, a warning against phytotherapy, commonly used to complement allopathic treatment in the Orinoco Delta (Wilbert 1996). In contrast to all but one of the previous images, she looks straight ahead but without engaging the reader, much less the ailing child, whom she seems to be dragging along by the hair. Bringing the teleological movement to completion, the last drawing pictures the clinic. These drawings are deterritorialized, placing figures on dry ground rather than the riverine and marshy landscape of the Orinoco Delta. Overlooking one of the major problems with access to health care, no form of transport—even a small canoe—is represented.

Like projections of doctor-patient communication, language is reduced to reference, bits of biomedical content that can be detached from the voices and bodies of nonindigenous professionals and attached—their didactic grammatical features still in place—to indigenous bodies. The pamphlet constructs biomedical content as moving transparently between languages, bounded packages of words and grammar. A copy had been given to the linguistic anthropologist María Eugenia Villalón; health officials had asked her to translate it into E'ñapa, a language in Amazonas State. The drawings, apparently, did not need a translation. Talal Asad (1986, 157) argued that an important way in which colonialism hierarchizes knowledge lies in projecting

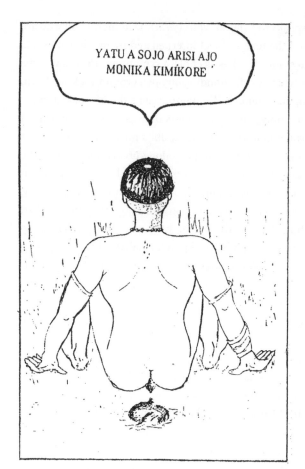

FIGURE 6.14. Guardia Nacional cholera pamphlet for delta, defecating patient

"institutionally defined power relations between the languages/modes of life" of colonizing and colonized peoples. Translations reproduce these hierarchical relations as they move content between the purportedly "weaker" languages of the colonized and the stronger languages of colonizers. One of the ways that Spanish is attached to modernity and citizenship in Delta Amacuro is by depicting it as the language of biomedicine. Warao, spoken by nearly all residents of the rainforest area and almost no people classified as nonindigenous, is projected as a language associated with "shamans" and belief in "spirits." As these associations were broadcast through local media outlets and in public meetings and policy discussions, racialized communicable profiling deepened and naturalized the forms of linguistic racism prevalent in Delta Amacuro State.

The pamphlet, which appeared only after many people had already died in the outbreak, was distributed in the clinics and temporary treatment centers where doctors, nurses, and community members were struggling to help scores of dying patients, who kept arriving around the clock. As witnessed by the physician Clara Mantini-Briggs, who worked in these settings during the epidemic, nonindigenous health professionals often inflicted linguistic racism on patients, denigrating people traumatized by death and illness if nurses judged them as having failed to understand instructions issued in Spanish (Briggs and Mantini-Briggs 2003, 81–97). By the time they got a pamphlet, patients already possessed embodied knowledge of cholera's symptoms and had viewed demonstrations of prevention measures. There was, in short, no new content in the pamphlet. More broadly, it naturalizes the legacy of colonialism and racism by medicalizing the cholera epidemic as caused by bacteria, adopting a narrow biomedical frame that directed attention away from structural factors that led to deplorable health conditions. The pamphlet reflected the magical formula of public health communicability: circulating biomedical advice through an invitation to communicability could magically end the circulation of bacteria—without providing sanitary infrastructures or improving healthcare systems, let alone responding to demands for political representation, housing, employment, and education. The point is not simply that pamphlets and news stories were smokescreens used to direct attention away from the political economy of racism; instead, their semiotic features did the ideological work of creating a more powerful, medicalized foundation for even more virulent racial inequities in the wake of the outbreak. For decades to come, this incommunicable stereotype rationalized withholding basic services in indigenous communities and the expropriation of funds allocated by the national government for the lower delta by corrupt party officials, even after they nominally aligned themselves with President Hugo Chávez Frías's pro-indigenous socialist government.

The pamphlet specified the cost of communicability: accepting this invitation to sanitary and communicable citizenship required accepting a denigrating stereotype. Echoing Fanon, the pamphlet said, in effect: "Look, a Warao!" It was a Tarzan-like work of constructing images of racialized incommunicable and unsanitary subjects and those of a nonindigenous, all-knowing doctor. The physician models the attenuated biocommunicable hierarchy that characterizes most interactions between Spanish-speaking physicians and their indigenous patients, as I documented in chapter 5: he only speaks, never listens. The pamphlet, along with news coverage in the local paper and radio stations, health policies, and healthcare practices, created an epidemic of incommunicability, of biomedically based racial subordination. Together, they created a new regime of incommunicability that would long outlast the presence of *Vibrio cholerae.*

Global Health

Health communication figures prominently in global health; analyzing how global regimes of communicability reproduce and extend hierarchies of knowledge and power is thus crucial for producing critical perspectives on global health. I noted that the unilinear, hierarchically organized model of communicability nearly always comes to the fore when designing programs to "reach" racialized or otherwise subordinated populations. Mohan Dutta's (2008) work richly analyzes how the production of incommunicability achieves global scale in public health. Global health communication programs portray North America and Europe—and the multilateral organizations, such as the World Health Organization, based there—as centers of knowledge production. North American and European global health programs recruit health workers from lower-income countries and train them as public health specialists. Health communication specialists from metropolitan centers employed by international health institutions and non-governmental organizations also travel to countries judged to have knowledge deficits to train health educators. This same hierarchization process continues in low-income countries as communicators produce materials, create websites and social media platforms, train local personnel, and conduct workshops with populations purportedly characterized by deficits of communicability. In short, global health communication creates a global chronotope, in Mikhail Bakhtin's (1981) terms, that envisions a unilinear, hierarchically structured transfer of knowledge. This process reflects the faith in scalability characteristic of global health, like capitalism: a preference for ideologies and interventions that can purportedly be moved from site to site with minimal modifications for differences of language, culture, and geography.

Two pathbreaking works in critical global health studies present remarkable ethnographies of the global dissemination of biocommunicability. Stacy Leigh Pigg's (2001) work places analytics devised by linguistic anthropologists at its core. Her article, a classic in medical anthropology, could fruitfully be brought by linguistic anthropologists to their students, as well. The essay foregrounds translation even as it pushes the term—in dialogue with Asad (1986)—beyond the more limited ways it is often used in global health. In the wake of the consolidation of knowledge about HIV/AIDS (Epstein 1996), Pigg traces how international health programs of the 1990s attempted to avert an epidemic in Nepal. Critiquing developmentalist global health inflections of the dominant biocommunicable model—here organized as much by geography as by professional status and race—she identifies a foundational language ideology that views "the task of international health education" as moving "bits of information from one social location to another." In good Lockean tradition, definitions of language are focused on words, attempting to achieve commensurability by matching the referential content of English scientific terms to "the right words" in Nepali (Pigg 2001, 483). Nepal was purportedly trapped in incommunicability due to the seeming ignorance of the majority of Nepalese of biomedicine and the lack of a communicable infrastructure for knowledge circulation due to prohibitions about talking publicly about sex.

In translating HIV/AIDS knowledge, Nepalese AIDS workers' efforts "to bend it, mold it, or force it to accommodate the contours of the Nepali social ground" involved code-switching into English, although many audiences lacked knowledge of the language (Pigg 2001, 482, 521). Why? Pigg carefully traces Nepalese participants' communicable models. The AIDS workers viewed English as the language of science and precision. Using English, particularly medicalized terms, indexed workers' positionalities within a global regime of HIV/AIDS biocommunicability. Scientific, affective, and sexual trajectories converged as English enabled workers to comply with referential demands to talk explicitly about sex and distance themselves simultaneously from displaying any affective connection to their words. This scientific interpellation and affective distancing seemed to be passed along, as evident in the acoustic materiality of voices "as an astonishing range of people would quote this information in the parrotlike voice of school rote learning" (497). These lexical, intonational, and other features thus marked the voice of biocommunicability. The performance of biomedical discourse using English terms produced the very incommunicability that it was supposed to eradicate.

Pigg (2001, 486) concludes that communication—here defined as biocommunicable models and the practices designed to make them seem real—constituted "one means (though certainly not the only means) by which a stable, internationally unified world of AIDS knowledge/intervention comes into being." Avoiding the reductionism that would analyze communicabilities as strategies that diverted attention from more political engagement with social inequities, Pigg documents the political and ethical effects of biocommunicability and the practices required to make it seem real, consequential, and ethically compelling. One of the difficulties in this export process was how it divorced biocommunicability—as imaginations of communication—from viral communicability: HIV/AIDS had not yet become the predicted "public health disaster" in Nepal (482).

Vinh-Kim Nguyen (2010) ethnographically explores the imposition of "international best practices" of HIV prevention in West Africa. He documents how a communicable regime traveled in unilinear fashion from US organizations to low-income countries and populations without embracing biocommunicable models. He details how international agencies sponsored workshops to train people to perform testimonials, disclosures of HIV-positive status, and illness narratives, thereby creating patient-activists who could elicit testimonials from others. Rather than transferring "expert" biocommunicable knowledge, "confessional technologies" (Hunt 1997) imagined discourse as emerging from the self, "made available as a *substrate* that could be examined, prodded, discussed, worked upon" (Nguyen 2010, 8). By mastering techniques for asking, telling, and listening, participants could transform other HIV-positive selves "into a powerful, life-giving force." Nguyen traces this communicable model and associated practices from social psychologists employed by the post–World War II US military to their adoption by business schools for training potential managers to their use in counterculture movements of the 1960s to US HIV activism to their global dissemination by HIV activists working for international agencies. This trajectory would warn us against positing any hasty or fixed correlations between particular communicable models and dimensions of power, hegemony, and "resistance." Although AIDS lay-activist communicability constituted a powerful force in the 1980s for critiquing and often opposing the CDC, other public health authorities, scientific research, clinical practices, pharmaceutical corporations, and "mainstream" news institutions (Epstein 1996), the particular form of lay-activist communicability that is seen as one of its trademarks became an important ideological tool for reproducing racialized global regimes of communicability inequity in the mid-1990s.

Nguyen (2010) also notes how testimonials intersected in West Africa with colonialism and contemporary evangelical ideologies. He suggests that government officials were as invested as international agencies in promoting this communicable model: testimonials provided both quantitative and qualitative evidence of the success of their programs and justifications for future funding. Workshops transformed activist communicability into models of egalitarian social relations of solidarity between West Africans and international consultants, a "hypothetical equality" not otherwise evident in the face of the massive social inequities signaled by the fact that consultants spent most of their time in five-star hotels (38).

Nguyen (2010) documents how existing African communicable models problematized the uptake of confessional technologies. "In a setting where one did not disclose intimate and painful matters in public," he writes, testimonials could be read as false claims performed for financial reward; they thus "could trigger suspicion rather than solidarity" (24). Tellingly, Nguyen describes how the founder of a youth group disclosed a young man's HIV status to him alone "because I was an 'outsider.' . . . The African feels that he can trust the White man . . . because they're not like us, they don't go around telling everyone everyone's secrets.'" Nguyen continued: "Whiteness meant being outside the network of rumor and gossip" (29). Ironically, confessional communicability—perceived as a quintessential embodiment of the whiteness of its promoters—induced West Africans to confess in public.

The two situations differ. International agencies promoted a medicalized form of communicability in Nepal and an anti-medicalized form in West Africa.[14] Likewise, the virus's communicability was vastly different in the two places, given the much more widespread seropositivity rates in Burkina Faso and Ivory Coast. Nevertheless, exporting communicable models drove a wedge between the entangled communicabilities of viruses and communicative practices in each. Nguyen (2010) reports: "Perhaps the most striking aspect of the response to the AIDS epidemic . . . was that although almost nothing was happening on the ground (clinics were empty, pharmacies bare, and prevention was limited to the broadcasting of public service announcements), workshops, seminars, and training sessions devoted to HIV and AIDS multiplied" (38). Adia Benton (2015) documents a vast gulf between viral and discursive communicability in Sierra Leone, where government and NGO efforts to depict HIV/AIDS as a dire threat drew the majority of health funding to HIV prevention. However, low seropositivity rates might suggest that other issues were more pressing. Nguyen argues that international agencies saw their mission not as providing lifesaving drugs but as producing confessionals. Despite humanitarian goals, inscribing dominant communicabilities onto the surfaces of vast differences in access to health care performatively produced health/communicative inequities in each case.

I noted in the introduction several studies that bridge linguistic and medical anthropology in illuminating issues of health communication, broadly defined. Here is an area in which linguistic anthropologists have much to contribute. Given linguistic anthropologists' interest in issues of scale (Carr and Lempert 2016), they could play a crucial role in analyzing how global health programs enable dominant communicabilities, interventions, and health/communicative inequities to jump scales. Dutta (2008) has carefully analyzed the crucial role of health communication ideologies and practices in maintaining geopolitical hierarchies and systems of dominance. He suggests that they often deepen the political-economic effects of international health agencies and NGOs, claiming moral high ground by infusing them with forms of humanitarian reason (Fassin [2010] 2012; Redfield 2013; Ticktin 2011). Given how ideologies of empowerment and agency are fundamentally contradicted by semiotic ideologies and complex, recursive pragmatics of discursive domination, health communication is much like the regime of international aid analyzed by James Ferguson (1990)—designed to fail but in such a way as to ensure its reproduction and serve the interests of elites all along the way.

A splendid article by T. S. Harvey (2011) points to how deep engagement with linguistic and medical anthropology can open up unexplored facets of health communication. During long-term fieldwork in the Mayan highlands of Guatemala, Harvey noticed how mobile Mayan medical salespeople gave health communication talks and demonstrations in open-air markets, town squares, and up and down the aisles of crowded buses. The subjects of their performances—given in K'iche, Kaqchikel, Tz'utujil, and Spanish—included prostate enlargement and cancer and reproductive health, even when these topics had no direct relation to the products they sold, which were mainly derived from local plants and animals. Harvey's insights from this work are of analytic and methodological importance. He notes that the long trajectory of research on Mayan health had largely focused on a binary between "'traditional' indigenous Maya healing and 'modern' Western bio-medicine" (51). Rather than drawing their legitimacy and authority from either, Mayan mobile medicine fashioned a space between them that critically engaged biomedicine and appropriated some of its terms without impinging on Mayan categories of disease and healing practices. Harvey argues that this a priori categorization prevented ethnographers from documenting Mayan mobile medicine as "localized forms of public health" (51) and as a widespread component of ecologies of health communication. In a move that parallels Eduardo Menéndez's relational approach (Menéndez and Di Pardo 1996), "a medically oriented ethnography of communication" (Harvey 2011, 50) provided Harvey with an ethnographic openness that enabled him to see the importance of practices that were erased by dominant models of communicability, both "biomedical" and "traditional," and had been dismissed as trivial manifestations of incommunicability.

Neoliberalism, Health Literacy, and the Rise of the Patient-Consumer

Until the 1960s, unilinear, hierarchically ordered biocommunicability dominated in the United States; media commonly exhorted patients to depend for health information exclusively on the family doctor (Lee 2007). In the 1960s, this model expanded to accord a role for journalists as participants in what is projected as its translation into popular registers and its dissemination, even if health professionals frequently complained that reporters "sensationalized," "exaggerated," or commercialized health knowledge. Recent decades have witnessed the emergence of a very different communicable model in the United States, which Daniel Hallin and I termed *patient-consumer communicability* (Briggs and Hallin 2016). Its complex and seemingly incompatible roots come from many sources. Many proponents of "back to nature" perspectives radically rejected biomedicine and looked to dissident scientists and medical professionals and explored complementary and alternative medicine. As Mark Nichter and Jennifer Jo Thompson (2006) document, the 1990s witnessed a massive increase in dietary supplements, including herbs and herbal medicines associated with the privatization and internalization of the governmental obligation to identify "risks" to one's health and, more broadly, a component of the technologies of the self (Foucault 1988) that sought to optimize "well-being" (also see Rose 2007). The rise of patient-consumer communicability was also fostered by the Ronald Reagan–era emphasis on "the market" and "individual initiative" as productive forces for change. Amid conservative efforts to reduce entitlement benefits and state participation in health programs, citizens were increasingly cast as patient-consumers who should take active roles in promoting their own health (Reid 2005, 94). Another factor that favored the rise of the patient-consumer modality was the deeper penetration of capitalism into medicine, and vice versa (Clarke et al. 2003; Sunder Rajan 2006), as quintessentially manifested in the pharmaceuticalization of health (Biehl 2007) and the advent of direct-to-consumer marketing by pharmaceutical corporations. Another crucial factor is the advent of evidence-based medicine, which positions the physician less as an "expert" with unique access to a clinically trained medical gaze than as a knowledgeable partner in sorting through relevant evidence and guidelines (Engebretsen and Baker 2022; Ødemark and Engebretsen 2022).[15] In October 2009, I visited my primary care physician, who was in his early sixties. He asked whether I wanted periodic PSA tests for prostate cancer. Trying to play the role of the expert patient (Dumit 2012), I responded: "I know the literature. I know the pros and cons. But if it were your body, what would *you* do?" "Oh, no," the doctor responded. "I never give my patients advice. I simply help them sort through all the information that comes their way" (Briggs and Hallin 2016, 53). Positioning me as the informed patient-consumer, *he* refused the biomedical authority model.

Rather than projecting laypeople as passive recipients of biomedical knowledge, patient-consumer communicability pictures laypeople as self-interested individuals who actively seek and consume health knowledge relevant to their "risk factors" and their particular goals for bodily and mental well-being. This type of communicability promises agency, casting individuals as endowed with rights but also governmental obligations to examine a wide range of sources, including mainstream media, social media, websites, advertisements, newsletters, friends and relatives, books and magazines, and other sources. Good patient-consumers must critically evaluate each source's validity and usefulness and decide which services to consume. One important factor here is access to professional medical publications. Reading the *New England Journal of Medicine*, for example, previously required access to a medical school library or a costly personal subscription. However, medical journals generally became available in digital, open-access form; search engines now include links to articles. Rather than excluding nonbiomedical modalities, patient-consumer communicability generally lauds efforts to use acupuncture, yoga, meditation, "natural" childbirth, and other modalities if they reflect rational, self-interested calculations that a nonbiomedical type of treatment is more likely to yield results. Laypeople, however, are projected not as producers of health knowledge but as knowledgeable, active, and agentive consumers.

A related but distinct form of communicability that challenged the exclusion of laypeople as knowledge producers grew out of numerous social movements and patient advocacy groups. Some of its sources were located in feminist, gay, BIPOC (Black, indigenous, and people of color), disability, and other social movement critiques of the biocommunicable status quo. Feminist critiques of male physicians' claims of expertise regarding women health, classically embodied in the Boston Women's Health Collective's (1971) *Our Bodies, Ourselves*, depicted women's reflexive understanding of their bodies as crucial means of knowledge production (Davis 2007). Patients with AIDS demanded active roles in the production of knowledge about the disease in the epidemic's early years (Epstein 1996). Deborah Heath, Rayna Rapp, and Karen-Sue Taussig (2004; see also Taussig, Rapp, and Health 2003) document several cases in which patients and their relatives actively shaped studies of diseases and conditions that affect them, challenging scientific findings, lobbying for research funding, recruiting scientists and clinicians, pooling findings, and creating alternative circuits for circulating knowledge. Georgia Davis and Mark Nichter (2016) document how women mobilized when they found that available biomedical nosologies could not identify or treat the symptoms they and their families were experiencing, later identified as Lyme disease. When confronted with doctors who confidently relied on inadequate diagnostic categories, dismissed their symptoms, and relegated them to the time-worn misogynistic image of the female hysteric, they turned to "vetting doctors who might become 'Lyme-literate,' locating scientists willing to collaborate with them, and gathering and sharing all manner of scientific knowledge" (218). This story suggests another important, albeit less visible, model that I would call *lay-activist communicability*, in which laypeople test the limits of biomedical authority *and* patient-consumer models in assessing existing biomedical knowledge; claim active roles in producing new findings; and shape research, treatment, policy, and health communication about a particular condition.[16] As numerous researchers have suggested, white middle-class laypeople are much more likely to gain such standing (Briggs and Hallin 2016; Davis and Nichter 2016; Epstein 1997; Reid 2005). I devote more attention to the role of social movements in challenging biocommunicability and pushing for alternatives in the interlude that follows this chapter and in chapter 8.

As the patient-consumer model gained force, communicability became more critical in racializing projects. As Hallin and I documented, health journalists most frequently pictured middle-class white people as ideal patient-consumers (Briggs and Hallin 2016, 180–83). Lifestyle and Health sections of newspapers often featured photographs of smiling white subjects meditating, taking yoga classes, jogging, biking, hiking, and the like. People of color appeared much less frequently. At the same time, health stories, billboards, and other sources that focused on nonwhite people or immigrants generally projected biomedical-authority communicability and positioned racialized subjects as passive recipients. Nonwhite subjects who assessed competing forms of treatment and accessed nonbiomedical modalities were commonly viewed critically, unlike white people. Claiming the individual agency associated with the patient-consumer role made it a more desirable subject position than the passive receiver of biomedical-authority communicability. Performing the former role was projected as the ability to make choices, rationally evaluate biomedical and other recommendations, and share the fruits of communicable efforts with others—in short, to make up their own minds.

Communicability thus became another form of white privilege. As was the case with housing, education, employment, and access to capital (Lipsitz

1998), white people—especially middle-class and urban or suburban ones—got credit for accessing patient-consumer communicability and being projected as communicable citizens or, at least, having the capacity to gain this status. Black, Latinx, and Native American subjects, trapped in biomedical-authority communicability, were most often treated by default as incommunicable subjects, ranked through projected degrees of disconnection and incapacity for remediation. It is thus crucial to complement the discussion in chapter 5 of how racialized inequities and biocommunicability operate in clinical spaces. The racialization of biocommunicability in health communication became another crucial vehicle for naturalizing health inequities, contributing to broader racialized stereotypes and structural forms of discrimination. Denise Ferreira da Silva (2022) suggests that violence and discrimination are authorized by a principle of necessity: they are required by conservative logics to protect (white) society and by liberal logics to help Black people achieve the sort of (white) subjectivity that would afford full inclusion in such categories as citizenship and humanity. Interventions, even if denigrating and debilitating, are thus authorized in advance and can generally withstand critical scrutiny, even if an occasional apology or manslaughter conviction is required. To paraphrase Shakespeare, so let it be with biocommunicability, where what are projected as the failures of individuals and entire populations seem to require constant surveillance and intervention. Incommunicability, in short, is a legacy of colonialism. To paraphrase Malcolm X's famous words, incommunicability is like a Cadillac: "They bring out a new model every year."

The cost of communicable citizenship has been rising for every US resident. Adele Clarke and her colleagues (2003) traced a shift roughly in the mid-1980s from medicalization, which Irving Zola (1972) characterized as the increasing extension of medical practices and forms of authority into wider spheres of life, to what they termed *biomedicalization*. They used this term to refer to the greater interpenetration of biomedicine with other social structures, such as industry, the state, and the mass media, and the proliferation and diversification of flows of biomedical knowledge through public channels. They emphasized how communicative and related practices and technologies go beyond representation to help constitute biomedicalized subjects and objects. The concept of "health literacy" points to ways that lay positionality in communicability has been complicated by biomedicalization. At the same time that health literacy promises to be a source of increased agency for laypeople by using communicative interfaces to navigate their travels through biomedical institutions and practices, the cost of this promise of freedom is new forms of communicative bondage. Successful fulfillment of the patient role has come to entail mastering a complex, shifting skill set: "Functional health literacy is the ability to read, understand and act on health information, including comprehending prescription labels, interpreting appointment slips, completing health insurance forms, following instructions for diagnostic tests, and understanding other the essential health-related materials" (Bulled 2015, 24).

Facing these tasks, whose complexity is now further exacerbated by their embeddedness in proliferating and constantly changing digital technologies, often produces feelings of frustration and failure. Today, it is common to admit defeat in navigating a website or "app" and call a helpline, only to be placed on hold for extensive periods and often cut off before a representative answers. The likelihood of and stakes for failure are far from equally distributed: the languages and registers used in digital platforms, the relative in/accessibility of technology and internet access, and vast differences in the "user-friendliness" of systems accessible to patients with expensive private insurance versus those who rely on Medicare, Medicaid, and other public programs increase health/communicative inequities. Decades of work in linguistic anthropology, sociolinguistics, and pragmatics on literacies could help illuminate the stakes for failing to negotiate telephone menus; electronic insurance forms and medical records; and online requests for doctor's appointments, prescription refills, and vaccines, as well as questionnaires that make access to work and other sites contingent on digital reports of symptoms and vaccination status. The rise of patient-consumer communicability, biomedicalization, and the digitalization of access to health care and medical records seem to offer liberation from the subordinate and powerless role of passive communicable recipients of health knowledge. Nevertheless, their false promises have created vast new possibilities for producing hierarchical regimes of incommunicability.

Rather than entailing a specific set of communicative practices, these expanding expectations form part of perhaps the most widespread domain for extending regimes of communicability, patient power and autonomy, and lay participation in biomedical knowledge production: "digital health." Defined by Patty Kostkova (2015, 1) as the "use of information and communications technologies to improve human health, healthcare services, and wellness for individuals and across populations," digital health becomes "an unprecedented opportunity to transform the healthcare sector and empower citizens in taking charge of their own health." A technological focus of digital health, beyond computers and smartphones, is wearable and tracking technologies, which some refer to as the "internet of things for smart healthcare" (Baker,

Xiang, and Atkinson 2017). A "smart bed" can now monitor your movements, breathing, and heart rate and then inform you each morning via your "smartphone" how long it took you to sleep, how long your sleep lasted, and how many minutes it was interrupted, among other measures. Digital health also embraces social media, health games, and health-focused apps, along with their interface with digital medical records, surveillance systems, and big data streams. Even as healthcare dollars are absorbed by creators of digital platforms and technologies, patient-consumers' governmental obligation to continually search for "information," technologies, and services yields massive digital advertising revenues. A crucial mediator for gaining access to health care, digital biocommunicability is thus a major component of the growing subservience of biomedicine to for-profit, investor-driven capitalist medicine (Waitzkin and Working Group for Health beyond Capitalism 2018). Susan Erickson (2012, 367) argues that electronic digital health information systems and the health statistics they produce and circulate crucially enable the restructuring of health as a global business enterprise, providing a "global administrative apparatus" for integrating health into commodity capitalism. In short, digital biocommunicability pays. As Graham Bodie and his colleagues (2009) and other scholars have suggested, e-health can amplify health inequities across scales, inscribing society and population disparities through individual usage of online health resources.

Proponents of digital health suggest that it promises to revolutionize communication between health professionals and laypeople, including using smartphones and social apps to enhance communicability by extending diagnostic data collection and providing health communication outside clinical interactions. Laboratory results are often quickly available to patients through their digital accounts. Another arena is efforts by public health agencies to detect public health "threats" through internet traffic and to extend "crisis and emergency risk communication" online and through social media. This new world of knowledge production and circulation reportedly requires a new "multidisciplinary domain" that "spans disciplines including computer science, engineering, information science, journalism, economy, clinical medicine, public health, epidemiology, and others" (Kostkova 2015, 2). Mark Khurana and his colleagues (2022, 2) argue that the COVID-19 "pandemic has accelerated the digital health trend," particularly by much greater use of telehealth and telemonitoring due to limited in-person access to healthcare providers. They suggest that medical schools add digital health components to curricula and integrate them more broadly into medical education.

Dennis Robbins and Patrick Dunn (2019, 154) argue that, "for these amazing technology breakthroughs to become reality, . . . there must be a shift from an emphasis on health literacy to digital health literacy." They suggest that exploiting this potential will require a shift from patient-centricity to "person-centricity," overturning a conception of "the passive and subservient, wounded and vulnerable" in favor of seeing people as changing, autonomous, agentive, and "free to self-determine their health future and journey to improved health and wellbeing" (154–55). This "entirely new paradigm" frees people from the patient role, even as the end goal is the same that dominates doctor-patient interaction: producing "positive health behavior" (154). The echo of long-standing instrumentalist, functionalist communicability reemerges. In the end, this seeming departure from linear, hierarchically structured communicability to digital extensions of patient-consumer communicability in a remarkably clear voice of neoliberalism that echoes settler-colonial rhetorics preserves teleologies and power relations associated with biomedical authority: "True engagement and behavior responsibility require continuously available, real-time, personalized and targeted nudging that is distinctive and meaningful to that person" (155). When it comes to communicability, it seems that *plus ça change, plus c'est la même chose.*

An ethnographic example can help reveal how communicabilities both structure and are structured by programs of digital health communication. It is drawn from a wonderful dissertation by Juliana Friend (2022) that examines how HIV/AIDS-oriented health communication programs and pornography circulate digitally in Senegal. Central to both is the concept of *sutura*, which Friend describes as an ethic of modesty or discretion that centers on shielding intimate aspects, such as sex, from public view. Failing to uphold *sutura* constitutes a loss of moral legitimacy and claims to Senegalese national belonging and full citizenship. Friend suggests, "Sutura brings into frame how the marginalization of particular bodily expressions and the marginalization of particular modes of communication happen in concert," even as the term highlights how communicative and health inequities are co-produced (9).

One of the major problems facing Senegalese HIV/AIDS education programs was how to protect *sutura* while at the same time breaking taboos against speaking about sexuality. The program Friend (2022) researched navigated this difficulty in two ways. First, it was conducted digitally, thus separating physical bodies from discourse. Program participants asserted that a digital format "would provide more sutura . . . than would handing out pamphlets in a hospital" (62). This assessment points to ways that ontologies of communication and embodiment are entangled. Second, health communicators had to shield the explicit talk about sexuality they initiated over public channels from communicative modes deemed erotic. Rather than seduction or erotic play, digital health communication had to increase knowledge about HIV/AIDS prevention and the likelihood that gay and MSM (men who have sex with men) Senegalese men would enact changes in sexual conduct in ways that program administrators could assess. An ideology of knowledge and discourse centering on "information" was critical. Providing information deemed "scientific" and "objective," mainly by pasting a paragraph that explained HIV/AIDS transmission, prevention, and treatment and testing biocommunicability, would structure exchanges about sex through the slogan "informer, pas draguer" (inform, not hit on). By being stripped of affect and arousal, "information" would transform digitally connected queer bodies into circulators of health communication rather than viruses.

The work of transforming biocommunicability into communicative acts, funded by an NGO, fell to eight individuals employed as digital peer educators classified as MSM. A classic unilinear, hierarchically organized biocommunicable model for the unfettered circulation of information to incommunicable subjects envisioned them as the ideal communicators. The educators could understand both the knowledge produced by scientists and the incommunicable social worlds inhabited by their interlocutors. The chosen venues—dating websites and Facebook—exacerbated the potential for violating *sutura*. Charged with presenting information alone, the educators challenged the premise that biocommunicability could be insulated from erotic play: an initial offer of "information" would fail to prompt a response, impeding health communication and preventing educators from achieving their quota of information-transmission events.

As a result, the educators devised—and attempted to hide from their supervisors—what they framed as efforts to entangle multiple models of communication, embodiment, and care. Dodging the administrators' biocommunicable "policing" involved creative movements between flirtation and seduction; evaluating the HIV/AIDS-prevention knowledge of their interlocutors; and pasting approved content that would fill in perceived gaps. It might seem as if the educators were disingenuous: as if incorporating other models and modalities resulted in the familiar teleology of biocommunicability in which a linear transmission of referential content and a promise to leave behind a life of incommunicability is all that mattered. Reworking notions of *sutura*, however, the educators redefined digital communication as "care in and of itself. *Sutura* does not only challenge the health/communication split;

it reimagines what constitutes care in digital health practice" (Friend 2022, 13). The educators engaged in what I might call *communicability-switching* (like code-switching) in such a way as to challenge the rigidity and monopolistic authority of biocommunicability. In the face of the stigmatization they faced as MSM, as potential threats to the health of the body politic, "digital dissidents leverage the very site of their marginalization—*sutura*—to promote health/communicative justice" (13).

Conclusion

This exploration of a range of health communication efforts suggests that they largely rest on a fundamental, sometimes fatal, contradiction. Projects take significant health problems—cholera, tuberculosis, HIV/AIDS, Ebola, dengue, metabolic syndrome, and COVID-19—and convert them into problems of knowledge and communication. By providing patients and populations that epidemiologists project as being "at risk" for these diseases with knowledge, the promise is that the incidence of pathologies will decrease and people will live healthier lives. Nevertheless, incommunicabilities are often produced and inscribed on individuals and populations in the process; in the case of racialized and other subaltern groups, being judged a biocommunicable failure increases stigmatization. The metrics required by state agencies, NGOs, and global health organizations (see Adams 2016) are projected as objective devices for measuring progress made toward biocommunicable citizenship. The assertion by the Senegalese health educators studied by Friend that such forms of assessment constitute biocommunicable policing seems quite apt. Scores on these incommunicability indexes can be used in shaping not only access to health care but broader rights to political participation, education, housing, and employment.[17]

E. Summerson Carr (2011) similarly documents how being deemed incommunicable vis-à-vis addiction treatment scripts can result in the loss of social services. The case she describes highlights the place of social class in assessments of in/communicability. Nadine Hubbs (2014, 37) suggests that middle-class professionals claim the role of the "narrating class: the analysts and experts, the language, representation, and knowledge specialists for the whole society" and, in her analysis, specifically of the white working class. I would go on to suggest that when white middle-class professionals assert their privilege as heirs of Locke to be the communicable class, they claim rights to define legitimate forms of communicability and evaluate the communicable status of individuals and communities deemed to fall into racialized and class stratified categories.

When researchers and media professionals use their privilege as members of the narrating class to portray the working class and racialized populations as impervious to communicable promises of rationality, they help transform social class into a matrix for a priori judgments of communicability and incommunicability. In the case of health communication, the result is the production of incommunicability, starting from the design of policies and programs, images contained in material and digital artifacts, performances of communicability by health workers, and the statistics that shape how communicable success is defined and rendered quantifiable. Health communication complements how provider-patient encounters and health media extend promises of communicability and produce incommunicability.

If cholera prevention pamphlets turned Delta Amacuro State into a territory of incommunicability, the health communication components of global health programs lock participants, places, countries, and institutions into particular positionalities on global maps of in/communicability. World maps of such stigmatizing diseases as cholera and HIV/AIDS and tables specifying which countries reported the most cases and deaths seemed to place the two sides of communicability—the circulation of pathogens and, inversely, of communicable discourse—into succinct graphic and statistical form. It seems small wonder that countries often construct "case definitions"—what counts as a countable case and death and who gets to count it—and distribute testing resources in such a way as to minimize their stigmatized position along both communicable axes (Briggs and Mantini-Briggs 2003, 256–68).

Ideological models of diseases, bodies, minds, discourses, and actions are always multiple, entangled, and shifting. Health communication generally reifies one model, making it seem naturally imbued with rationality, science, ethical virtue, and the agentive potential to vanquish all rivals by converting them into forms of incommunicability. I suggest, following Menéndez, that forms of care undertaken by laypeople outside the clinic often get erased or stigmatized by professionals. Similarly, the myriad forms of health communication and knowledge that laypeople undertake within their families, workplaces, schools, peer-support groups, and so forth, like the mobile Mayan public health presentations documented by Harvey, become invisible or identified as sources of incommunicability and ill health. As we saw from the Nepalese and Sierra Leonean cases, epidemiology and communicable goals are often mismatched, focusing funding and personnel on the priorities of state, multinational, and NGO goals that are not at the top of the list of health problems. The production of incommunicability hides deep ties to colonialism and race, class, and other inequities even as it can, as in the cholera example, make addressing structural factors unthinkable.

I frame these observations as an analytical wake-up call for structural issues that emerge in the design and implementation of many health communication programs. To be sure, painting everything that goes under this label with the same broad brushstroke would be most unfair. Health communication specialists are no less varied in their perspectives and practices than physicians, and many wrestle with the sorts of contradictions that I have discussed. Moreover, clinging to unilinear, hierarchically ordered models does not indicate that practitioners have conservative political views or are comfortable with the status quo of health inequities. My research in Cuba suggests that revolutionary efforts to provide free health care and train doctors who treat patients with respect can go hand in hand with biomedical-authority communicability and a skeptical view of lay reception of health discourse (Briggs 2011). In the end, supporting optimistic spaces that critique dominant communicabilities and explore alternatives is essential. The interlude that follows this chapter calls attention to efforts that push health communication in very different directions. Together, these efforts demonstrate that biocommunicable hegemony and its false claims of transparency and efficacy are not the only possibilities.

Social Movements and Incommunicability-Free Zones

Clara Mantini-Briggs and I spent months traversing the vast Orinoco Delta in 1994–95, working closely with Tirso Gómez, a healer who knew the delta like the back of his hand. Starting at dawn, we traveled to the next community and met with residents. We began by asking about current health conditions and offered to see patients who needed attention. When no nurse was available, I assisted "Dra. Clara." We drew from the stock of medicine kept in boxes in our boat, occasionally seeing as many as a hundred patients in a day or two. We then asked to meet with anyone interested in talking with us, first about current health conditions and then about residents' experiences in the cholera epidemic, including their efforts to save the lives of community members and their interactions with clinicians, healers, and health officials. Collectively we produced a popular epidemiological count of cholera deaths. Afterward, we shared ideas about prevention, learning from a range of healers and other residents and collaboratively thinking about different approaches to healing. We then moved on, continuing until night fell, hanging our hammocks and cooking a simple meal in a borrowed corner of a house in the last community we had visited. A good part of the exhaustion we felt was psychic, the impact of listening to myriad accounts of deaths that need not have occurred and seeing at firsthand continuing deep health problems.

One day, after more than a month of this nonstop work, Clara needed to rest. I thus set out at dawn with Gómez. At midmorning, we reached Waku-hana, a community with just over forty inhabitants. We began, as usual, with our survey of health conditions. The response from the community representative and *wisidatu* healer Eulalio Torres astounded us: recent outbreaks of measles, whooping cough, chicken pox, and other diseases had not appeared in Wakuhana. When I asked about the cholera epidemic, Torres reported: one case and no deaths. Delighted and surprised, I asked him why Wakuhanans had been so fortunate. Wakuhana lies near the small rural hospital in Curiapo, the municipal capital. Having heard from other communities how quickly cholera can kill, residents took the infected man immediately to the hospital, watched the treatment the doctor provided, and listened carefully to him. (Torres understands Spanish well.) Upon returning to Wakuhana, Torres made a threefold announcement: first, residents would boil every drop of water they consumed; second, no one would be permitted to travel to other communities as long as cholera was present; and third, as the community's *wisidatu* healer, he would consult with the *hebu* that caused cholera and then hold a *nahanamu* ritual to ask them to leave Wakuhana alone. Our conversation with Torres took place two years after the epidemic. No additional cases of cholera appeared, and no one, according to his account, had been infected by the other diarrheal diseases that claim so many children's lives.

Wakuhana exemplified the first alternative to biocommunicable hegemony—one that I term *multiple, laterally organized communicabilities*. Torres did not view biocommunicability skeptically. He took the physician's description of the disease and prevention guidelines seriously, relayed the essential stipulations to other residents, and ensured that they carried them out, even after the epidemic ended. Wakuhana became, in this sense, a biocommunicable community. At the same time, he placed the disease within the communicable model that he, as a *wisidatu*, controlled, opening up a circuit to invisible pathogens and including other Wakuhanans, through palm starch gathering, dancing, and celebration, in events that underscored the need for a community-wide effort to prevent cholera. To be sure, this amalgamation of multiple communicabilities did invest more power in one man.

When I next visited the headquarters of the Regional Health Service in Tucupita, I suggested that the approach adopted in Wakuhana of multiple, laterally organized communicabilities might provide an excellent model for collaboratively building health communication programs with delta residents. The only response was scathing laughter. To officials, it was inconceivable that biocommunicability could achieve a respectful, balanced relationship with other communicabilities rather than seeking to extirpate or, at least, subordinate them. Indeed, their origin story of the cholera outbreak asserted that trusting "shamans" and believing in "spirits" precludes any engagement with biocommunicability or effective participation in clinical encounters— and, indeed, that it was one of the major "causes" of the outbreak in the delta. The step I recommended thus would have undermined their efforts to draw attention away from the structural factors that led to such massive morbidity and mortality and their failure to prepare for the outbreak. It also would have undermined how politicians were seizing on this culturalist origin story in extending racial domination in the face of an indigenous social movement that, sparked by the "500 Years of Resistance" to colonialism movement of 1992, was growing. Given that racial domination and exploitation of the delta's people and resources was the political goal, even thinking about inviting a rapprochement with other communicabilities was, for them, laughable.[1]

The Wakuhana example opens up other modalities for health communication. When he relayed the doctor's words, Torres echoed the prose used by the doctor in the hospital, translated into Warao. In calling the *hebu* he deemed responsible for cholera, however, Torres used a rattle containing small stones capable of healing, a small bell, and his voice, its power amplified by strong tobacco, a collective version of the type of healing performance I analyzed in chapter 5. As the *hebu* took over Torres's larynx, Wakuhanans could hear the fearful voice of the pathogens and their messages about prevention. The two communicable registers were thus contrastively marked by the semiotic expansion evident in the *hebu* song, opening up acoustic modalities that called for different modes of listening—and that engaged both human and nonhuman audiences.

Steven Black's (2019) excellent ethnography of a South African Zulu gospel choir named Thembeka suggests how musical form and expressive bodily engagement can be infused in biocommunicable registers. The reach of Black's training is impressive, including not just linguistic and medical anthropology but also psychological anthropology and ethnomusicology, in addition to years as a jazz saxophonist. He presented Thembeka as a "biospeech community" where members are connected by their HIV-positive and biocommunicable status: sharing a biosocial identity (Rabinow 1992) based on a biomedical diagnostic category and their commitment to disseminating biomedical HIV/AIDS discourse. Their investment in biocommunicable hegemony was complicated, however, by how Thembeka's members "transposed," in Black's terms, speech about HIV/AIDS into genres of joking and singing. The ludic exchanges, which took place during rehearsals, drew on multiple linguistic codes that crossed between English and Zulu, and they contained lexical items tied to biomedical, Christian, and alternative Zulu explanatory models of disease. Even as choir members displayed alignment with biomedicine and a critical relationship to "traditional Zulu understandings" (Black 2019, 54), joking routines confirmed their positionality within multiple communicabilities and their ability to entangle them.

Thembeka's primary modality for performing biocommunicability—song—provides an excellent example of a different way of complicating biocommunicability. Like the previous example, it did not involve overt critiques of biomedical authority (Black 2019, 152). Here the move involved muting the demand for referentiality in biocommunicability through *semiotic transformation and aesthetic elaboration*. Thembeka members embodied biocommunicable alignment by synchronizing vocal cords, lungs, bodies, and minds (23). Beyond transposing HIV/AIDS biocommunicability into a shared aesthetic engagement using the acoustic materiality of voice and instrumentation, the process linked the members' bodies not just through their viral status but through forms of stepping, swaying, and gesturing that kept time with the music. The central demand for referentiality associated with biocommunicability was thus perceptually placed in the background, even as explicit references to HIV/AIDS largely gave way to indirect modes that, similar to joking, opened up space for other communicabilities.

Black extended his analysis to trace how Thembeka's commitment to biocommunicability positioned the choir in relation to global health institutions. The group gained modest income and international recognition by performing at medical conferences and in the course of tours designed to raise funds for South African clinical facilities that treat HIV/AIDS patients. In an ethnographic sketch of their performance at an HIV/AIDS conference, Black perceptively noted that Thembeka's members were presented in colorful "traditional" costumes even as conference members performed their status by wearing professional attire. Rather than being invited to participate in producing and debating knowledge about HIV/AIDS testing and treatment—based on their status as people living with HIV who enjoyed deep knowledge of patient populations and had engaged extensively with biomedical knowledge—Thembeka's role was limited to performing its music onstage. In the eyes of the health professionals, bodily adornment and temporal and spatial containment marked the precarious and limited biocommunicable positionality of the members. In addition, conference organizers imposed biocommunicable containment by asking the choir members, especially when they were performing for international audiences, to sing "traditional Zulu" rather than gospel songs and to forgo the use of sound equipment, drums, and keyboard in favor of a cappella singing. Particularly, for US audiences invested in stereotypes of Africans, African bodies, and African music (Black 2019, 85), this traditionalization (Bauman 1992; Briggs 2021) process seemed to suggest that Thembeka was valuable to biocommunicable regimes insofar as members' seemingly foundational incommunicability provided the backdrop for performing limited inclusion in biocommunicable worlds.

Steven Epstein's brilliant *Impure Science: AIDS, Activism, and the Politics of Knowledge* (1996) takes us squarely into the realm of critical engagement with the logics, modes of knowledge production, and claims to authority of biomedicine. Examining the role of the gay men's social movement—and particularly the highly visible ACT-UP organization—during the early years of the HIV/AIDS epidemic, Epstein explored how the nosological category of AIDS and the identification of HIV as its causal mechanism gained credibility. Building scientific and medical credibility was challenging due to the time it took to establish the cause of AIDS and develop effective treatments; no cure or viable vaccine is still available. Moreover, given that millions of persons worldwide were already infected raised the stakes during a fearful time in which scientists, physicians, and laypeople were cast into incommunicability. Paraphrasing Dante, health officials, scientists, and journalists cast three stigmatized groups—homosexuals, Haitians, and heroin users—into the seventh realm of incommunicable hell (see Farmer 1992). Gay activists worked to transform their positionality from "victims" or "patients" to that of experts who possessed the ability and the right to contribute to emerging scientific and medical knowledge. They also challenged anti-gay biases on the part of scientists, journalists, and politicians. Their remarkable interventions exemplify what I refer to as *biocommunicable appropriation as patient activism*.

As a body of scientific discourse about AIDS emerged, activists—with the help of doctors, nurses, and scientists within gay communities—embarked on a massive self-education program to gain detailed knowledge of relevant dimensions of virology, immunology, and epidemiology (Epstein 1996, 8). They also claimed expert status through embodied knowledge, presenting their personal experience of AIDS as providing a basis for authority (63). Activists developed a thoroughgoing critique of AIDS discourse, including basic research, clinical trials, treatment protocols, health communication, and media representations. Regarding media representations, activists developed strategies for critiquing extensive mainstream media coverage of AIDS, sending their press releases and statements to reporters and developing newsletters and other venues for circulating critical and alternative perspectives (202). Even as they sought to claim positionalities within biomedical AIDS biocommunicability, they went much further: as Epstein traces, activists claimed some degree of control over it and thus the ability to help shape its content, how knowledge circulated, and how particular perspectives gained credibility. Their program for what Epstein refers to as the democ-ratization of knowledge production confronted standard participation struc-tures and their hierarchical organization: they went beyond claiming expert status to question the expert-layperson binary itself (3).[2]

Through a range of strategies that included making alliances with dis-sident scientists who were themselves deemed incommunicable, creating grassroots archives regarding clinical trials, demanding research on issues and treatments excluded from hegemonic biocommunicable channels, and conducting "underground" drug trials, activists went on to multiply AIDS communicabilities, shape their intersections, and contest biocommunicable authority. Countering mainstream public health campaigns and their roots in stigmatizing views of gay sexuality, grassroots AIDS organizations drew on emerging evidence regarding sexual transmission and the effectiveness of condoms in challenging assertions that AIDS prevention required monog-amy. They instead counseled that sex, pleasure, and multiple partners were perfectly viable as long as HIV-prevention guidelines were followed (Epstein 1996, 96–97).

Epstein went on to analyze how AIDS activism led to important changes in science, clinical trials, medical practice, doctor-patient interaction, and who can make claims to possess and contribute scientific knowledge. Nev-ertheless, he stressed that the story he was telling was not a romantic tale of resistance. Gay activists' ability to convert stigmatizing incommunicable status into forceful roles within biocommunicability drew on their status as white, largely middle-class men; he notes that efforts by women and com-munities of color faced more uphill battles (Epstein 1997). Critical engage-ment, moreover, did not displace dependence on scientists and clinicians for lifesaving treatments. Ultimately, challenging professional monopolies on knowledge production and asserting the ability to evaluate scientific cred-ibility came at the cost of adopting more conventional, positivistic under-standings of science (232–34).

A final example, provided by Alondra Nelson's exemplary *Body and Soul: The Black Panther Party and the Fight against Medical Discrimination* (2011), similarly examines how health communication can be transformed when it emerges organically from within social movements. The Black Panther Party's creation of no-cost community-based clinics and free breakfast programs for children provides a model that I call *integrative critical transformation*. Like the AIDS activism that Epstein describes, the Panthers advanced a thoroughgo-ing critique of biomedicine, challenged the expert-versus-layperson binary, and emphasized lay experiences of illness as a central basis for participation in the production and dissemination of health knowledge. Rather than focusing on a single nosological category, the Panthers' revolutionary health program embraced a wide range of health, social, and political-economic issues.

The Panthers' health program was rooted in their broader ideological and political project, informed by intense collective readings of the work of Mao Zedong, "Che" Guevara, and Frantz Fanon. The Panthers drew in particular on *The Wretched of the Earth*, cited by the Panther member Eldridge Cleaver as "the Black bible" (quoted in Nelson 2011, 67). They used Fanon's analysis of how colonial medicine formed a tool for racialization, oppression, and control in Algeria to advance an "analogous critique of the U.S. medical–industrial system as an instrument of social control" (67). The Panthers similarly followed Fanon in using diagnosis not simply as a means of identifying pathologies in individual bodies but as broader forms of political diagnosis, identifying the structural roots of illness and how these factors escape the medical gaze. Nelson credits the Panthers with developing a "social health" perspective that linked health and social justice across scales through a Marxist-Leninist critique of capitalist medicine while drawing simultaneously on a long history of Black efforts to provide health services.

The Panthers recruited health professionals to work in their clinics, including Black professionals and others who shared leftist and justice-oriented perspectives. They drew on this specialized knowledge for providing clinical and laboratory services and teaching Panthers, staff, volunteers, and community members about diagnosis and treatment. Here biocommunicability was extended in such a way as to challenge hierarchically organized roles and forms of professional boundary work. At the same time, the Panthers' goal of challenging biomedical authority and integrating health care into a broader revolutionary program led to the requirement that physicians and other health professionals participate in their political education, including studying Fanon, Mao, and Guevara. In other words, the Panthers incorporated biocommunicability, but only after they had stripped it of unilinear, hierarchically organized, and capitalist underpinnings. Moreover, this transformation included the demand that everyone entering the space of the clinic—including health professionals, Panthers, volunteers, and patients—be considered collaborators in producing forms of knowledge. The Panthers and their collaborators drew on visits to China and Cuba to open additional communicable channels, including those associated with acupuncture and other nonbiomedical forms of healing.

The Panthers liberated health communication from unilinear, hierarchical forms and an instrumentalist focus on changing patients' understandings and behavior. Jumping scales, health communication, like prevention and treatment, became a crucial means of confronting racial, class, and gender inequities and contributing to revolutionary transformation and justice. Beyond exchanges in the clinics, the Panthers' health communication strategies extended to their newspaper, other leftist media, and interactions with journalists reporting for local and national newspapers and television channels (Rhodes 2007), as well as presentations in churches, homes, parks, and elsewhere (Nelson 2011, 6). In short, they both appropriated dominant communicable circuits and built their own. Inside and outside the clinic, health issues were de-medicalized. "Patient advocates" assisted with housing, legal, economic, and other needs. They urged patients to demand greater agency in shaping the care they received and to take active roles in questioning doctors and challenging clinicians who were condescending or disrespectful (88).

The Panthers' focus on sickle cell anemia provides a fascinating example. As researchers and policy makers largely overlooked the disease and its tremendous impact on Black communities, the Panthers launched a massive program of screening, health communication, and advocacy, resulting in greater funding and mainstream attention. They reframed sickle cell as part of a campaign of genocide against Black people that included inadequate and discriminatory health care, reproductive violence, medical experimentation, police violence, unequal housing, the massive availability of illegal drugs in predominantly Black neighborhoods, and the small and large injuries of racism. Even as engagement with genetic and other scientific evidence on sickle cell partly medicalized their approach, the Panthers attacked interpretations of the disease as evidence of Black biological inferiority and cast it "as a somatic sign of the fortitude of slave descendants" (Nelson 2011, 135).

Even as the Panthers' health program resonated with those of other social movement-based organizations, they made a trenchant and unique contribution to transforming the place of biocommunicability in health communication and in clinical practice. As I discussed in chapter 5, evidence shows that physicians sometimes profile Black (and Latinx) patients as ipso facto incommunicable—as less likely to understand what their physicians tell them, change their conceptions of disease and treatment, and enact recommended behavioral changes (Smedley, Stith, and Nelson 2003; Van Ryn and Burke 2000). The Panthers, in essence, created incommunicability-free zones. They expelled health professionals who engaged in the sort of hierarchical and denigrating patterns of interaction with patients identified by Fanon. Even as experiences of illness and oppression on the part of Black and poor patients became a major source of insight for transforming care and communication, the Panthers embraced biocommunicability and medical treatment—once they had radically democratized them.

The examples compiled in this interlude illustrate what Barbara Tomlinson and George Lipsitz (2019, 13) call spaces of "insubordination," where oppressed people "turn many of the tools used to subordinate them into technologies for liberation." The authors argue that the "acts of improvisation and accompaniment" that emerge in such spaces "fuel the creation of new social relations and new social realities" (14). I have argued in preceding chapters that biomedicine—sometimes unwittingly and against its practitioners' foundational convictions—plays a crucial role in fashioning spaces of oppression through the production of incommunicability. This interlude has traced just a few of the ways that people who get stigmatized as incommunicable or find themselves descending into incommunicability turn their experiences and ways of sharing it with others into practices of improvisation and accompaniment. The Panthers' contributions to exposing the central role that health inequities play in anti-Black racism also demonstrated how crafting incommunicability-free zones forms a crucial step in transforming health into a central locus for achieving justice. Through an examination of the COVID-19 pandemic in the United States, the following two chapters seek to demonstrate that everyone, including health professionals, will live healthier lives if we join each other in demanding that all of us live in incommunicability-free zones.

PART III

*Communicable Contours of the
COVID-19 Pandemic*

7

PANDEMIC ECOLOGIES OF KNOWLEDGE

In Defense of COVID-19 Conspiracy Theories, Sort Of

The phrase "COVID-19 is 'the big one'" served as the leitmotif of the pandemic-industrial-complex assemblage of scientists, military planners, security experts, public health officials, politicians, journalists, and writers and producers of germ-thriller movies and books. They warned for decades about the "threat" of widespread death caused by a bioterrorist attack or a novel virus (Caduff 2015; Lakoff 2017). And lo and behold, a form of the SARS virus has caused nearly seven million officially reported deaths worldwide and upended healthcare systems, economies, schools, and lives. The US Centers for Disease Control and Prevention (CDC) massively funded training courses and "exercises" or "scenarios" in which the actors mentioned earlier (except popular culture producers) practiced using its principles of "emergency and crisis risk communication" in carefully orchestrated coproductions of discourse for lay publics. The H1N1 ("swine flu") pandemic of 2009 proved to be the graduation exercise, and most journalists and public health officials gave one another high marks. The H1N1 virus itself was the spoiler, refusing to cause the scale of death and severe illness envisioned in pandemic-industrial-complex imaginaries. By contrast, COVID-19 is the big one for both sides of the biocommunicability equation: the circulation of discourse and of pathogens. After declaring COVID-19 a pandemic, the World Health Organization (WHO 2020) declared an associated "infodemic," which it defined as "an overabundance of information, both online and offline," specifying that it included both "mis- and disinformation" that constituted "deliberate attempts to disseminate wrong information to undermine the public health response and advance alternative agendas of groups or individuals."

Nevertheless, even as the COVID-19 pandemic resulted in perhaps the most massive circulation of discourse and viruses in world history, there seems to be broad agreement in the United States that the pandemic-discourse-production assembly line failed. A significant minority of US residents rejected official COVID-19 discourse, along with masks, social distancing, and vaccines. Most explanations map a political opposition between "conservatives" and "liberals" onto an opposition between "anti-vaxxers" versus people who take the disease and its mitigation seriously, articulated early in the pandemic through a moralized binary between such categories as "lockdown warriors" versus "superspreaders" (Caduff 2020, 478). Nevertheless, even many people who took public health warnings seriously later began tuning out reports of possible surges of new variants and warnings about the need to enact health officials' recommendations (Qu, Saffer, and Austin 2023), often claiming "pandemic fatigue." A standard charge—presented by people classified as belonging to both camps—is that the pandemic was disastrously "politicized." Two scapegoats continue to hold preeminent rhetorical value. Many who identify with former president Donald Trump denounced Dr. Anthony Fauci, director of the National Institutes of Health's National Institute of Allergy and Infectious Diseases, as authoritarian and as displaying so much inconsistency as to rank him, as one of my interviewees put it, somewhere between incompetent and "a clown." Trump opponents equally viscerally blamed the former president's proclamations for prompting the rejection of public health measures; mistrust of doctors and scientists; and the highest reported rates of infection, hospitalization, and death worldwide.

In keeping with the notion of the infodemic, a common mode of explaining what went wrong was pointing to the internet and, particularly, social media, given COVID-19's status as "the first pandemic of the social media age" (Viswanath, Lee, and Pinnamaneni 2020, 1744). K. Viswanath and his colleagues suggest that "the extensive global penetration of social media provided a fertile ground for the spread of information, misinformation, and disinformation. Information on COVID-19 has spread unhindered at a great speed with limited gatekeeping from usual filters such as editors, advocates, and interest groups." They conclude that "social media have contributed to the *spiral of amplification*" of mis- and disinformation (1744, emphasis in original). Such projections often conflate the vast, complex pragmatics of contemporary biomediatization with the ideological work undertaken using biocommunicable models. Luc Berlivet and Ilana Löwry (2020, 533) examine this relationship by suggesting that "'biocommunicable cartographies' (Briggs and Hallin 2016) have become even more intricate since Charles Briggs and Daniel Hallin started to lay out the concept of 'biocommunicability,' 10 or 12 years ago." Public health professionals, particularly those most deeply identified with the pandemic-industrial-complex assemblage, often complained that their years of planning did not enable their voices to shape discourse about COVID-19. In an interview published by her alma mater, the Yale School of Public Health, Rebecca Katz, a COVID-19 adviser to President Joe Biden, suggests, "Maybe the important lesson is that we need to yell louder and make sure that we are collectively heard when we talk about the importance of preparedness" (quoted in Mendenhall 2022, 244). My analysis suggests that more insistence on pandemic biocommunicability may not be the answer.

The preceding chapters open up different analytical strategies for thinking about why COVID-19 has had particularly catastrophic effects in the United States. Rather than accepting the pandemic as "the imaginary of an unprecedented event" (Kelly 2018), seeing it as a repeat of nineteenth- to twentieth-century pandemics, or as just another effect of neoliberalism, I would argue that the roots of what is taking place go back several hundred years—to our physician-philosopher John Locke. Epidemics and pandemics have—especially after they came to be characterized in the nineteenth century as caused by infectious microbes—formed influential sites for reifying in/communicable models in ways that define the positionality of states, elites, and subaltern populations. In this chapter and the next, I explore how the viral trajectory of COVID-19 in the United States emerged from a clash of two dominant communicable models and one that presses against them from the margins. They are the unilinear, hierarchically structured biomedical-authority model that provides a key infrastructure for the pandemic-industrial-complex; patient-consumer communicability, which projects laypeople as agentive, self-interested individual consumers of health knowledge and care; and lay-activist communicability, where patients claim active roles in evaluating and producing biomedical knowledge.

I argue that demands by public health professionals that laypeople temporarily surrender claims based on patient-consumer and lay-activist communicability and fully embrace the passive, trusting position that sustains the biomedical-authority model of biocommunicability jeopardized the viability of COVID-19 public health discourse. The effects of this clash of biocommunicable models in the pandemic were exacerbated by how they had become racialized. I further suggest that analysts need to broaden their categories of knowledge and care to appreciate the complex and contradictory relations between what I term *pandemic ecologies of knowledge* and *pandemic ecologies of care*, which, respectively, form the foci of this chapter and the next. In this chapter, I use the notion of pandemic ecologies of knowledge to shift the discourse beyond a narrow focus on COVID-19 biocommunicability, meaning assessments of who grasps biomedical and public health discourse about COVID-19 discourse, who has failed to assimilate it, and who has rejected it. I examine a broad range of efforts by laypeople to contribute to knowledge about the pandemic, as well as how most people—including many health professionals—experienced a descent into incommunicability. I analyze how the prolonged experience of incommunicability pushed some to reject dominant COVID-19 perspectives, practices, and technologies; others to quit professions (from health care to teaching to trades); and still others to inhabit COVID-19 incommunicabilities in critical and transformative ways. I thus use the term *pandemic ecologies of knowledge* to help bring positionalities that are generally seen as diametric opposites into dialogue.

The stakes for getting a better hold on COVID in/communicabilities are, I think, high. Beyond the differential impact of the circulation of SARS-CoV-2 and mitigation measures on different populations and how "vaccine refusal" continues to affect epidemiological patterns, the effects of COVID in/communicabilities have resulted in deep and acrimonious social divisions. These rifts fracture families and worksites as much as electorates. Clara Han (2012) argues that researchers must become attuned to the singularity of lives to grasp how precarity gets woven into the fabric of people's experience. To press beyond vast pronouncements about "the pandemic" or broad categories of people it has affected (such as "essential workers," "Trump supporters," physicians, nurses, and laypeople), I draw on my interviews in these two chapters to look closely at specific people's experience and at parallels and contrasts between them. Dissecting COVID in/communicabilities can, I suggest, help us understand these toxic politics more deeply and imagine better futures.

Pandemic Ecologies of Knowledge

As Michel Foucault famously taught us, producing knowledge creates what is projected as nonknowledge (Geissler 2013), casting other ways of knowing as ignorance, superstition, and the like. Scientific and medical professionals conduct what Thomas Gieryn (1983) calls "boundary-work," efforts to police the borders that demarcate scientific and other approaches and practices. Unlike perspectives framed as religious, economic, or political that assert no relation to science, discourse produced by people who are not scientific or medical professionals that either claims to add to or criticize scientific and medical formulations can turn boundary-work into moral indignation, anger, or ridicule from scientists. Here, the use of the most reductionist and denigrating labels—conspiracy theories and misinformation—indicates strong negative assessments. A vital premise of the CDC's manual *Crisis and Emergency Risk Communication: Pandemic Influenza* is that a pandemic "will generate immediate, intense, and sustained demand for information from the public, healthcare providers, policy makers, and news media" (CDC [2006] 2007, 5). A central goal of the manual, not surprisingly, is to maximize biocommunicability: to provide principles for translating biomedical "information" about a pandemic into popular registers, circulate it as widely as possible, and induce "the public" to assimilate it and enact designated "attitudes" and "behaviors." A second goal is to detect "rumors" or "misinformation." According to the CDC, a critical mistake would be to "leav[e] myths, rumors, and doomsayers unchallenged or corrected" (2002, 11). Pandemics, in short, imbue remarkable regimens of discursive control with not only state legitimacy but also moral and medical force, demanding that professionals and laypeople alike foster the circulation of discourse embraced by biocommunicability and actively repress alternative forms, especially those that actively contest it. The COVID-19 "ordinary ethics" (Das 2015; Keane 2016; Lambek 2015) that required a constant ethical praxis of calculating space, intimacy, and viral contagion everywhere beyond seemingly safe "bubbles" or "pods" (Trnka 2021) also required an ordinary ethics of discursive surveillance, classification, and passive assimilation or overt suppression.

In other words, Locke's teleology is alive and well here: perfect pandemic biocommunicability is required, first, to disseminate what counts as knowledge and, second, to stamp out incommunicability, defined as the circulation of discourse generated outside the pandemic-industrial complex as well as laypeople's failure to assimilate pandemic biocommunicability. Massive efforts to identify and counter "misinformation" and "disinformation" suggest

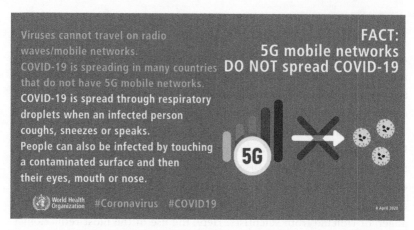

FIGURE 7.1. World Health Organization, Mythbusters, slide on 5G conspiracy theory

that what is framed as "information" is not neutral, autonomous, or apolitical but is constantly relationally constructed as a projection of its nefarious opposites. Again harking back to Locke, a third feature of pandemic biocommunicability is the need to manage problematic "public" emotions, which "range from terror and shock to blame, anger, and guilt." Using the CDC guidelines can restore "a sense of control . . . by modeling optimistic behavior" (CDC [2006] 2007, 8). As projected in biocommunicable formulations, the incommunicable trajectory leads from misinformation to mistaken beliefs to wild emotions to behavior that jeopardizes public health. In short, conspiracy theories, myths, and misinformation can be at least as dangerous as pathogens. Just as the circulation of public health discourse is projected as inversely correlated with the circulation of SARS-CoV-2 viruses, a direct viral-discursive correlation links the movement of misinformation with viral transmission.

What sites and forms of ideological labor produce oppositions between COVID biocommunicability and incommunicability? Here we might look to the WHO. After declaring an infodemic, WHO created a "COVID-19 Mythbusters" website that offers downloadable slides that position each "myth" on one side and medico-scientific knowledge meant to counteract it on the other.[1] Figure 7.1 focuses on a widely disseminated "conspiracy theory": the assertion that the pandemic emanated, literally, from 5G mobile networks.

This seemingly simple slide performs a great deal of ideological labor aimed at creating a binary between biocommunicability and incommunicability. First, it reduces complex, heterogeneous, shifting, globally distributed discourse networks and practices to what is framed as their essential refer-

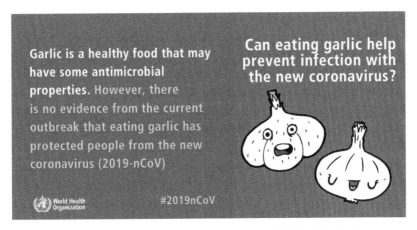

Garlic is a healthy food that may have some antimicrobial properties. However, there is no evidence from the current outbreak that eating garlic has protected people from the new coronavirus (2019-nCoV)

Can eating garlic help prevent infection with the new coronavirus?

World Health Organization

#2019nCoV

FIGURE 7.2. World Health Organization, Mythbusters, slide of garlic talking heads

ential content. "Myths" are often presupposed in the WHO slides, projecting that audiences are already familiar with them and, perhaps, a fear of iteration (Derrida ([1977] 1988), the idea that repeating these assertions might inadvertently help them circulate. The infantilization of viruses and circulation routes in these graphic representations, which share the space of "myths" in the drawings, is much more pronounced in some slides, such as in the anthropomorphized (and sexualized) garlic heads in figure 7.2. Here we see a reflection of the process of stigmatization and infantilization pinpointed by Frantz Fanon (see chapter 3), where the graphic features of the "myths" seem to echo projections of a similar lack of sophistication on the part of people who purportedly embrace them, contrasted with the Lockean rationality and scientific status of the text on the left. Research on "conspiracy theories" related to COVID-19 and people who circulate them suggests that this simplistic mode of representation gets things wrong. Elisa Sobo and Elżbieta Drażkiewicz (2021, 70) note that they "are fluid networks of ideas," adding that "what appears as one conspiracy theory on the surface may contain several versions of something proximally the same, but different in terms of the ends desired and the lifestyles represented" (82). Based on years of research on previous social movements centered on vaccine rejection, these authors importantly show that COVID-19 "anti-vaxxers" (who often reject this label) come from a wide range of social classes and political and ideological affiliations. Thus, WHO's simplistic representations of "myths" and their purveyors are very unlikely to interpellate those who circulate them.

The Mythbusters slide's binary between scientific biocommunicability and mythic incommunicability separates seemingly purely communicative phenomena ("misinformation") from scientific and medical knowledge. Nevertheless, the slide's ideological labor simultaneously undermines the medical versus communicative opposition, suggesting that biocommunicable discourse is directly tied to biology and projecting that the "infodemic" shapes epidemiological patterns by augmenting the virus's circulation. Even as it projects ideologies of science and communication, the slide illustrates how in/communicable models attempt to regiment the pragmatics of discourse, often in equally simplistic ways. Stopping the "infodemic"—and thus slowing the pandemic—apparently requires pairing specific examples of knowledge and ignorance. Once laypeople learn the "facts," they will stop circulating "myths" and perhaps even actively challenge them. In short, we return to the Lockean politics of knowledge and in/communicability that has helped increase inequities for more than three hundred years. As Sobo and Drażkiewicz (2021, 72) suggest, "debunking" is ineffective as a strategy for rewiring lay communicabilities.

Mythbusters and other simplistic biocommunicable representations of scientific discourse contradict fundamental principles of how science evolves—and are particularly at odds with scientific and medical work on COVID-19. Science offers complex processes for producing, contesting, and reformulating evidence and interpretation rather than simple pronouncements like those projected by Mythbusters. The SARS-CoV-2 virus is very tricky, and it has constantly challenged efforts by clinicians, laboratory scientists, and public health professionals to represent, as much as control, it. In other words, the WHO slides mythologize COVID-19 science as much as popular discourse. The organization itself was "suffering from a crisis of reputation affected by the contradictory messages during the initial phase of the pandemic" (Entradas 2022, 7). Moreover, social media bashing by WHO and other public health agencies might well be seen as disingenuous, given that WHO and many national health ministries partnered with Facebook and Google to become hubs for authoritative COVID-19 discourse. Beyond all of these parties' stated goals of enhancing biocommunicability and countering "misinformation," Earvin Cabalquinto and Tanja Ahlin (2021) suggest, these alliances helped burnish the often tarnished reputations of these social media giants and boost their profits during the pandemic.

For readers who lived through the pandemic, I hardly need to recite the fundamental shifts in scientific, medical, and public health knowledge about SARS-CoV-2 and COVID-19. A key question—how it is transmitted—moved from a concern with surfaces and droplets emitted through coughs and sneezes to generalized aerosolized transmission in indoor spaces. Many questions emerged: Does COVID-19 endanger only particular age groups and people with specific underlying conditions? Can previously healthy people, even young people, need hospitalization and even die? If children and youths only get asymptomatic or very "mild" infections, why did significant numbers end up in hospitals? After full COVID-19 vaccination was touted as protecting all but a small fraction from infection, "vaccination breakthrough cases" became common. Can fully vaccinated individuals transmit the virus? How long does COVID-19 infection or vaccine provide protection? Tying biocommunicability to a totalizing chronotope of SARS-CoV-2 gave way to concern with the fractured chronotopes of new variants: B.1.1.7 from the United Kingdom; B.1.351, first identified by scientists in South Africa; B.1.617.2 (known as delta) in India; omicron or B.1.1.529, also first identified in South Africa; and now BA.2, BA.2.12.1, BA.4, and BA.5.

The scientific penumbra of post-acute sequelae of COVID-19 (PASC), more commonly known as long COVID, entered the heart of scientific and medical uncertainty about COVID-19. Some scientists and physicians treated long COVID skeptically, attributing it to nonphysiological origins; others deemed it to be the product of mental illness (Phillips and Williams 2021). Another group of researchers and clinicians mapped the complex and extensive ways SARS-CoV-2 affects multiple organ systems after the acute infectious period ends.[2] What are its symptoms? Are any treatments effective? Should the Occupational Safety and Health Administration require employers and workmen's compensation plans to cover long-term disability resulting from job-related COVID-19 infections? Is it a temporary problem, or might PASC affect the labor market and increase healthcare needs for decades? As Carlo Caduff (2020) argues, public health measures—particularly the lockdown approach that heightened social inequities—were often based on scanty scientific evidence and false assumptions. Public health professionals counter that pandemics require rapid responses: waiting for systematic evidence would further endanger lives. When asked to reflect on whether the emergency communication strategy for H1N1 had been *too* successful, given that the virus had much less impact than initially suspected, Richard Besser, then the interim director of the CDC, responded, "You only have one chance to get out ahead of a new outbreak. You have to hit it hard, hit it early, and then you can back off."[3]

Time—like space, population, and nosological categories of disease—is part of the epidemiological infrastructure that afforded the statistical pandemic imaginary unfolding daily on the "dashboards" of local, state, and national public health offices; WHO and other international public health organizations; leading media outlets; and the Johns Hopkins University Coronavirus Resource

Center. One of the most frequently recurring sources of disenchantment for interviewees from all political and viral persuasions was chronotopic: how linear temporalities projected early in the pandemic gave way to cyclicities and feelings of spatiotemporal dislocation. Classes from kindergarten through high school would be suspended for only two weeks, which turned into a year for many students. A dominant chronotope suggested that lockdowns would "flatten the curve." Many people accepted initial measures that seemed exaggerated due to the promise of the teleological horizon for all these temporalities: a return to "the normal." When "the normal" seemed almost visible on the horizon, along came a new variant with yet another "surge" and a new pandemic chronotope. Montana, which became a site of deep anger against masks and COVID-19 vaccines, imposed a statewide lockdown under a Democratic governor during an initial period in which only a tiny number of cases emerged. When hospitals later filled to overflowing, resulting in decisions to "ration care," many residents vehemently rejected masks and mandates. These temporalities, constantly reified by "unleashing a pandemic of scary charts with exponential curves" (Caduff 2020, 473), relied on what Caduff referred to as "a trust in the power of mathematical disease modeling" (471). As Hanna Garth (2021, 105) tellingly points out in a provocative discussion of how COVID-19 and Black Lives Matter protests intersected, temporal projections were both medicalized and highly selective: "While the COVID-19 pandemic fueled a political drive to 'flatten the curve' in Los Angeles, little effort has been made to flatten the curve of increasing inequities."

And then we come to what one interviewee, a university administrative assistant, described to me as "the yo-yo game." A skeptic of COVID-19 public health discourse and mitigation measures, she used this expression to criticize official recommendations that masks were not needed, followed by masking mandates, then lifting mask mandates, later suggesting that masks are not required for the vaccinated. The spatialization of interpersonal relations shifted with the "six feet" rule, as measured by a pair of skis or three vegetable or fruit crates. Floor signs in the San Diego Airport in June 2022 declared "one surfboard apart: Because the only wave we want to ride is at Sunset Cliffs." Here material measures of "social distancing" merged with mathematical modeling. Does "social distancing" apply everywhere or only indoors? Then we learn that you were exposed if you were three feet or less away indoors for fifteen minutes. What kind of test do you need? How long does it take for a positive result to show up? When can you trust a negative result? Do you need to quarantine for fourteen or ten or seven or five days? Do you need a negative test to be released from COVID-19 purgatory? Moreover, if most US residents are using over-the-counter antigen tests at home and not reporting positive results in 2022, what do COVID-19 statistics mean anymore?

Constant acrimonious exchanges among parties who accused one another of COVID incommunicability, along with skeptical, even parodic, revoicings of scientific, medical, and public health discourse, became part of the cultural fabric of US pandemic life. Conflations of categories and binary oppositions proliferate: scientific and medical knowledge versus conspiracy theories and misinformation is joined to anti-vaxxers versus lockdown warriors. A major problem with these logics is how the extensive, heterogeneous, and complex range of types of discourse produced outside of biomedical and public health professional sites got stuffed into a residual category of "conspiracy theories" and "misinformation."

From "Conspiracy Theories" to Illness Narratives and Collaborative Knowledge Making: Violating the Knowledge-Production Monopoly Mandate

The attempt to enforce a professional monopoly on knowledge production regarding COVID-19 faced a significant constraint in the United States: the decades-long movement from biomedical authority to patient-consumer communicability that I traced in the preceding chapter. Rather than projecting laypeople as passive recipients of biomedical information that health professionals deem essential for them to know, patient-consumer communicability pictures laypeople as self-interested individuals who seek out and consume health information related to their "risk factors" and their desire for bodily and mental wellbeing. The tremendous heterogeneity in the ranks of COVID-19 "anti-vaxxers" and the logics they deployed connected implicitly with the remarkable diversity evident in the history of patient-consumer communicability.[4] Thus, even as some of the roots of patient-consumer communicability lay in progressive and revolutionary social movements, they also included conservative, antistate forms of heightened individualism and the rejection of collectivist public health ideologies and efforts to shape thought and behavior as teleological requirements for individual and community health.

As Daniel Hallin and I emphasized, biomedical authority and patient-consumer forms of communicability do not form a neat binary. In *Making Health Public*, we examine how a health news story can weave complexly between the two (Briggs and Hallin 2016). Stories commonly start with discovery of a new drug and then moving to advise viewers or readers to determine whether individual "risk factors" or health conditions might suggest, in the words so often repeated in television commercials for pharmaceuticals, that *you should ask your doctor for advice about whether it might help you.* Moreover, demands for individual agency are not evenly distributed across health issues and medical fields. Individuals who vehemently reject biomedical authority in some areas—such as masking and COVID-19 vaccination—often happily become recipients of scientific and medical knowledge concerning other health issues (such as elective surgeries and life-threatening chronic conditions). The heterogeneity of the roots of patient-consumer communicability becomes apparent when one examines how particular "influencers"— including politicians, celebrities, media stars, and physicians and scientists with popular followings—promote the rise of patient-consumer communicability in domains formerly dominated by biocommunicability. These different routes toward embracing patient-consumer communicability affected how laypeople in the United States positioned themselves in relation to the COVID-19 pandemic.

Efforts to prompt laypeople to turn off patient-consumer communicability and become faithful passive receivers of authoritative biomedical and public health knowledge in pandemics were repeatedly tested by what many construed as pandemic false alarms, where H1N1 provided the most striking example. The prediction that "swine flu" would sicken and kill substantial numbers of US residents did not match what unfolded. Massive epidemics of avian bird flu, Middle East respiratory syndrome coronavirus (MERS-CoV), and Ebola did not take place in the United States. US audiences thus increasingly refused to surrender their preferred communicable model, particularly given that it had become for many a primary modality for performing the self. Prophesies of annihilation and "a culture of danger" (Caduff 2015, 5) associated with biosecurity infrastructures had fractured; more serious challenges to them were to emerge in the COVID-19 pandemic.

Although relatively few people have read the CDC's pandemic biocommunicability manual, it would be hard to live in the United States during a health "emergency" without becoming attuned to its textual, affective, and bodily features. As I noted earlier, public health; Homeland Security and elected officials; clinicians; journalists; and others were trained through CDC courses and manuals and well-funded "scenarios" or "exercises" to use a single set of metapragmatic principles in producing discourse for media sources and mass audiences in times of pandemics. A checklist titled "Basic Tenets of Emergency Risk Communication" in the CDC manual includes:

- Don't over reassure.
- Acknowledge uncertainty.
- Express that a process is in place to learn more.
- Give anticipatory guidance [regarding possible negative outcomes].
- Acknowledge people's fears.
- Express wishes. "I wish we knew more." ([2006] 2007, 15)

The guidelines attempt to metapragmatically regiment (Silverstein 1993) not only the referential content of discourse but also questions of "tone" and the display of emotions that shape affective projections of identification with lay audiences. Richard Besser, who was the CDC's interim director during the beginning of the H1N1 pandemic, constructed health communication, like medicine and public health, as ideally evidence-based, as a linear process in which publics are constructed for statistically verified knowledge already existing in specialized biomedical domains.[5] The process aims at shaping and standardizing performances by trained and rehearsed "spokespeople," other (including potentially dissident) public health professionals, scientists, clinicians, politicians, and journalists. The goal is to train this diverse set of actors to use a common set of metapragmatic principles, often embodied in recurring phrases, resulting in a process that Briggs and Hallin (2016) call biomediatization, the coproduction of public discourse by integrating diverse professional logics, personnel, and sites. The CDC manual identifies "bad communication practices that contribute to a poor public response":

Mixed messages from multiple experts, . . . messages that are over-reassuring, recommendations to the public without a reality check, leaving myths, rumors, and doomsayers unchallenged or corrected, spokespersons who engage in improper behavior, exhibit a lack of affect, or use inappropriate humor, public power struggles and confusion. (2002, 11–12)

The CDC suggests that "the goal should be to produce an informed public that is involved, interested, reasonable, thoughtful, solution-oriented, and collaborative" (18).

Trump violated these principles systematically, fracturing the illusion that politicians would dutifully perform pandemic biocommunicability, as President Barack Obama had done in 2009. Trump offered a classic example of over-reassurance during a press conference on March 15, 2020: "Take it easy. Just relax. Relax. We're doing great. It all will pass." He displayed anger and defiance rather than establishing an affective relation of sympathy for seriously ill patients and the families of those who died. Trump proudly refused to wear a mask or practice "social distancing," shaking hands like never before. Trump highlighted the discrepancy between his pronouncements and those of the physicians on his Coronavirus Task Force, particularly Fauci.

Trump created a palimpsest of competing communicabilities almost daily as he either changed the script that had been prepared by his science/medical advisers or simply ad libbed at the podium. Trump's press conferences and tweets amplified statements promoted by just the sort of conservative media and political figures that WHO deemed to be promoting "mis- and disinformation." He rejected the authority of epidemiologists and the power of their statistics, again in concert with conservative media figures, both in initially downplaying the virus's pandemic potential, only to later declare, "This is a pandemic. . . . I felt it was a pandemic long before it was called a pandemic" (quoted in Rogers 2020). Trump declared that official counts of cases and deaths were exaggerated, even as CDC director Robert Redfield told reporters, "Our best estimate right now is that for every case that was reported, there actually were 10 other infections" (Aubrey 2020). During a campaign rally in Tulsa, Oklahoma, that violated social distancing guidelines, Trump proclaimed to supporters, "When you do testing to that extent, you're going to find more people, you're going to find more cases. . . . So I said to my people, 'Slow the testing down, please'" (quoted in Freking 2020). So much for relying on evidence-based public health.

In one of the most famous examples, Trump racialized SARS-CoV-2 by using "one of his signature Sharpies to cross out the word 'corona,' changing the phrase to 'Chinese virus'" in the script provided him for his daily coronavirus briefing, to the chagrin of infectious disease specialists standing next to him (Crowley, Wong, and Jakes 2020). He also referred to SARS-CoV-2 as the "kung flu." Facing "a growing chorus of criticism that [the term *Chinese virus*] is racist and anti-Chinese," reported Katie Rogers, Lara Jakes, and Ana Swanson (2020) for the *New York Times*, Trump countered, "It's not racist at all." He then explained his rationale: "'It comes from China, that's why.'" Trump went on to say that "he was attaching 'China' to the name of the virus to combat a disinformation campaign promoted by Beijing officials that the American military was the source of the outbreak," suggesting that the latter assertion could stigmatize the US military. Note the power of the "disinformation" label: Trump could reframe remarks that departed from the biocommunicable script given to him by his scientific advisers as legitimate by positioning his words as countering Chinese "disinformation."

Here linguistic anthropology can join with medical anthropology and history in analyzing the ideological labor performed by these statements. Jane Hill's foundational work suggests that linguistic racisms rely on implicit connections that enable words and phrases to indexically conjure racist lexicons and stereotypes with deep historical roots. "Yellow peril" discourses have been a prominent means in the United States of mustering anti-Asian, and specifically anti-Chinese, xenophobia (Espiritu 1992) and, frequently, of catalyzing hate crimes. Note that in World War II, US citizens of Japanese descent—but not of German or Italian heritage—were summarily rounded up and place in "relocation camps." As Natalia Molina (2006), Nayan Shah (2001), and other historians have documented, "yellow peril" discourses have projected what are classified as Asian bodies as potential sources of contamination for white people. Connections that are generally missed by studies of linguistic racism involve how health and language ideologies have been coproduced and how they have been transformed into such governmental apparatuses as zoning restrictions, health statistics, reports, and policies, and highly visible racialized quarantines during disease outbreaks. Labeling cholera in the nineteenth century "Asian cholera" or "Indian cholera"—similarly justified by claims that pandemics began in Asia—helped transform structures of colonial domination and exploitation into claims of the moral and biological inferiority of the colonized and justifications for repressive measures (Arnold 1993). Just as microbes travel, these colonial discourses followed migrants from colonies. During the pandemic, the nineteenth century reached into the twenty-first as anti-Chinese linguistic racism associated with COVID-19 helped catalyze a rise in anti-Asian hate crimes (Gover, Harper, and Langton 2020).

Mythbusters and other simplistic, hierarchically ordered and hierarchicalizing discourses are by no means the only ways that health professionals engaged laypeople during the pandemic. The approaches adopted by some local and county public health agencies were based on years of experience in listening to laypeople and clinicians and building relations of trust and cooperation. Substantial funding for health education, particularly as focused on building strong vaccination rates among racialized minority populations, was given to community-based organizations. Some of the most impressive were carried out by Native American health professionals and lay collaborators, including in places such as the Diné or Navajo Nation, which had some of the highest COVID-19 rates of infection in the United States. As a result, some Native American nations had vaccination rates that approached 100 percent.

In my interviews and observations, which clearly could not begin to chart this vast and still-emerging set of experiences, I often learned of nonwhite professionals who saw themselves as transmitters of biomedical and public health knowledge and yet avoided stereotyping their interlocutors as incommunicable. Interviews suggest that, in some cases, professionals engaged community leaders and activists not as producing knowledge about SARS-CoV-2 but in learning together about the challenges facing particular populations and figuring out how to collectively confront them. In these instances, communicable models were complex, less hierarchical, and more dialogic. As such publications as *The Long COVID Survival Guide* (Lowenstein 2022) suggest, long-hauler activists were able to recruit some physicians and scientists as partners in knowledge production and dissemination and in the development of treatment options. It would be difficult to summarize these results here, and the discussion would take me beyond the role of these chapters in adding more depth and substance to the incommunicability approach; I thus leave this task to future publications. I do want to suggest, however, that collaborative, community-based efforts to document communicable experiments that emerged in the pandemic would have a great deal to offer us in developing and implementing alternatives to dominant communicable models and associated practices.

Long COVID, or, How Patients Are Forced to Start from Scratch

Now it is time to slow things down, to move from charting broad features of COVID-19 landscapes to listening to the details, as seen from people's accounts of how they became dots on pandemic maps and numbers on dashboards. I start with myself.

I developed a broad range of COVID-19 symptoms in late March 2021, one month after being fully vaccinated. The message at the time was that the fully vaccinated had only a minimal risk of infection. A call to my physician's office resulted in a conversation only with the administrator, not a health professional, who assured me that it was doubtful that I had COVID-19. I must have the flu. (There were virtually no flu viruses circulating in the area that spring.) "Nevertheless, you should get tested," the administrator said. I did: negative. I was a classic vaccine-breakthrough case, but the term was not in public circulation then. It was not widely known that fully vaccinated symptomatic individuals often had viral loads that were low enough to produce a negative PCR test. For two weeks I was the sickest I had ever been, except for one nasty flu in graduate school. My symptoms, which resolved in a month, never entered the inflammatory phase and thus didn't require hospitalization. My COVID-19 symptoms forced me into incommunicability, trying to connect what SARS-CoV-2 was telling me and what I could—or couldn't—learn from health providers, journalists, websites, social media, friends, and relatives.

The demands for engagement in knowledge production forced on me by an early vaccine breakthrough infection were, however, dwarfed by what is required by people experiencing the complex and diverse symptoms of long COVID. I have learned a great deal about long COVID from people whose lives have been upended by its disabling effects. Those facing the symptoms of long COVID confronted a sparse, shifting, and perhaps begrudging ecology of biomedical knowledge. Just learning to live in a long COVID world requires participation in knowledge production that is perhaps as tiring as coping with the effects of cohabiting with SARS-CoV-2 and its effects on multiple organ systems, including the central nervous system. I turn to the testimony of Pato Hebert, who knows this world all too intimately.

Pato Hebert, Artist and Professor

I got what seemed like a fairly innocuous sore throat. Then I started feeling pretty substantial flu-like stuff. That started to seem a little bit like the symptoms I was seeing on the news. But as I hadn't traveled, I thought, "This is just a winter flu." I had a really, really bad cold in November 2019—I probably was on the edge of pneumonia—so I was comparing it with what I'd gone through then. I remember feeling "I'm pretty wiped out," and I could barely get up. By then I was starting to really wonder. And then within a week, I was having trouble breathing. By late April, I was long hauling.

Somebody I was with tested positive and had the courtesy and love to call me and tell me that, so then I had a mechanism for testing, because nobody could get tested at that point, at least in LA. I got a test on the second day they were available in the county, so I was one of the few people in that early wave who was able to get a test diagnosis. I realized quite quickly while trying to interface with health systems how vital having the positive diagnosis was. Even still, if I were at some point to need to apply for disability, [I would need] that diagnosis. Many other people in that first wave between March and May 2020 who never got a diagnosis were playing head games with themselves. It was really intense for them, and I didn't have to play the head game. I was like, "I know I had it." That gave me something, like, first of all, I knew that I'd been sick. And second of all, I knew as soon as I started comparing notes with what other people had, we came to understand ourselves as long-haulers. I had some science behind it. That was helpful. It was really, really helpful.

I tested on the twenty-fourth [of March], and I got the call [with the results] on the twenty-sixth or twenty-seventh. I told my closest friends and family that day. The next day, I went public. I think I did that for a couple of reasons. One is that I have an almost thirty-year history of HIV community and know how complicated the question of disclosing one's status is in HIV. I had a kind of framework and language for disclosure, as different as the two viruses are. I understood the importance of having been an HIV veteran of why people should document their own stories. I knew what it meant to train and support one another to be our own experts and advocates but also to access the care and expertise and health and support we need. I'll never know what my life with COVID would have been like without that. Also, there was so much misinformation circulating and so much denial and so much downplaying, particularly from the federal administration. There was just so much confusion and not knowing that I just felt like making it transparent. I wrote, "I'm doing this to make it grounded and to make it feel real." I was the first person that most people in my network knew, just because I was so early and I went public immediately. I didn't yet understand COVID. It was exhausting my own capacities to process information, and I'd be like, "Why am I so tired? I've only had three calls today, or I've only responded to thirty texts." And now I know, "Oh, yeah, yeah."

By late April, I was starting to write through social media posts that your corporeal compass can skew. I thought I understood what the body was doing, or saying, or teaching, or asking for, but I didn't always know how to hear, and I didn't understand what it was saying, because I was trying to go on previous experience. I was like, "Wait a minute. I've been in bed for three days," then needing midsentence to stop. "I cannot speak and I can't understand what you're saying." Or the physical version of that: "I have to lie down right now." Maybe if I'd had other experiences to draw on, but I had the ableist privilege of having a very healthy life. I was an athlete and mostly able-bodied to that point. I would have to take sleep whenever I could take it, whenever it would come. The fractured sleeps of two hours or three hours or four hours at night were horrific. Sleep had unfriended me, no matter how much NyQuil and melatonin I offered in seduction and supplication. One night I had taken NyQuil, knowing I needed to sleep, but my breathing was so tight that I couldn't. I was in a horrific clusterfuck where one part of my body was shutting down from the NyQuil and another part was forcing me to stay awake to try to get oxygen. I would say those are some of the four or five ways I was learning in the first month.

There were certain parts of my bodily symptoms that did get better, and then tons of shit would emerge. So for the first year, I did a typical ableist thing: "If I just do X, Y, Z, I get to go back to being able-bodied, right? If I rest more, if I hydrate better, if I take out the inflammatories from my diet, if I go see a neurologist. . . ." I stopped doing that. My angle isn't like this is somehow going to get better. And I have to pivot here to managing and to learning all kinds of language and skill sets that I don't have, like pacing, more familiarity with the practices and skills that folks with multiple sclerosis (MS), myalgic encephalomy-elitis / chronic fatigue syndrome (ME/CFS), or lupus have developed. The challenge I had was having to teach my people, my networks who weren't sick, that their ableism was not helpful for me. I don't need to be told about fucking positive thinking. I remember explicitly a family member saying, "You know, it's been over three weeks. This is quite concerning." And it was truthful and loving. Other people were unable to put me in the limited frameworks that the press was providing for us—or, frankly, the CDC. And it wasn't disbelief exactly. It was more fear and concern that I was hearing and feeling from people. But I was like, "I can't go up the stairs without losing my breath. So I'm not fucking making it up. This is real in this body. I may be an exception, but this is real." And then, because of the Body Politic Slack group and the Patient-Led Research Collaborative for long COVID, I was aware there's a ton of really smart politicized and very seriously ill people, some of whom were scientists and doctors themselves, and I was not alone.

When the gyms were shut down by public health, I needed a way to be in my body, so I started walking in Elysian Park. And I'm not a walker. I have tended not to like to walk because if I'm going to exercise or sweat, I want to swim or do something else. The walking became really great, and I was really grateful for it. I had just begun it as a week or two in practice when I got sick, and it turns out that the place where I got my test was in that same park. The park became really important.

Returning to that park, for a very short, slow walk was incredibly vital. I had been working super hard on the equivalent of two books coming to press at the same time. That got stopped before they came to light. But what I had was this thing called a smartphone. I was able-bodied enough to walk super slowly with limbs that kind of worked and lungs that were trying to find their way. And I was seeing detritus all through the park—these being the masks, people still had gloves on, people were still using wipes. Our human kind of imposition on the land was all over. Every fifty yards I might see a mask. And it became kind of like a Where's Waldo? game for me. I started documenting it because I was seeing it. It was a way to stay creative. I'm just always making pictures kind of compulsively, and I journal a lot for myself. Those two practices were really easy to put together, because they didn't require, you know, for instance, stretching canvas or getting paints ready or heavy lifting physically. They were scaled to what the body could do.

I feel like Alexandra Juhasz and I were in some ways doing the cultural production art side of things before very many other people were, a kind of real time COVID cultural production. I actually became more of a public-facing writer in COVID than I had ever been. I did have a lot of anxiety about whether it was art. I wasn't sure what I was doing. A lot of art spaces were not interested in it, and I didn't need that. Because of my community experience, plenty of other people were happy to have language and images circulating in their lives as ways to begin to process what was happening to us through this pandemic. It was really helpful because it was work that I thought was relevant to what I was trying to explore for myself. I learned a lot of new things and tools and places where I could work, but I also had to just keep it super-manageable. And there's a kind of modesty that's required of the process. Yet because I've been making work for years and years, I have, I guess, the practice and discipline to know what practice and discipline are, even as there's having to know what chronic illness pacing is.

Pato Hebert, in his own words, "is an artist, teacher and organizer" who "works across a range of media, including photography, installation, sculpture, language, light, temporality and graphic design."[6] Hebert, who uses his work to explore and effect interconnectedness, teaches in the Department of Art and Public Policy at New York University. In March 2020, Hebert found himself in the frightening and uncharted realm of early US COVID-19 cases.

As he tried "to be [his] own nerdy epidemiologist" in tracking both unfolding symptoms and how he might have been infected, he looked to the news media, material available from the CDC, and his prior experience as a patient with both previous influenzas and "a really, really bad cold" contracted the previous winter. It is, in part, Hebert's characteristic generosity that prompts him to interpret a call from a friend who had tested positive as an act of courtesy and love. An odd gift, the call enabled Hebert to obtain a positive COVID test, positioning him in a biocommunicable trajectory that provided him with a biomedical basis to frame his experience and assistance in requesting biomedical care. Like other people I interviewed who are deeply involved in HIV/AIDS worlds, he had a community-based framework for understanding testing, informing others that they had been exposed, and public disclosure of disease status that gave these actions a very different, very much more positive feel than most individuals who lack this experience.

Hebert's narrative could be characterized as a poetics of long-hauler in/communicability. Not only did he immediately inform his "closest friends and family," but he "went public" by launching a practice of journaling shared through social media posts, mostly on Instagram. "It did go into university and education worlds, and it did go into grassroots organizing worlds that were also global, because I had been doing global HIV for a long time," he said. "And it went into art worlds. There aren't many people who would have that weird particular mix. And so quite quickly reporters would find me." His words were designed to counter failures of official communicability and "so much misinformation circulating." His motivation captured a basic tenet of communicability: "just making it transparent." Nevertheless, his work did not reiterate biomedical discourse and public health guidance. Instead, it attempted "to make it grounded and to make it feel real" by charting his own embodied experience. Given that most people in his network had not yet felt symptoms or listened to other individuals who were experiencing them, he also designed his words to introduce others to intimate worlds of COVID-19 and appeal for the forms of care and love that would enable him and others to make it. His narrative unfolded heteroglossically in three ways simultaneously: as a dialogic text produced in the interview, as a parallel track to his social media journaling, and as a verbal layering of his visual art production.

The poetics of Hebert's narrative did not follow either biomedical authority communicability or the self-interested individualism of patient-consumer varieties. His response was, rather, shaped by the sorts of social movement logics I traced in the interlude, that he had gained through decades as an HIV community organizer and activist. As he found himself adrift in the uncharted waters of long COVID, Hebert transformed his body into a site for the production of knowledge that he could not find in media, biomedical, or public health sources. His public journaling framed it as collective knowledge, meant to reach out to others facing an unfamiliar world. Despite differences between HIV and SARS-CoV-2, AIDS and COVID-19, he placed the pandemic in the space of the commons that had been opened up by HIV lay-activist communicability. Making his journaling public reconnected him with City University of New York faculty member Alexandra Juhasz, with whom he had collaborated on HIV-related projects. The writing became a dialogue in which Hebert and Juhasz used a space of art and reflection to enfold discussions of symptoms and efforts to obtain biomedical care into a set of broader reflections on COVID-19 worlds as Hebert asked, "What is a COVID body? Who is a COVID person?" (Juhasz and Hebert 2021, 2). He wrote that "the virus and pandemic are at once abstract and visceral, everywhere and nowhere, immediate and endless. And, of course, isolation. Ghosting. Care that is essential and not enough. The limits of the human" (4).

Georges Canguilhem ([1966] 1978) argues that a prolonged illness imposes new forms of bodily experience that cannot be adequately grasped or described through forms of knowledge and articulation associated with preceding "normal" states (see chapter 4). Hebert went much farther, exploring "the limits of the human." Like those of other long-haulers, his efforts to obtain assistance from clinical professionals also involved a difficult process of confronting a lack of scientific knowledge about post-acute sequelae SARS-CoV2 infection. Some physicians doubted the existence of long COVID or attributed symptoms to other diseases or to mental illness, thus sealing off important sites for producing pandemic knowledge (Phillips and Williams 2021). Hebert reports that his first clinical encounter in an urgent care facility produced "pretty intense stigmatization and fear coming from the provider." Noting that he lacks overt linguistic and bodily markers of Latinx identity, he suggests that the issue was not racialized medical profiling but discomfort on the part of the health professionals he encountered in treating patients during the early days of the pandemic. Hebert joined forces with other social movement communities in redefining the positioning of laypeople in knowledge production, care, and disability.

Hebert initially tried to draw on his previous experience of being "an athlete and mostly able-bodied" to chart a linear trajectory toward a return to normality. He later reversed this projection by viewing his prior bodily experience as an ableist orientation that had left him devoid of the skills he needed to survive. Contra Canguilhem, his process of "learning all kinds of language and skill sets that I don't have" was collective. Even as he drew on HIV community organizing, he embraced "the practices and skills" already possessed by people with MS, ME/CFS, and lupus. Seeing that long COVID patients were facing similar uncertainties and roadblocks, a number of patient organizations opened their virtual doors to support long-haulers. Like so many other long-haulers, Hebert participated in online patient-activist collectives, particularly the Body Politic Slack support group and then the Patient-Led Research Collaborative for long COVID that grew out of it.[7] Like other patient-activist organizations (see Davis and Nichter 2016; Heath, Rapp, and Taussig 2004), the group worked with scientists, clinicians, medical associations, and public health agencies (including WHO and the CDC) to influence policies, provide patient-generated ideas for research, and fund work on long COVID. Hebert used a "loving" rather than a confrontational approach to teaching friends and family about the effects of imposing ableist perspectives on him with their naïve linear trajectories.[8]

Hebert's narrative opens up a fascinating dimension of lay participation in the production and circulation of knowledge about the pandemic. He was never hospitalized, and, unlike many freelance artists who depended on art galleries and exhibitions, he did not lose his income. Nevertheless, his mode of connecting to the world through artistic production suddenly vanished. Several major exhibitions and two books that were nearing publication suddenly went up in smoke. Carrying canvases or sculptures and focusing for extended periods on mixing and applying paint became impossible. He couldn't sustain his body through gyms and swimming pools. He thus found solace through walks in Los Angeles's Elysian Park, the city's oldest public park, which lies in the heart of the city. His immersion in the world of COVID-19 and his photographic vision began to converge there as he discovered pandemic landscapes as signs of biocommunicable engagement turned into "detritus" in the form of discarded gloves and masks. His long COVID body/mind became a Lévi-Straussian bricoleur, using the tools at hand—a cell phone—to find a way to make new interventions. The images he took during slow, gentle walks captured COVID worlds in fragments of park landscapes. He used inversions of color to capture "'how askew COVID makes us feel'" (Talmor 2022, 13). These ethereal images, including the image of an Elysian Park landscape with a suspended surgical mask that graces the cover of this book, convey the bewildering incommunicability experienced by long COVID patients and a communicable power to bring in viewers who lack this embodied knowledge.

Hebert thus found different ways to engage in producing knowledge about the pandemic, which he juxtaposed with the words he used to convey the world in which he and people around him were living. He observed a fallen eucalyptus limb in the park, dragging a limb home to carve. His uncle, artist Tom Henscheid, taught him to produce spoons, exploring a new subject and medium. Why spoons? Christine Miserando (2003) proposed "the spoon theory" to help people understand how daily tasks deplete energy for persons living with debilitating diseases—in her case, lupus. Each daily task, no matter how small, uses a portion of very limited energy, symbolized by a spoon. A series of carved spoons, each of which took twenty-five to forty hours to produce, gave a material form to his efforts to teach himself and those around him about the challenges posed by living in a long-hauler body/mind. He shared his remarkable ability to use art—words, images, and objects—to explore his COVID world in an exhibition in 2022 titled *Lingering* (Talmor 2022).

When we spoke in October 2022, Hebert suggested that some symptoms had improved even as sleep and neurological problems were worsening. Viral infections, including those caused by other corona viruses, can invade the central nervous system and damage nerve cells, possibly leading to autoimmunity disorders (Desforges et al. 2014). Amy Proal and Michael VanElzakker (2021) note that SARS-CoV-2 can linger in particular tissues after acute infection has ended, injure one or more organs, reactivate other neurotrophic pathogens, and interact with microbiome/virome communities. They propose that it can cause autoimmune problems due to molecular mimicry between pathogen and host proteins. Not only was none of this information available to Hebert in April 2020, but, as for many autoimmune and other poorly understood diseases, attempting to gain access to biomedical knowledge, diagnosis, and recognition was its own struggle. Even as new COVID-19 vaccines and medications continue to come online, treatments for the significant percentage of patients who develop COVID-19 post-acute sequelae symptoms—that is, millions of people in the United States alone—lag far behind (Bach 2022).

Learning to Listen to the "Anti-Vaxxers": Finding Fellow Travelers in Lay Knowledge Production

I would guess that many readers found Hebert's intervention inspiring, as it certainly is for me. Now I would like to introduce you to an individual who, for some, might inspire a much more distant reaction—perhaps even an angry one. In addition to interviewing journalists, physicians, nurses, public health officials, legal professionals, and others who largely trusted medical and public health discourse about COVID-19, I spoke with people who viewed pandemic biocommunicability with deep distrust. I conducted fieldwork in California counties where Trump flags were common and masks were rare. I have also interviewed San Francisco Bay Area residents working in classically "liberal" spaces who, often hesitantly at first, critically engaged biomedical and public health discourse about COVID-19. My learning curve was highest and most challenging during a month in rural Montana, an intense and acrimonious COVID-19 "battleground," in the words of one of my interlocutors. I interviewed ranchers, retirees, priests, ministers, doctors, dentists, journalists, hospital administrators, and others. Although I found a wide range of perspectives on COVID-19, many of the people I spent time with could be easily classified as quintessential exemplars of the looming figure of white, Trump-supporting "anti-maskers" and "anti-vaxxers," who were often blamed for filling hospitals and keeping COVID-19 infection rates high. This fieldwork took me beyond what provides the liberal comfort zone for most anthropologists (Açiksöz 2020; Mazzarella 2019).

In juxtaposing Hebert's testimony with that of my next interlocutor, Frank Miller, I make no attempt to achieve commensurability or to paper over the vast differences that separate them. I only ask for a bit of openness to consider how people who start from very different premises and end up in contrastive pandemic positionalities might assist us in destabilizing entrenched assumptions and sensibilities, thus helping us all figure out how COVID-19 has turned into boundaries that empathy, understanding, and researchers are seldom able to cross. I do not position Miller and other interlocutors classified as "Trump supporting anti-vaxxers" as exotic curiosities; nor do they simply provide me with just another element of the matrix of COVID-19 communicability. Instead, I see the challenge their words offer as particularly useful ways to bring into focus the implicit assumptions that inform my work on and relation to COVID-19, medicine, science, public health, media, and communicability and that of many other anthropologists, health professionals, journalists, and educators. In the end, listening to people who are Othered by the middle-class professional "narrating class" (Hubbs 2014) has much to teach us about biocommunicability and the production of incommunicability.

Frank Miller, Midsixties, Rural Montana

I started watching all the news. Very quickly, I stopped watching most of it, because whether you were watching ABC, CBS, NBC, or even the conservative news channels, all they're doing is putting down, contradicting, saying something different every night. So basically, pretty much I gave up on it. When I first heard about it, it sounded like typical politicians attacking the other party, saying, "This guy didn't do this. This guy will do this." Right off the get-go, it didn't seem like they were being honest about what was really going on. So when it first started out, I said, "Well, gosh—they know it's coming. Why don't they *do* something about it?" Basically they've made up stuff from day one. They don't really have the knowledge to have somebody get in front of a camera and say, "This is what we need to do; this is what you need to do to be safe," because they don't really know. And the conclusion that I come up with, why I think they don't know, is because they keep changing their mind. There's nothing scientific, in my opinion. You get the same guy who—everybody thinks he's a joke, that's Dr. Fauci—gets up and he says one thing one week and the next week it's an about-face. How can you believe that until they're ready to say what is real, leaving the politics out of it? I don't want to hear about how they say Trump caused it because he didn't do anything. It's just politics. Leave that part out. Let's get down to the scientific facts of what needs to be done.

Stop shoving medicines, pharmaceutical stuff, vaccines down people's throat until they make something up that they know is going to work. Don't use me as a guinea pig; don't use everybody else. But if they do want to do that, don't tell [people] they *have* to do it. Should be your choice. They can say, "I highly recommend it." Don't say, "We're going to fire you from your job if you don't get a vaccine, or we're not going to let your kid come to school." It's *our* choice. If I want to die, if that's what they think is going happen, that's my choice. No, I don't want to die. But I have a God that I trust more than a pharmaceutical company that is in business to do one thing: make money. And that's bottom line. That's what they're doing. My good friend Johnnie, they're saying he's going to lose a job because he's taking a stance on vaccination. I think he should back off just because of the consequences of it for his family, but I understand totally his stance. Don't tell him to do something, because it's not right. It's not. I think that if it were a law, he'd bitch about it till the cows come home, but he'd go do it. But it's not a law.

But don't shove your beliefs on me. If you want to wear a mask, if you feel comfortable, that's your business. My personal opinion? I think it's silly. I'm not a doctor. I haven't studied stuff like this. But I know how germs spread. Usually it's from saliva that comes out of your mouth or germs on your hands that you transmit by them touching what you touched. There's simple things you can do. You're going to wash your hands once in a while, [keep them] away from your face. You're going to cut your chances of spreading something to yourself just by being careful. Simple. Don't need a law for that. You've got to educate people, but you got to educate them with the correct information. That's the biggest problem.

It's no more dangerous than anything else we've had. And yes, I got sick. I was pretty down for a couple of weeks. You don't want to be sick and have to figure out what to do, because you got a gazillion different opinions of what to do. And I don't think the few things that they said were really important. I know, from past experience, number one thing when you're sick, you have to have rest, and you have to get a lot of fluids in you—way more than you really want to have. And that's pretty much how I dealt with it. I mean, you could ask my wife: there were some days I didn't do much. I'd get up and try to have my coffee and I'd feel maybe fair when I got out of bed, and within an hour or so I was just wiped out. I still have effects, but it didn't kill me. I don't think I have any respiratory issues from it, which I've heard that I could have got. But I was lucky, evidently. You know, it's probably just like flu. It was a different strain, and I didn't get all the bad effects, but I got enough sense to know that I was sicker than a dog. You didn't really hear on the news what your symptoms were. They just told everybody to go get tested: get in a cattle-line drive-through and have somebody that's never touched a syringe in their life poke you or stick a swab up your nose and then wait. I mean, how do you know? You don't know what they're doing with those swabs. When you walk away from it, you're done. You don't know whether you were positive or not positive.

I'm real careful about diving into conspiracy theories. When you first start reading, and until you really look into it, it sounds real convincing. I had a gal from our church, and she's very conspiracy theorist, I guess is a word. Sends a message—"You got to read this!"—and it's saying something that the senators voted one thing. And then you start listening to it and then it becomes radical. It's just fabricated. You can't believe it—and I didn't want to believe it. But, you know, there's some truth to it. What you hear, you have to trust that the person that's providing that to you is knowledgeable and has done their homework and verified the information they're giving you.

I spent many days and evenings with Miller and his wife, Linda, in October and November 2021. They hold similar political and religious orientations: white, evangelical Christian Trump supporters who reject masking, testing, and vaccination. Both were infected with COVID-19 in May 2021, probably at a church activity that led to the infection of many congregants and the death of one. When I observed these services the following October, I was the only person wearing a mask. You might, at first glance, take Miller's statements as a rant and, perhaps, as evidence of ignorance. However, I urge you to look more closely and consider how Miller positions himself along multiple in/communicable borderlines.

In the early days of the pandemic, Miller was open to biocommunicability, as is evident in how he increased and broadened his consumption of "mainstream" and conservative television news. Although he soon rejected medical and public health guidance on COVID-19, that did not amount to a complete disavowal of biocommunicability. Contra the stereotype that is so often touted for so-called anti-vaxxers and anti-maskers, Miller was not and did not become anti-science or anti-medicine. Indeed, he shares with most scientists and physicians a quintessentially Lockean view of biocommunicability. Public health and medical guidance, he suggests, should be based on evidence, resting solely on "scientific facts." This objective, again in Lockean fashion, should preexist communicative acts and be carefully, completely bounded off from "politics." Communication then becomes a straightforward, mechanical process of putting someone with "the knowledge . . . in front of a camera" to translate "scientific facts" into simple, clear, unequivocal guidelines. This is precisely what the CDC advises, even as it leaves more room for scientific uncertainty (on which, more later). Miller then embraces what is commonly referred to as "knowledge translation" in science and medicine: turning knowledge into actions, technologies, and materials that constitute "do[ing] something about it." He thus shares what John Ødemark and Eivind Engebretsen (2022, 2) critique as a reductionist view of notions of translation in medicine that "take translation and knowledge transmission as a phenomenon for granted, and accordingly downplay the complexity of translation as an entangled material, textual and cultural process." Precisely in line with the CDC's projections of lay reception, Miller emphasizes that pandemic biocommunicability rests on trust in and the credibility of spokespeople, suggesting that violating the "Great Divide" between science and politics (Latour [1991] 1993) led him to conclude that "there's nothing scientific" in mainstream discourse about COVID-19.

What was the basis of his assessment? Miller shares a widespread language ideology that identifies particular social roles with specific registers, seen as lexicons and speech styles that perfectly embody the particular status that individuals are claiming. Politicians are thus clearly distinguished from medical and public health professionals through their speech. When health officials purportedly "sounded like typical politicians attacking the other party," they lost scientific credibility for Miller. The binary opposition between these roles and registers also discredited political officials who brought COVID-19 discourse into political debates during a presidential election year; they betrayed public trust by politicizing science. I discuss later why Miller did not place Trump in this category. Note once again that the CDC's training for pandemic spokespeople lines up with Miller's construction, providing techniques for constructing a credible and trustworthy scientific persona by using a standardized "crisis and emergency risk communication" register by stressing "facts," the goal of performing actions to minimize suffering and death, avoiding contradictory "messages from multiple experts," and keeping power struggles and confusion out of laypeople's view.

Presenting a stable relationship among scientific, medical, and public health personas and registers faced a number of destabilizing forces. One was that Robert Redfield, the CDC's director at the beginning of the pandemic, was not a handsome, well-rehearsed, media-savvy person like Richard Besser. Another was that the Trump administration chose to strip the CDC of its role as the leading stage for disseminating pandemic discourse, positioning it in the quintessentially political arena of the White House. Further, as I noted, Trump not only refused to perform according to CDC metapragmatic guidelines but systematically violated them as he rewrote or simply dismissed scripts provided by the White House Coronavirus Task Force. But more structural factors were also at play.

First, Asif Agha (2005, 2006) greatly complicates this commonsense view of register. Rather than fixed relations between roles and speech forms, "enregisterment" involves reflexive processes that draw on "metapragmatic stereotypes" (2005, 46), even as communicative acts bring "entextualized figures" (41) into being, construct utterances that animate them, and align them in particular ways. Moreover, this process is shaped in each instance by entextualization (Bauman and Briggs 1990), the overall structure of formal discursive features, and by unfolding indexical orders. Enregisterment similarly is affected by processes of uptake, such as Miller's, in which interlocutors, viewers, or readers evaluate these constructions on the basis of their own social and linguistic repertoires and experiences and contexts of reception. In the process, "register models undergo various forms of revalorization, retypification, and change" (Agha 2005, 38). The year 2020 came after four years in which Trump systematically upended "metapragmatic stereotypes" of politicians—to the delight of his supporters and the horror of his opponents. Pandemic discourse also unfolded in the middle of an election year and in the midst of widespread antiracist protests over the publicly broadcast murders of Black people and violent white supremacist mobilizations. Relations between social categories and discursive constructions were particularly unlikely to be stable or neatly bounded at the time.

Second, although Miller did not and would not consult the "WHO Mythbusters" site, he shared the ideological construction of science that it projected. When health officials knew that COVID-19 was "coming," they should have had a clearly defined set of "scientific facts" in hand; refrained from revising or contradicting earlier formulations; and told people immediately that "this is what you need to do to be safe." A contradiction is thus evident in Miller's construction of the biocommunicable role of health professionals: even as he accuses scientists and physicians of arrogance, he also wants them to project perfect transparency and certitude. I am tempted to think about this response psychoanalytically as the desire for the good parent who can be trusted to provide a clear, reassuring answer in an extremely chaotic and anxious time. When scientists and health officials were judged to fall short of filling this role, the reaction was often not only distrust but rejection and anger.

Providing clear, reassuring answers, as I have emphasized, was impossible. Even the line between scientific "information" and "mis- or disinformation" was not static. Eivind Engebretsen and Mona Baker (2022, 30) reproduce a WHO tweet that contains a "FACT CHECK" slide similar to the Mythbusters image that asserts that "COVID-19 is NOT airborne. The virus that causes COVID-19 is mainly transmitted through droplets generated when an infected person coughs, sneezes, or speaks. These droplets are too heavy to hang in the air. They quickly fall on floors or surfaces." The slide suggests that people keep one meter of distance from others, disinfect surfaces frequently, and wash their hands regularly. The airborne status of SARS-CoV-2 soon shifted from being misinformation to a fundamental tenet of COVID-19 biocommunicability. The Mythbusters 5G slide that I analyzed earlier (figure 7.1) thus counters what is framed as misinformation with what the WHO later came to view as misinformation. I am not asserting, like Miller, that changing formulations and guidelines provide evidence of ignorance or prevarication. The problem is that ideologies of science that envision distanced, stable sets of scientific facts and formulas rather than the more dynamic, unstable, competitive relations among social actors, materials, technologies, modes of inscription, and interests documented by society-technology-society scholars (Latour 1987) were particularly ill equipped to prepare audiences of lay-people to grapple with efforts to sort out COVID-19.

Moreover, Miller's disenchantment with science and medicine reflected a shift in how evidence was disseminated and how the pandemic was biomedi-atized (Briggs and Hallin 2016), meaning how representations were jointly pro-duced by scientists, clinicians, journalists, and laypeople. Rather than follow-ing up on press releases that focused on articles published in the *Journal of the American Medical Association* or the *New England Journal of Medicine*, many stories reported studies that had not yet been peer-reviewed but, instead, had been posted online. Coverage of debates among scientists and health profes-sionals about COVID-19 was common. As K. Viswanath and his colleagues (2020, 1744) observe, "Science[,] as an enterprise, is usually conducted in rela-tive obscurity in the labs or the field but is now occurring under intense and constant public scrutiny." As Mark Nichter (personal communication with the author, 31 March 2023) suggested to me, we could frame these developments in a positive light as a democratization of science. Nevertheless, they ran afoul of how lay audiences interpreted biomedical-authority communicability.

The associations of social personas and registers against which Miller plot-ted his own relationship to COVID-19 did not lie exclusively with distant fig-ures of scientists, doctors, and politicians. Instead, they also lay with positions he attributed to friends and relatives. Miller placed his brother, who formerly worked in health care, as one pole on this map, as a passive lay receptor who parroted official COVID-19 biocommunicability.[9] The second positionality is that of his wife, who is deeply immersed in an evangelical worldview. She as-serts that COVID-19 is a smokescreen invented by the devil, whose servants—politicians, mainstream journalists, and health professionals—enacted mitiga-tion measures to carry out the devil's orders by using prevention measures to isolate people and fill them with anxiety, thus making them more susceptible to diabolic influence. Scrutinizing COVID-19 discourse has become a cen-tral part of a process of religious knowledge production in which she engages each Sunday, continuing daily as she uses her well-worn Bible to identify rel-evant details of pandemic debates and analyze them in locating hidden aspects of divine revelation. A third positionality is that of a fellow church member whom Miller classifies as "very conspiracy theorist," whose posts he judges to be "fabricated." John Bodner and his colleagues (2021) may well be correct in suggesting that religious beliefs may significantly increase people's suscepti-bility to "conspiracy theories." However, the differences between Frank and Linda Miller and the "conspiracy theorist" in their congregation suggest that causal arrows should be invoked here with caution. Finally, the last indicator on his map is taken by his closest friend, Johnnie Owen, who angrily accepted an economically disastrous early retirement as a maintenance worker at a California community college because he refused to get vaccinated. "I think he should back off," Mr. Miller suggested, "just because of the consequences of it" for his family's economic precarity.

Miller identified his own positionality in opposition to these four entextualized figures as he carved out a shifting space among them. He particularly contrasted his views with those of Owen: "He's radical about it, you know, and he's radical about a lot of things that have to do with politics." Frank Miller, whose "vaccine hesitancy" is connected with his fear of needles, constantly weighs evidence that might push him toward the complete rejection of vaccination embraced by his wife and Owen or toward the sense that he might someday decide to get vaccinated, as his brother frequently urges. With his wife, Owen, and the conspiratorial co-congregant, Frank Miller shares, in Sobo and Drażkiewicz's (2021, 73) words, "an emphasis on free thinking," "the sanctity of free choice," and a "distrust of authority," but it does not lead him to identify with their positions on COVID-19; nor has it induced him to trust YouTube videos by dissident scientists and physicians or social media posts. Miller's relationship to COVID-19 discourse and prevention and treatment measures thus follows from his reading of these four figures, each of which is defined by what he sees as a contrastive relationship to COVID-19 biocommunicability. With Mikhail Bakhtin (1981) we could say that Miller's voice is not isolated, monolithic, and simplistic, as is often projected for what are characterized as Trump-supporting anti-vaxxers, but is shot through with those of these four contrastive entextualized figures, as well as the COVID-19 biocommunicable discourses that he rejects.

Miller's rejection, like that of many others I spoke with, of masks and COVID-19 vaccines and his negative view of health professionals who promote them does not rub off on other areas of medicine. Miller had a knee replacement in February 2022, and after carefully weighing different treatment strategies in consultation with urologists, he chose to be operated on for prostate cancer. Herein lies a crucial difference: for patients with access to health insurance and sufficient resources to cover copays, such as Frank Miller, such procedures are framed—by doctors and patients—through patient-consumer communicability. There Miller is in the driver's seat, encouraged to explore "options" and make self-interested decisions.

Let me return to why Miller did not place Trump in the camp of politicians who politicized science. Miller instead identified with Trump's extension of patient-consumer communicability into a commonsense lay communicability.

As Miller reacted against both biomedical-authority pandemic biocommunicability and the entailed prohibition against laypeople relying on patient-consumer communicability, he saw Trump as a fellow traveler. Miller deemed a half century of reception of public health discourse and physicians' recommendations, along with his experiences as a patient, as having taught him "how germs spread" and the "simple things you can do" to prevent infections and provide self-care. Here we return to Eduardo Menéndez's analysis of *autoatención*, of the central role of lay efforts to prevent, detect, and treat health problems outside the purview of the clinic—and to decide when health professionals are needed. Miller, as I noted, is very attentive to issues of hygiene and quite observant of factors that affect health. His reliance on self-care and embrace of patient-consumer communicability led him to perform a speech act analysis on health professionals' pronouncements. Doctors who respect patient-consumer communicability are judged in positive terms as giving recommendations, but health professionals who insist on biomedical-authority communicability get classified as trying to "shove your beliefs on me" and "shoving medicines, pharmaceutical stuff, vaccines down people's throat."

Patient-consumer communicability, after decades of its promulgation through clinical visits, news stories, pharmaceutical and health system advertising, and, more recently, social media, has become for many laypeople a habitus, in Pierre Bourdieu's ([1972] 1977) terms, a deep, enduring, conscious and unconscious, embodied, automatic way of being in the world. By contrast, COVID-19 biocommunicability steered as far away from patient-consumer communicability as possible. Social distancing was presented not as a recommendation but as a requirement; that rules often were not enforced in public places does not change the framing. Then came the ultimate condensed symbol of the negation of patient-consumer communicability: the *mandate*. For the Millers and many other interlocutors, the word *mandate* constituted the performative utterance that brought the new boundary line into full swing, separating people who imposed and followed mandates and those who realized that mandates were bringing the world as we know it to an end.

Conclusion

In discussing Frank Miller's testimony, I have attempted to push beyond stereotypes of anti-vaxxers as "conspiracy theorists" who occupy fixed, simple positions that reject science and medicine. I argue that he is navigating a very complex borderland, even as he responds critically—and often angrily—to biocommunicability. Joining him at his church one Sunday as the only masked, and very likely one of the few vaccinated, participants, I probably became an embodiment of the mandate. During our conversations, many of which took place in remarkable Montana landscapes, it was hard for me, as a left-leaning medical anthropologist, to avoid moments in which Sigmund Freud's uncanny emerged within me like a flash of recognition. Miller's critiques of the effects of capitalism ("greed," in his terms) and the bureaucratic and depersonalizing dimensions of government health policies and for-profit healthcare systems on care often converged with my own, even as our logical infrastructures and ultimate conclusions diverged. The way he distinguished forms of state power as embodied in laws, mandates, recommendations, statements, and policies might interest a political anthropologist.

It may be the case, as Marta Entradas (2022, 7) and so many critics suggest, that "social media served as a powerful means to amplify misinformation, rumors, and conspiracies that circulated widely early in the pandemic . . . and was significant in the increase of the online anti-vaccine movement . . . and anti-masks groups." Ethnographic work on reception with the Millers and others suggest that the situation might be a bit more complicated. I sat with them evenings as they flipped through social media on their cell phones before watching a movie (given that they no longer spent time watching news programs). My observations suggested, however, that social scientists' frequent projections of passive, unquestioning assimilation of "conspiracy theories" and "misinformation" may not stand up to media ethnography. When new items related to COVID-19 popped up on their phones, they stopped to read aloud or summarize them or passed the phone along to their spouse. As with other families and gatherings of friends, I found with the Millers that subsequent discussions more often took the form of debates than collective assent. The presenter placed the item in one or more interpretive frameworks, then paused and looked up. Some posts—such as those reporting protests against mitigation measures and rollbacks of mandates—often generated immediate consensus: "Damn right!" Nevertheless, many sparked periods of disagreement as Frank Miller rejected his wife's biblical interpretations or Linda Miller challenged her husband's claim that COVID-19 policies sprang from greed on the part of politicians and drug companies rather than diabolical intervention. In short, they actively examined and debated communicable models as much as facts and guidelines.

Professional projections of ecologies of pandemic knowledge were largely medicalized, focused on SARS-CoV-2 and how it circulated, how it affected bodies, and how it should be treated and prevented. In recounting in interviews ways the pandemic affected them personally, health professionals provided detailed accounts of how they undertook the same sorts of improvisations in their residences, relations with family members and friends, food procurement, and the like as was required of laypeople. They registered profound uncertainties about their decisions, especially during the beginning of the pandemic, and worried that acting based on minimal knowledge might endanger their families. Nevertheless, this commonality did not lead any of the physicians I interviewed to recognize that they shared spheres of knowledge production with laypeople. It did not challenge how they mapped biocommunicability or assessed what they projected as lay incommunicabilities. Even as some were much more open to listening and responding with "evidence" to patients' questions, concerns, and assertions, they lumped together efforts by laypeople to engage in the production of knowledge about COVID-19 as forms of incommunicability that disrupted provider-patient interaction, augmented their greatly overburdened workloads, and cost lives.

I hope this chapter makes two things clear. First, I suggest that laypeople who have been classified as good sanitary citizens; contentious long COVID activists; "anti-vaxx" and "anti-mask" Trump supporters; and nefarious spreaders of germs, disinformation, and conspiracy theories all contributed to and were relationally linked in broader pandemic ecologies of knowledge. Second, I argue that, although lay contributions often led to very different decisions, the ways that they overlapped with biocommunicable logics are much deeper and more extensive than professional versus layperson and biocommunicable subject versus "anti-vaxxer" might suggest. Two primary examples, chosen from more than eighty interviews and mountains of other material, cannot do justice to the vast and varied cartographies of lay knowledge production. I am left wondering how differently things might have unfolded if the "we are all in this together" motto had been applied not only as a rationale for demanding fidelity to COVID biocommunicability and mitigation measures but for generating an inclusive, more democratically organized process of sharing the burden of pandemic incommunicability. It is like the well-prepared student who has their hand up so they can contribute to a class discussion but never gets called on to speak—and is always ordered to erase the blackboard, straighten the desks, and empty the trash. This discussion of lay knowledge production brings me to the massive gulf between ecologies of knowledge and ecologies of care, the subject of chapter 8.

8

PANDEMIC ECOLOGIES OF CARE

Care is essential and not enough.
—PATO HEBERT, artist, educator, and long COVID artivist

A crucial reason that laypeople sought to open the door to participation in knowledge production was that it seemed necessary for survival. Ellen Block and Cecilia Vindrola-Padros (2021) rightly argue that shortages of reliable knowledge, personal protective equipment (PPE), and effective drugs and a vastly expanding burden of care required health workers to engage in extensive innovation. The same could be said for laypeople. Indeed, a vast and deep contradiction emerged as the pandemic-industrial-discourse complex demanded that laypeople locate themselves exclusively in the passive receiver position in unilinear, hierarchically organized biocommunicability and simultaneously demanded that they contribute massive amounts of care. Self-isolating and providing self-care for weeks in a multiperson household and assisting ill family members required learning, observation, reflection, and creativity. In small multigenerational and often multifamily dwellings with limited resources, the challenges often seemed insurmountable. In some parts of the United States and other countries, officials made vacant motels available to COVID-19 patients and provided food assistance, but most of the infected—unless they required hospitalization—were largely on their own.

In this chapter, I look at forms of care provided both by health professionals, including emergency room (ER) and intensive care unit (ICU) doctors and nurses, dentists, paramedics, infectious disease physicians, epidemiologists, and others, as well as by a range of laypeople. I de-medicalize forms of COVID-19 care by examining how the broader ecology of pandemic care relied crucially on forms innovated by laypeople in negotiating the challenges of work, education, and daily life. I trace how biomedical knowledge gaps not only complicated efforts by health professionals to treat patients but often left them feeling uncertain, anguished, and vulnerable. I document vast needs to innovate ways of coping with pandemic restrictions outside clinical spaces, suggesting that health professionals faced these dilemmas just like nonprofessionals. By listening to people reflect on their experiences, we learn how these challenges were woven into the grain of people's lives, including ongoing issues not directly related to COVID-19. Indeed, I argue that there was no single pandemic. Each person experientially constructed a different pandemic as COVID-19 was inflected and refracted by fine details of their daily lives.

How to transform domestic, work, and other spaces in managing space, air circulation, food, childcare, and the movement of material items was exceedingly complex. We are only beginning to realize that a viral pandemic exacerbated a broad range of health problems, including chronic and other acute issues. Many conditions went undiagnosed and untreated by health professionals, and such prevention measures as ordinary vaccinations, mammograms, and pap smears were missed due to reduced access to health care and, for many, fear that just entering a clinical space would result in COVID-19 infection. An endodontist I interviewed in Montana traced how routine dental visits plummeted early in the pandemic; only patients with acute pain came to him for root canals. Once they reopened, dental offices were buzzing with a backlog of patients; his practice was overwhelmed with referrals. The pandemic also produced a mental illness pandemic as fear of dying or losing relatives and friends to COVID-19, sudden restrictions on movement and loss of access to exercise and entertainment venues, visits with friends and relatives, travel, and much more came crashing down. Increases in depression, eating disorders, agoraphobia, and domestic violence emerged as mental health services were pushed online and failed to keep up with mushrooming needs. Such in-person rituals as wakes, shiva, funerals, memorial services, and family gatherings were largely unavailable for those who lost friends and family to COVID-19 or other causes, even as others experimented with online funerals. Balancing needs for food and other "essentials" and avoiding infection involved figuring out how to negotiate social distancing and masking requirements and how to "wipe down" purchases—in short, developing new ways to classify safe and unsafe spaces, people, objects, and practices that were not mapped by biocommunicable circuits.

For low-income populations, acute food scarcity often seriously jeopardized mental and physical well-being. Actual or threatened losses of jobs and housing created tremendous challenges, which—as usual—were most exacerbated for BIPOC and low-income populations. Their members often faced simultaneous surges, so to speak, in the life-threatening effects of health care, housing, employment, transportation, and food inequity. Recall Hanna Garth's (2021, 105) observation that flattening the curve of mushrooming racialized inequities was not a top priority on most official agendas. Carolyn Rouse (2021, 362) trenchantly contrasts how social distancing rules were differentially policed, literally, on Black and white people: while Black New Yorkers were sometimes violently arrested, police offered free masks to mostly white residents sitting in a park. Interviewees who filled jobs that did not become remote during the pandemic perceived official proclamations and guidelines—especially as embodied in "lockdown" measures—as designed by and for middle-class professionals without listening to the perspectives of the most impacted populations.

Even before ERs and ICUs were full, care was in short supply. Figuring out how to locate and access scarce resources and how to confront language barriers, immigration status, and the like required extensive, creative, and frenetic efforts at knowledge production and its laterally organized exchange. When vaccines were in short supply and primarily accessible only through online portals slammed by the volume of requests, remarkable knowledge production and exchange systems emerged as people called, texted, or emailed relatives and friends and told them where appointments were available. When issues of language, access to digital technologies, internet accessibility, and website-navigation experience prevented many older BIPOC and other people from getting appointments, younger relatives and volunteers helped connect them. Drawing on Merrill Singer and colleagues' (2017) concept of syndemics, I argue that COVID-19 is less a singular, bounded pandemic than an assemblage of inequities that have assaulted oppressed populations. This chapter goes on to suggest that how racialized populations were constructed by regimes of communicability formed a crucial component of lethal syndemic configurations.

One of Frank Miller's main beefs, as discussed in chapter 7, was the contradiction between knowledge production and care. When he and his wife, Linda, became symptomatic in May 2021, he called his brother, who once worked in the healthcare field. Miller didn't say he was asking for advice, but he was certainly interested in thinking about care options. I have been friends with Miller and his brother for years; I have helped Miller fix houses, including that of our friend Johnny Owen, his figure of the most "radical" opponent of vaccination. Our families have spent time together enjoying remarkable landscapes. His brother asked me to call Miller and "tell him to go to the doctor and get tested—and then tell all the people he may have exposed." I knew that if I passed along these suggestions, Miller would not trust anything I had to say. On a speakerphone with a physician on board, Dr. Clara Mantini-Briggs, I gave Miller a list of warning signs of serious illness and asked him to head to the ER if any of them appeared. While I spoke, there was dead silence—he was listening. I immediately sent him an oximeter, which he and his wife used. I kept in touch with him frequently during their convalescence. These conversations—and knowledge of Montana's demographics and complicated response to COVID-19 mitigation measures—led to my request to visit them in October and November 2021.

How Miller tackled the task of figuring out how to care for himself after contracting COVID-19 sprang from having tuned out news sources and his sense that, in a COVID-19 landscape, available varieties of biomedical care seemed to amount to impersonal forms of state knowledge production disguised as care. I interviewed several community health center physicians who reported that although they tried to keep patients who had tested positive or were in isolation out of clinic spaces, they directed staff to call all COVID-19 patients periodically to check on symptoms and provide guidance on care. They also delivered packages with everything from chicken soup packets to a pulse oximeter. If patients lacked food, the clinics purchased groceries and meals and had them delivered. The ER physician whose story I present later in this chapter noted that she gave nonacute COVID-19 patients a list that included signs that their symptoms might be entering the acute phase as well as advice on isolation and activating networks of friends, family, and coworkers to provide groceries and other essentials.

Nevertheless, most of the laypeople I interviewed reported that testing was the only medical service available to them if their symptoms were less than acute (before COVID-19 vaccines and treatments such as Paxlovid were available). Getting a positive test did not generally afford greater access to care, except in acute cases, or even much additional guidance. However, a positive test often produced a call from a contact tracer. Virtual armies of people who were not health professionals—some displaced from their jobs by the pandemic's economic impact—were rapidly trained and employed. An online program urged trainees to tell interlocutors, "I'm calling to see how you are and to help keep you, your family, and your community safe." Miller and many others who rejected public health discourse about COVID-19 saw contact tracing as a confessional technology, requests by strangers trained to use a personalized voice of concern to elicit details regarding "contacts," people and public spaces with whom the patient had intersected following what the tracer calculated to be the beginning of the infectious period. As Alan Brandt (2002, 1099) notes, some contact tracing programs shifted "from a public health approach based on police powers of the state to one that emphasizes community social engagement and support." Although a good contact tracer might have helped the Millers work out a care plan, in view of Miller's criteria for deciding who could provide credible knowledge about COVID-19, a Health Department worker who was not a health professional who cold-called was the last person he would trust.

Miller complained that reaching out to his doctor, getting tested, and getting a call from a contact tracer would place him in a biocommunicable network designed to advance knowledge-gathering activities that served state interests in statistical projections, not patients' needs for care. Like other interviewees who rejected vaccines and masks, Miller specifically pointed to contact tracing—like mandates—as a point of rupture. What seemed to be an offer of care from a stranger, he complained, turned out to be a practiced enactment of a caring voice uttering scripted phrases that only suggested phone numbers for overburdened agencies that would be unlikely to provide resources. Miller later extended this logic to his decision about COVID-19 vaccination, believing that it had more to do with governmental control than a genuine offer of care.

Even for individuals who did not reject COVID-19 biocommunicability, facing pandemic challenges involved accessing knowledge production and exchange networks, including friends, family, mainstream and social media, websites, health authorities, pastors, rabbis, priests, and others. No one could get by simply as a patient-consumer of existing knowledge: every individual and household situation and shifting local ecology of care required reading changing circumstances and anticipating possible future changes. Many people who could not work remotely devised elaborate rituals to erect viral borders between their place of employment and home and to facilitate reincorporation from the former into the latter. Similar to many accounts that emerged in my interviews, Block and Vindrola-Padros (2021, 314–15) report a routine worked out by a COVID unit nurse and her husband, who worked from home and cared for the children:

When I'm coming home, I take my scrubs off at the hospital, put on pants and a t-shirt. I have a tracker thing where my husband has me share my ETA on my way home. He likes to get the washing machine going, and the thing is already open and the water and soap already in so I don't touch anything. The basement door is open, everything's ready to go. So I leave my shoes in the car I come inside. I put the t-shirt, the pants, my scrubs and the canvas tote all right in the wash. I have a bleach spray for my phone. And then I have to run upstairs naked, take a shower and then he's fine.

Block and Vindrola-Padros use this lovely example to illustrate improvisations (Livingston 2012) undertaken by health workers, but it seems to grant at least as much agency and power in devising this elaborate ritual to the layperson, the homebound husband. Even once routines had become reasonably well established, viral surges, food or other shortages, and the like prompted additional improvisation.

One of this book's central concerns has been how health professionals claim monopolies on biocommunicability and how this process can produce incommunicability and obscure lay contributions. I have also been concerned with how these hierarchically structured ecologies of health knowledge intersect with ecologies of care. In chapter 5, I drew on Eduardo Menéndez's classic work on *autoatención*, the work of care performed by laypeople outside clinical settings. I argued that by limiting definitions of care to the forms *they* provide, health professionals produce their own ignorance of the broader ecologies of care in which their patients dwell and miss vast opportunities for collaboration. In the pandemic, even as health professionals focused on narrowly defined dimensions of prevention, quarantine, isolation, and self-monitoring for danger signs, professionals passed along a massive burden of care to laypeople. Some doctor's offices, like mine, virtually closed. As hospital services were suspended, health systems asked patients to put many other health complaints aside or to bring them, if life threatening, to the ER.

This chapter makes three primary contributions to debates about pandemic care. One is to analyze the central role of this gap between ecologies of knowledge and care in producing pandemic angst; widespread distrust of health professionals; and a backlash against recommendations and mandates concerning masking, vaccination, and "social distancing." I argue that these effects were predictable, emerging as if by design. Second, by listening closely to grandparents, college students, firefighters, nurses, farmworkers, physicians, epidemiologists, and others, I trace the impressive depth and complexity of the daily improvisations required of laypeople and health professionals just to make it through the pandemic. Third, I hope that listening closely to the pandemic testimonies of firefighters/paramedics, nurses, physicians, and laypeople will disrupt homogenizing, distorting, and distancing barriers, including health professionals' views of people like Frank Miller and how laypeople often construct health workers through dominant images, whether as heroes or as arrogant, insensitive autocrats. It turns out that even their friends and family members, not to mention their patients, seldom took the time to listen to them talk about their pandemic lives. Health professionals faced the same challenges in giving and getting care; just making it through another day; and imagining futures not poisoned by pandemic fears, frustration, and anger. Although they claimed a privileged position within COVID-19 biocommunicability, it turns out that this status did not vaccinate health professionals against some of the painful incommunicable dilemmas faced by others.

Even as laypeople faced massive burdens of care, the labor of keeping acutely ill COVID-19 patients alive sometimes was more than health professionals, particularly ER and ICU nurses and doctors, could manage, even when they were willing to work practically around the clock. Thanks to journalists and social media, this is now a familiar story. By listening closely to their accounts and placing them in dialogue with one another—and even with the COVID-19 skeptics who sometimes despise them—this chapter breaks new ground by documenting people's attempts to navigate uncomfortable borderlines between biocommunicability and incommunicability and face painful failures of care.

From "Unprecedented Pandemic" to Viral Amplification of Existing Burdens of Care

Rosette Smith, Professor and Grandmother, Northern California

When her marriage fell apart, my daughter moved in. The twins were one, and another baby was on the way. They've been more or less under my care, at least part of the time, since they were born. My daughter moved into the downstairs apartment, but I took two of the kids upstairs with me. So it was a multigenerational, multistory family. The big difference before COVID-19 is that the children were nine and seven, so they were in school. That gave me a good chunk of the day to not have to think about their welfare and their activities. I was the Friday person. But the rest of the week, I felt that I could do my priorities, mostly my professional priorities, in an orderly way, and then in the evenings do dinner, then put them to bed. At eight o'clock, I could be my own person again. I could go back to work. I usually found myself crossing the country about once a month to give a lecture or attend a conference or work for the government reading applications and things like that. So there was a lot of travel. We found a way to make that work. We had a group of high school kids and a couple of university kids who would come in the evenings and help. I had no big complaints. Before, each day was different, but it was a stable system.

Then COVID happened. My daughter, an ER physician, of course was immediately informed about how it spreads and all the knowledge about it. She was very worried about herself because she was in contact with COVID-infected people whenever she went to work. So we took the kids out of the apartment and brought them upstairs—all of them. We even closed off the air vents to the apartment so that there's no air going between the two units. She waved at the kids through the window. They had entirely become my responsibility. In those days, they were eating four meals a day, so I was preparing and cooking and cleaning up after and doing the laundry and all that, which I had been doing; it's just that there was a lot more of it, plus the homework and helping the kids with their projects of all kinds. Sometimes in the middle of one of my [online] lectures, they would float in the background and ask me when I would be available to help them or something. It made my teaching, let's just say, more informal.

After a lot of quietness for many decades, many of my neighbors decided that this was the time to gut and renovate their houses, and the church behind me decided to build a house. So the sounds of construction surrounded us all the time. I tried to teach, tried to lecture, but it was sometimes hard to shout over what was going on. I would look with a certain envy at students who would be coming to class with their earphones on in a quiet place, and I'd be thinking, I can't put on earphones because I have to listen for the kids. I had to be in the middle of the house, in the middle of the action, because otherwise I wasn't doing even a bad job of looking after the kids. The students got acclimated to the fact that there would be these children kind of floating around. You know, for you and me, we can delay lunch for an hour, an hour and a half. It wouldn't be a big deal. But for these little guys, you know, it's their due, right? They're growing. I mean, they've grown six inches since COVID started. They waved at the students and students waved at them. And they came to faculty meetings. I mean, there was no way they could not if they felt like passing through the room, which they did.

Then, in October 2020, my daughter got COVID-19, and that was really scary. For her, of course, it was scary because she was alone and she couldn't breathe. We put up a baby monitor so I could hear her. She couldn't lie down because if she did, she couldn't breathe, so she had to sit up. To hear her suffering was hard. By Christmas she was feeling better, but it took a long time for her to feel 80 percent. That was really hard.

Thank goodness, the kids were old enough to be good readers. We would order books at the library and pick them up. They don't let you hang around, but you can pick up a stack of books. They consumed an enormous number of books. We're very fortunate I have a backyard. It's not very big, but it has a little deck, and we hung off the deck all sorts of things to climb on and swing on and stuff like that. And we put up a tent with a table under it so they had an outdoor place where they could study or play a game or something like that. And they created a pack. They turned my living room into kind of a tree house at one point—made tents out of blankets and rooms out of chairs and stuff. I mean, they really colonized the house, and I let them do that. I'm a pretty good cook, and they like it, so they look forward to meals and to helping. The youngest learned how to make ice cream, and they all can make lemonade now from our lemon tree. We have a garden, and our big project last summer was to build a critter-proof garden structure. We got some recycled redwood and built this structure with the screening down into the earth, so the tunneling creatures couldn't get in. The kids became very much like little farmers with me. And I arranged for them to each have a Zoom meeting with one of their buddies once a week, and they felt that was quite special.

I must admit to having felt a sense of awe when I listened to Smith describe her pandemic life. Her account immediately contradicts projections of COVID-19 as "unprecedented," as a fundamental rupture with a "normality" that preceded it. Her story centers on continuities and discontinuities of care; the need to sustain the lives of three grandchildren even as the sudden loss of support from their mother, school, and babysitters placed full responsibility on her shoulders. In a calm, understated way, she reports that the pandemic just extended the labor of care: "It's just that there was a lot more of it." Viral vulnerabilities transformed familial roles: even as the daughter's job as an ER physician made her much more likely to be infected, the possibility of losing a mother in her seventies or a child to COVID-19 suddenly displaced the daughter from a central role in sustaining affective relations and household labor to a simultaneously distant and proximal figure.

Of importance here is a forced digitalization of life. The children had no experience with computers, and the family had distanced the children from television, videos, and, except once a month, movies. Digitalization posed challenges: keeping four persons on Zoom entailed bandwidth limitations, working out technical difficulties, and facing the acoustic challenges that emerged as the neighborhood became a construction zone. Digitalization also afforded pandemic workarounds, as Smith could give guest lectures across the country without leaving home, and the children could experience weekly connections with friends. The "Zoomification" of life both reshaped and was shaped by how care unfolded in space, restricting Smith's ability to claim any degree of privacy (at least until the children went to bed at 8 p.m.). Boundaries between work and family life blurred for the grandmother as the children appeared in classes, lectures, and faculty meetings. (The latter must have certainly been a fascinating experience for them.) Interpersonal relations expanded as the three children became part of students' and colleagues' lives, and the children waved at Smith's students (but seemingly not at faculty members).

These transformations of care, work, school, food preparation, gardening, and leisure required creatively turning the fine details of daily life into sites for improvisation and engagement. An adultist perspective would attribute these emerging designs for pandemic living exclusively to Smith. This view, however, would overlook the three children's agency in transforming family relations: how "they created a pack," imaginatively reconfigured the space of the living room, claimed active roles in cooking and gardening (but perhaps not washing clothes and dishes), reterritorializing the backyard, and turning reading into a way to reduce their grandmother's work of care. As a result, Smith reports, "they have never said they're bored." Their bodies asserted their own claims of agency, turning alimentary needs into a force that resisted demands to allow Zoomified work to dominate temporalization entirely. A significant part of the labor here was affective. Smith reports, "I didn't want them to feel they were in prison. I wanted them to feel—here is an opportunity." Engaging in household labor, entering into their grandmother's work life, and transforming domestic space helped create sites of experimentation, connection, and agency. Rather than claiming any heroic status, Smith was quick to point out forms of privilege enjoyed by a white family with two professionals who own a home with a backyard in a relatively affluent, generally quiet, safe small city with ample parks, including one almost next door (where I conducted the interview). "We're much more fortunate than most people," she said. "We've been able to make it work. Other people had it worse."

Even as her measured tone and description of carefully worked-out pandemic routines projected a sense of calm and order, the soundscape that she depicted pointed to acoustic, social, and material chaos that would not stay within borders. The juxtaposition of the three chronotopes (Bakhtin 1981) that emerge—pre-pandemic relative order, the collaborative search for new forms of care and intimacy, and the daughter's subterranean movement from watchful physician to severely ill patient—fracture the orderly narrative and infuse the sense of resilience with a strong feeling of precarity. Behind her voice of calm and fortitude lay the shadow of fear, a central force for reorganizing care. "One of the hard things about these two years is a family friend did die of COVID," she said. "At this point [February 2022], like 900,000 Americans have died. Everyone must know someone who has. Or knows someone whose kin has. And, yeah, that is sort of fearsome." Her ER physician daughter constantly warned of COVID-19 precarities, shaping what grandmother and children could and could not do, even when she was in quarantine and then isolation. We'll hear the mother's story a bit later. The grandmother's account highlights this movement among optimism, resilience, and precarity poignantly in the image of listening to her seriously ill daughter's breathing through a baby monitor. She appears to be in control of both the story and, with the collaboration of the three children, the creation of novel pandemic routines. Nevertheless, the physician's voice from the basement allows biocommunicability to seep into her narrative as the daughter constantly vets the details of everyday life to weed out potential sources of infection.

My question, "What do you think was hardest for you about the pandemic?" elicited a surprising response: "Well, it was this thing about having colliding obligations—obligations that couldn't be reconciled. It meant that I was disappointing someone in a big way, not doing what I should be doing. And I don't remember feeling that way before." Smith worked to maintain her remarkably high standards as an academic, doing far more than her share of service and administration at a research university, publishing, giving lectures, and supporting students as their research plans and career expectations collapsed. Her offhand comment about caring "badly" for her grandchildren points to her lofty expectations of what care entails, as did her regret at not being able to attend in person—due to travel restrictions—to her dying father on the East Coast. Then she faced helping her daughter confront her fear that she would die and abandon her children. Remarkably, the one challenge Smith felt incapable of overcoming was the expectation that she would accomplish all of these roles perfectly and simultaneously. Ordinary ethics emerge here not as a unified set of practices but as discrepant, irresolvable conflicts among competing ethical commitments. Rather than asking for heroic status, Smith not only expresses what she sees as the limits of her ability but, with particular relevance to the broadened cartography of care I am developing here, helps chart parameters of the work of care that laypeople assumed. Her testimony makes it clear that care went far beyond issues of COVID-19 symptoms and treatments.

Smith's testimony provides an example in which biocommunicability—emerging both from mainstream news consumption and taking detailed instructions from her physician daughter—went hand in hand with an elaborate set of care practices that reshaped the fine details of her life and her grandchildren's lives. Biocommunicable citizens, including health professionals, journalists not affiliated with conservative media, and laypeople, often claim that individuals who reject COVID-19 biocommunicability and vaccination turned their backs on mitigation measures. The Millers, discussed in chapter 7, fairly closely embodied this generalization. Nevertheless, Clara Mantini-Briggs and I interviewed Polly Weaver (PW) and Dave Strong (DS) in September 2021 in a small community in the Sierra Nevada foothills of Amador County, California. In their sixties, they are avid Trump supporters who engage daily with Fox News, AM radio conservative talk shows, and social media. At the same time, many of the forms of care they enacted during the pandemic do not fit "anti-vaxx" stereotypes.

Polly Weaver and Dave Strong, Sixties, Amador County, California

PW: We were scared to death. The news really scared us to death. We listened to all of the news—CNN, MSNBC, Fox. . . . A lot of Fox. A lot of CNN, trying to figure out what was going on. I would jump back and forth. It was very scary. You go to CNN, and all the figures [are] to the side: the number of people dying every day, every day throughout the world, throughout the United States. I even follow a map from the *New York Times* and religiously, like twice a day, I check that map to see—it tells you how many cases, how many people had died, how many people had died that day. I said, "You know what, people? This isn't sci-fi—this shit is real!"

In the beginning for me, it was like total fear. I wouldn't go out of the house. I wouldn't go into stores at first. Then, you know, it's like, just sit at home and do nothing or—. So then we started going out to stores with our big mask on, then we'd have bags of alcohol rags. Yeah, everything that came in our house sat in the garage until it was wiped down with alcohol. Our hands were constantly washed. We'd throw our clothes in the washing machine. All kinds of stuff. I mean, we just, I don't know, it changed our lifestyle.

DS: We didn't go out as much and stuff.

PW: It was all closed. You couldn't go shopping. You could only go to a grocery store.

DS: You didn't go out as much, so I had to do the errands all the time. And she would make sure that I was totally supplied with all the, you know, antibacterial/viral—[*interrupted*]

PW: Well, we had heard that men don't get COVID as much as women. They're not as susceptible to it. That's what we had heard.

CB: During this time, did you talk to your relatives and friends very much about COVID and what you were doing?

PW: My sister. And we both said, "Stay home! Wear a mask if you go out. Carry plenty of alcohol rags. Don't put anything in your cart without wiping everything off." That's how we lived. I do believe that whoever is out there and doesn't want to wear a mask and they're protesting against it, they're nuts! Because if you are the right person with the wrong type of blood or the wrong type of some ailment in your body, you're dead, you're dead with COVID. I'm wearing my mask from now on with this variant. Dave, you should see the numbers coming out of California every day.

Mostly, a lot of it is like, for me, how it changed my life was my life with my grandchildren, too. They would come over, or we would go over there, like, usually once a week, and I was teaching them how to bake, you know, how to do a lot of different things. It all just abruptly came to an end. And it's devastating. It makes me want to cry. The day that ended and we couldn't see each other was devastating. Dave and I would drive up at night. We would meet at Starbucks, in the parking lot. All our masks on, the girls would stay in the car and sit on the gate that goes down on the Toyota RAV4. They were so afraid they were going to kill grandma, you know? Because of the unknowingness, thinking they were going to kill their grandparents. I just feel like we lost, like, almost two years.

[The youngest grandchild] was . . . four and a half or so when this started, and she would come over and swim and grandma would take care of her, and Dave would swim with her, and this would happen like every weekend. The water balloons, the fun we had. And that all just abruptly came to an end. She treats us—Dave and me both—sort of like strangers now. It's weird, but she was so young.

Dr. Fauci says that masks don't work. Well, he did at first, and now he says you should wear two masks. So that was very confusing. I'm sure the news is very confusing to everybody. Well, you know, President Trump: I thought he was trying to do—I think he was sincere and he really wanted everybody to get healed. And, you know, he wanted a vaccine. I think during the pandemic, he really tried his best. I mean, you can't fault him there. He got all those companies, big amounts of money, you know, to get the vaccine done and apparently they did it.

DS: I lost a lot of trust—in everything. I mean, one month it's this and one month it's the other, and that's the new protocol. Contradictory information instead of as we go along, we'll learn dah, dah, dah, dah, dah. No, you must do this and this and this is the way it would always be, but then it changes. Boom [*snaps fingers*]. Just like that. You know, for one thing, we still don't know the truth of the origins of COVID-19. We still don't know the truth, and it's being hidden. No one knows; even if they think they know, they don't. Personally, it's an opportunistic thing that fell in the lap of the Democratic Party to do what they want to do to the future of this country—turn it into a socialist state for one world order. And you already see the signs that always in every other country have led to that. Yep, overspend governmentwise, create debt, overtax the wealthy—you know, I can go on and on—and create divisions of poverty and wealth.

PW: My theory is different. I think that China did a biological war on us. That's how I feel. All the facts are there, if you really study it. They sent it here. They sent it all over the world. Five hundred and fifty thousand flights flew out of China—the worst day of the pandemic, and they flew all over the world. Why? Highest airlift day ever in the history of China. It's the start of taking over America. I mean, I don't believe it's the Democrats. I really don't.

I'm not vaccinating, and I will never be vaccinated. I don't think the vaccine is working, and I think the vaccine can do more harm to people than it can do good. Women are dying of heart failure. People are dying from that shot. They are. They're dying. I'm not saying that they are trying to do depopulation. Some people believe that within two years everybody that has been vaccinated will either have lung problems or heart problems. . . . I just don't like the fact that it changes your DNA, your whole DNA—you are not the same person. I don't want my grandchildren to have the shots. It causes reproductive [problems]. I don't know. Nobody even knows. I just say, "Oh, I don't want them to die from it." But I don't know. No, it's not for me to say. I have no idea about anything, really. I just blame the Chinese, that's all.

Despite embracing just the sorts of pandemic reasoning that the WHO attempted to discredit as "myths" and "mis- and disinformation," Weaver and Strong continued to take COVID-19 mitigation measures quite seriously and to use them in shaping day-to-day activities. Reporting being "scared to death" did not give way to a twenty/twenty hindsight verdict that Weaver's "total fear" was unfounded. They reported initially using the same sorts of systematic sanitizing protocols adopted by many "liberals" who accepted mainstream COVID-19 explanations, and they adopted masking. Weaver still masked when entering spaces in September 2021, although Strong had begun to vary his masking practices according to his perception of the demographics of particular public spaces. I read her aside to him about "the numbers coming out of California every day" in September 2021 as trying to convince him to return to a more consistent masking practice. Based on my observations of businesses in the surrounding communities, he still used masks more than most residents.

Weaver's devotion to prevention measures went as far as to jeopardize what she most values in the world: interactions with her two grandchildren. She cried as she recounted losing almost two years with her grandchildren. Talking, masked, in a Starbucks parking lot did not replace babysitting, pool parties, and shared culinary pursuits. Now, more than a year after the interview, she is rebuilding a relationship with the granddaughter whose pandemic distance had led her to treat them "sort of like strangers."

The interview with Weaver and Strong confounds simplistic, stereotypical conclusions about how COVID-19 biocommunicability and forms of care intersect. Even as she rejects vaccination and embraces the anti-Chinese COVID-19 origin story that would seem to be indexed by Trump's assertions about "the Chinese virus," she characterizes people who choose not to wear masks and protest against mask mandates as "nuts." Strong and Weaver do not simply live in an alien world whose texture emerges exclusively and transparently out of Fox News broadcasts or right-wing YouTube videos and Facebook posts, even as their pandemic experience includes them. The couple's pandemic story involves a complex web of sanitary practices designed to confront a deeply incommunicable and scary reality. Their rejection of scientific views of the emergence and spread of SARS-CoV-2 did not lead them to tune out biocommunicability. Unlike Miller, they still avidly watched news coverage of COVID-19 on multiple channels, including CNN, which most conservatives vilify, a year and a half into the pandemic. Miller would seem to line up squarely with Wagner and Reifegerste's (2023, 1015) observation that the "flood of information and the surrounding debates on the COVID-19 pandemic occurring in both mass media outlets and on social media make it more difficult to interpret a situation and to form an opinion about the evolving events." Nevertheless, both Strong and Weaver seemed to feel perfectly able to navigate this wide range of sources and use them to decide what to trust and what to do. For Miller, COVID-19 testing and the circulation of statistics proved that government agencies were interested only in surveillance and control, not care. Weaver, however, not only checked pandemic statistics twice daily but visited what conservatives generally see as the epitome of "liberal" media—the *New York Times*—to use its website to track COVID-19 and structure her activities beyond the home. They used these sources, as well as consultation with her sister and a registered nurse relative, in devising a detailed mitigation plan, which the couple followed consistently.

At the same time, their co-narrated account of pandemic life is heteroglossic, such that these mundane details are shot through with traces of hidden narratives. Even as they enter into the "conspiracy theory" territory that Frank Miller discounted and their secular worldview left no room for Linda Miller's fundamentalist Christian logic, their reductionist logics of Chinese and Democratic COVID-19 plots exhibit features associated with so-called conspiracy theories. Nevertheless, Weaver's disclaimer—"No, it's not for me to say. I have no idea about anything, really"—is hardly in line with the claims of pervasive control, agency, and totalizing effects that have been cited as the hallmark of "conspiracy theories."[1] Adding further complexity, their acceptance of masking and disinfecting practices were woven together with ways of participating in global networks of knowledge—sending texts to friends and relatives with links to YouTube videos that feature physicians who challenged scientific and medical findings. They consider their position as emerging not from passive acceptance of what others would label "conspiracy theories" but from "research" they conducted in positioning themselves as active contributors to a network of people fighting a losing battle to preserve communicable freedom by countering liberal, state, corporate, and media efforts to impose censorship and authoritarianism. We could consider the "I'm doing my research" leitmotif that is so vilified by the biocommunicable faithful as a way of signaling the rejection of a passive lay receiver position in biomedical authority communicability and a claim to be a participant in the lay production of knowledge about COVID-19. Strong and Weaver complained vociferously about what they saw as the suppression of anti-mainstream, conservative views on Facebook and YouTube, citing numerous examples of what they depicted as posts that had been taken down almost immediately and individuals—including some friends—who had been placed in "Facebook jail," meaning that their accounts were deleted.

Like Miller, the couple is not anti-science or anti-medicine. Weaver consulted multiple physicians to see who might best perform a highly complex knee replacement, settling on a leading medical school and hospital. Strong suffered a heart attack and spent four days in the hospital in early 2023. Unfortunately, he succumbed to another cardiac event that summer. Their views on vaccination, Fauci and Trump, and the provenance of SARS-CoV-2 may have estranged some readers even more than Miller's more hesitant and calibrated perspective. I hope, however, that their testimony complicates any hasty generalizations about relations among biocommunicability, care, and media ideologies and seemingly direct correlations with political leanings.

Silvia Montaño, San Joaquín Valley, California

In January 2020 I was in New York City for my friend's book launch. I was like, "Great! I need time off; need time to dance." That was lovely and amazing. At that moment I was feeling very hopeful about a lot of things. One, I was beginning to sense that I might need to change my job, really remembering the value of being connected to community and doing work that was meaningful. "I want to be able to enjoy the work that I'm doing," I was thinking. "I want to know that it makes an impact on people's lives. I want to have a little bit of creative control over the work that I do. I don't want to just be dictated to me top-down." So there were all these things that were floating through my head, my own personal things. And coming back home, I was like, "OK, we've got to start working on the garden again, because now I'm living at home again."

But definitely that changed pretty quickly. I think it was just watching the news, what was happening at a global level, and telling my husband,

Jerry, "This isn't looking good at all. I don't think it's going to stay contained. It sounds like it's very infectious. It sounds like there are a lot of questions." So for me, it was like, "There's something else going on here. I don't exactly know what it is." That was February, early—maybe middle February. We had some community garden activities planned in March, and I just told Jerry, "We're canceling them." He asked me why. "Because I see what's coming," I said, "and I don't think we're going to be safe here." It was being discussed, like, "Oh, yeah—we're in the United States where it's not gonna come to us. It's not gonna hit us here." I was like, "Nah. I don't buy it."

So my birthday's in early March. I didn't plan anything: "We're not getting together, we're not celebrating." I think my mom was upset because I didn't want to celebrate my birthday, which I don't normally celebrate. She always wants to celebrate it. I was like, "I don't want to make a big deal, but we're definitely not doing anything. We're not gathering." So there were a lot of things going on, like a birthday that we didn't get to celebrate now for new reasons—sort of scary, unknowing reasons. We heard about this disease in the news. We don't know how widespread it is. Apparently, contact with anything and everything can expose you. So it was overwhelming. My aunt had just been taken to the hospital, and they found a brain tumor. So she spent the entire month of March in the hospital. That was really hard, especially as shelter-in-place orders came in. The hospitals were closed. I was telling my mom: "The hospital is not the best place for you to be right now, because dad is high-risk, and to a degree you are, too, because you've had these health conditions in the past, and I just don't want you to be exposing yourself." And she's like, "No, it's my *sister*. I *have* to be there!" And she would get upset with me because I wouldn't go to the hospital. I didn't see my aunt until the very end, the week before she died. So I was dealing with a lot. I had to start looking for a job, but I had a husband who was depressed because he had just lost his job. My mom was going through a crisis, and all of this was happening at the same time [*crying*].

So I'm thinking that we've got our families to take care of. My parents don't have enough food resources, so I'm shopping for them and delivering food to them and to my husband's family and my sister while making some of those resources also available in the community. My husband and I actually started very early on, particularly when shelter-in-place came in and I had a chance to go to the store and see the shelves empty, we actually did some house-to-house delivery for people who were disabled, seniors. We did that for a little while, until local churches began to do that work, and we didn't feel that obligation as much.

My aunt died at the end of that month, and we didn't have a funeral, I think, until June. That was hard, too, because we had family visiting. It was the first over 100-degree day that year, and here we were outdoors in the heat, and, with all the venues closed, all restaurants closed, there was nowhere anyone could go. So then my husband and I said, "We can't let my eighty-year-old uncle be out in the heat. We'll invite him over here. We'll invite our family over here." We had about, I don't know, thirty people in here. And I said, "Once the party's over, we're going to make sure everything is cleaned and disinfected. Then we go into quarantine, because we don't know." We put ourselves in quarantine because we consciously made that choice to invite our family—my family—over, so we would make sure that we stayed home the whole time.

We were at home. By the time that the shelter-in-place orders came in, I remember feeling relieved, because I didn't want to go to work anymore. By the end of March, I was notified that my position had been terminated. That was my first month of the pandemic!

If we accept a narrow, medicalized definition of COVID-19, Montaño's testimony might not count as a pandemic story. When we spoke in October 2021, neither Montaño nor her husband or any of her close family members had displayed symptoms or tested positive. The couple had recently moved back to their hometown to provide the care needed by their parents, siblings, and extended family, whose economic and health precarity had demanded more attention than they could extend while living elsewhere. Before March 2020, providing groceries and meals and attending to healthcare needs for two sets of parents and other relatives formed a big part of the couple's daily routine. They were first-generation college students and the only professionals in two extended families; their access to the resources needed to sustain this network was disrupted precisely at the beginning of the pandemic due to job losses.

Montaño's narrative, like Smith's and so many others I heard, separates two chronotopes: pre-pandemic and COVID-19 space/time cartographies. Nevertheless, the latter is not medicalized, structured by biomedical features. The arrival of COVID-19 did not cause the couple's sudden loss of economic security: both dismissals were due to other factors. We have become familiar with pandemic narratives of how mitigation measures and their economic effects led to job losses; with Montaño's story, we have to think more broadly and look more deeply. The pandemic enters the couple's routine when Montaño sees that the shelves are nearly bare in the only grocery store in town, complicating the work of providing for extended family members and prompting her to survey food scarcity issues for the entire community and locate resources to meet them. An old conflict with her mother resurfaces in Montaño's refusal to throw herself a birthday party, even as she attributes her position to "new reasons—sort of scary, unknowing reasons." Then the expected forms of care and closeness among siblings are disrupted when Montaño's mother cannot visit her dying sister in the hospital, and the daughter fails to fulfill the mother's expectations. As pandemic restrictions closed in, the focus of care shifted to a small, bounded stage: caring for a husband trapped at home by joblessness, a pandemic, and depression. The pandemic chronotope is thus woven out of a narrative rearrangement of the principal threads that characterized the couple's lives before March 2020.

If we do not view Montaño's story as a pandemic narrative, however, then we need to discard not only a medicalized definition of "the pandemic" but the very concept itself. Certainly, COVID-19 is a protagonist here, a specter that haunts events and affective relations starting in January 2020, turning a feeling of optimism and new possibilities into a "scary" premonition. However, the disease becomes a presence only after it is woven into the fine details of everyday relations, obligations, and disruptions. Rather than constituting a distinct, medicalized landscape of care, COVID-19 seeps into the fabric of events that are not of its making. Refusing to host a birthday party becomes an act of COVID care, part of the work of protecting the lives of vulnerable relatives. While COVID-19 does not take the beloved aunt's life, the pandemic infects the binational extended family's ability to care for the aunt and one another. The approaching death prompts Montaño to define care as avoiding contact with her aunt and extending the work of care to the broader family circle. As Lawrence Cohen (2020, 543, 547) usefully argues, definitions of care during the pandemic shifted in ways that framed *not* visiting or touching vulnerable relatives and friends as forms of care that "can feel perverse," engendering "the feeling that to care is to an extent to abandon." What ensued was less a new consensus about care than an acrimonious debate that engendered hurt feelings and multiple incommunicabilities.

This partial demedicalization of COVID-19 might reflect the status of Montaño's account as a lay pandemic narrative. However, it is not: she is a health professional. I strategically omitted a crucial sentence in her prediction regarding COVID-19's pandemic potential: "I had already been at the Health Department when H1N1 broke out and had to deal with that." She holds a master's in public health and a doctorate and served as a county epidemiologist in 2009. Afterward, she became the director of a food bank and broadened its agenda into documenting and addressing food scarcity issues rather than providing meals alone. She thus catalyzed a regional approach that included the creation of community gardens and a more active role for schools in addressing food scarcity in a region—California's San Joaquín ("Central") Valley—where they are far too familiar. This work, which earned her a major award from a leading university, emerged in her account of the need to cancel a community-garden event in March 2020 and her ability to call on old networks to address suddenly more pressing problems of food scarcity. At this point in the book, you may have sensed that Montaño claimed biocommunicable clairvoyance, even as she cast coworkers and unnamed others as nationalistically incommunicability: "Oh, yeah. We're in the United States, where it's not gonna come to us." Her voice shifts here in grammatical and intonational features to construct an uninformed subject. When she quotes her inner speech (Vološinov [1929] 1973), by contrast, her careful reasoning and ability to put together scattered details in a comprehensive way is given voice. Her narrative thus complicates any easy categorization of health professional versus lay lives, responses, and narratives. In short, Montaño's pandemic, no less than Rosette Smith's, is woven from the threads of the intimate details of daily life that surrounded her and, in particular, her ongoing obligations of care. As it did for Smith, COVID-19 enters the stage through the back door, fitting itself into existing relations, intimacies, and struggles, even as it sometimes changes their course.

Conditions in many areas of the San Joaquín Valley are generally dismal, as documented by Dvera Saxton (2021). Seth Holmes's (2013) ethnography of conditions facing West Coast agricultural workers, many of whom are indigenous immigrants from Mexico and Central America, powerfully describes the overcrowded, substandard conditions in which they are forced to live, labor processes that wear out laborers' bodies by the time they are forty, and the gaps in health care and worker protections.[2] And then along came COVID-19. Beyond the failure of growers and the managers of fruit and vegetable packing plants to provide adequate PPE, interviews revealed that bosses often told workers who called in to report COVID-19 symptoms that they would lose their jobs if they did not show up for work, multiplying infections and deaths in these sites. Research on the impact of the pandemic on farmworkers and their families documented the many ways that COVID-19 and mitigation measures deepened long-standing oppressive health, housing, work, and other conditions (see Bade, Ramirez, and Saxton 2021; Ramirez, Mines, and

Carlisle-Cummins 2020). The very people who pick and pack a considerable portion of the food consumed in the United States and beyond faced the acute food shortages that Montaño describes.

Visiting predominantly agricultural communities in the San Joaquín Valley was tremendously disheartening, as I learned how deep oppression runs there and how much the pandemic had exacerbated misery. At the same time, I stood in awe of a host of grassroots movements that transformed the pandemic into a site for advancing the health and rights of workers in the fields and packing plants. A remarkable interview I conducted jointly with Anai Ramos, an undergraduate student at UC Berkeley in December 2022, featured Roselia Bustos, who lives in the Salinas Valley, west of the San Joaquín Valley. Here she describes her work as a lettuce picker, her experience of the pandemic, and how she became involved with a group I will call Luchadoras del Campo, an activist organization formed by women who work or formerly worked in the fields. Bustos describes efforts by members to protect workers during the pandemic, including writing a series of letters to California governor Gavin Newsom and his wife.[3]

Roselia Bustos, Former Farmworker and Luchadoras del Campo Member

I'm from Jalisco [Mexico]. I came here at ten years old, and at fourteen I started to work in the lettuce fields. I am a mother of four: three boys and a girl. My parents worked in the fields, so I starting working with them, and I kept at it.

At first I didn't pay much attention to COVID. I didn't think it would be so serious until I starting seeing that relatives were dying. I became scared, because I just didn't know. You heard about it everywhere, but you heard that no one knew what it was like. They said one thing and then another, right? We got COVID, like, in October [2020]. When I got infected, honestly, I was panicked. My aunt got infected at the same time that a cousin died, and I think that's how we got infected. She felt like she couldn't breathe, and she thought she was dying.

Farmworkers just kept going, like always; there were no restrictions. And there were no options. People couldn't just stay home because they had to keep working. Like always, the supervisors want the work done quickly. They don't care. They were supposed to take precautions, to keep workers distanced, but, honestly, in the fields people are all piled up. Where I worked, you are packing and the cutter is right next to you, so there is no way to maintain distance. When workers reported symptoms, there were some supervisors who said, "Just keep quiet and come in to work." Some people didn't have symptoms and they infected everyone else. I think that by now there are very few farmworkers who can say, "I didn't get COVID." I think that getting infected was inevitable. Some people were frightened, even anxious, and I think that they protected themselves better. I have relatives who said, "You can't come to visit." They washed their hands; they washed and disinfected everything. But there were people who said, "If I get infected, I am just going to get infected, that's it." The economic effects impacted all of us, because prices were rising. I know people who are getting evicted from their homes because landlords want to rent or sell them. Food prices are really climbing, especially for me, with my four kids.

I joined Luchadoras del Campo. All members of Luchadoras are farmworkers who work or worked and are relatives of people who work in the fields, so I think it's easier to get the message across because you connect with people. You're in the fields; you're working; and you're talking about what Luchadoras is doing—about our rights, about how you can exercise your rights here in our community, how you can ask for help from agencies. One of the challenges we faced was when people started buying up everything. Nothing was left in stores. Prices were high and wages were low. I was hearing from people who didn't have diapers for their children, things like that. That's why we starting working with organizations that were distributing diapers and food. We delivered hot meals with the United Farm Workers.

We started to take doctors to the fields so that they could talk directly to farmworkers: explain the situation with COVID and encourage them to get vaccinated so they wouldn't be in danger, because us farmworkers, we don't tend to go to doctors much. We get information secondhand, when a friend or a compadre says, "If you get it, you are going to feel like this." That's why we saw the need to take experts to the fields so that people would receive the information firsthand and not have to get it secondhand; so that they wouldn't have to trust what people say but [could hear] what the experts are saying. At first people were surprised, because doctors don't visit the fields. But I think that it was a very good experience, especially after people started conversing with the doctors and started to open up and ask questions. I think it was very spontaneous. The doctors were dressed in casual clothing. We also organized a vaccination clinic. I think that we gave almost three thousand vaccinations.

We decided to write to the governor because we were hearing a lot of things. People said, "We can't go to the store because we're afraid of getting infected." We sent a letter to the governor to request that stores set up a special time for essential workers to visit, as were being established for senior citizens and healthcare workers. We were hearing about people's needs, so we decided to put forward in the letter eight ways that we could help our community. The vaccines we distributed were sent by the office of the governor.

I particularly like being part of Luchadoras because I have had the opportunity to learn so many things. When we have educational meetings, we invite different agencies, and I'm like, "Wow, I didn't know that!" Before, I was very shy. If I had been speaking with you before I would have been saying, "Um, yes. No." I am going to tell you a story. One day I was in the meeting that we had in the Office of the Governor. I had the opportunity to be part of that meeting. And I was thinking that Roselia Bustos, who didn't get an education, who worked in the fields cutting lettuce, is speaking in the Office of the Governor. I was like, "Wow!"

In her account, Bustos confirms what I heard many times in the San Joaquín Valley and other agricultural areas from farmworkers and employees of fruit and vegetable packing plants. Not only did supervisors not implement COVID-19 prevention measures and very rarely provided more than minimal PPE, but they told workers who called to report that they were experiencing symptoms that they would have to come to work or get fired.[4] Luchadoras del Campo was organized precisely through a lateral, egalitarian form of communicability through practices of listening to fellow farmworkers, responding to their concerns, and building alliances with local and state agencies and nongovernmental organizations to confront the immense obstacles farmworkers face. Some activist organizations medicalized their responses to the pandemic, adopting mitigation measures but maintaining their focus on other issues, including working conditions, wages, gender discrimination, sexual abuses in fields and homes, political representation, and building leadership skills. Luchadoras, however, immediately responded to the pandemic's economic, material, and health impacts. Letters to Governor Newsom decried the lack of COVID-19 health education by health professionals for farmworkers, the inaccessibility of health care, and the scarcity of food and other essentials. Luchadoras also asserted the need for "essential worker" hours in stores and delivering boxes that met basic needs to the fields, packing plants, and dairy farms; providing access to unemployment and stimulus funding for the undocumented; protecting basic rights; stopping the rising tide of gender violence; and providing temporary housing. The organization's members knew how difficult it would be for farmworkers, who often work seven days a week and face obstacles of transportation and communication, to sign up for vaccination appointments and travel to vaccine sites. They accordingly organized a vaccination program that provided shots in the fields.

One of the group's primary goals is to develop leadership and advocacy skills among farmworkers. Indeed, Bustos crafts her account as a teleological narrative that reflects a movement from incommunicability and timidity through events in which she gained knowledge and understanding to the emergence of a strong, confident voice. Hampered by the lack of a supportive educational environment in schools and at home as a child, Bustos reflects eloquently on her personal transformation—the growth of her knowledge base, communicative skills, and self-confidence, as manifested in speaking at a meeting in the office of the governor. Her narrative orchestrates a complex web of contrastive voices, such as of people who strictly embrace COVID-19 protocols and others who projected a fatalistic incommunicability. The first-person plural—*nosotros*, the masculine form, for farmworkers and *nosotras*, the feminine, for members of Luchadoras—enables her to position herself within both farmworker and female activist communities. It thus undergirds her claim to be in the perfect position to close a biocommunicable gap between doctors who do not usually go to the fields and farmworkers with limited access to health services.

Indeed, a striking feature of her testimony lies in the biocommunicable model that shaped her efforts to bring health education and health care to the fields. The Luchadoras' position as activists and practices of listening to and learning from fellow farmworkers did not lead her to reject a unilinear, hierarchically ordered biocommunicable model of health education. She instead echoed dominant discourses about Latinx populations in depicting some farmworkers as viewing disease fatalistically and citing what seem to be personal decisions rather than access issues, medical profiling, and translational problems as limiting access to health care. Rather than seeing farmworkers as partners in producing knowledge about health and health inequities, she characterized lateral exchanges as producing defective secondhand information. In short, without intervention farmworkers are incommunicable, as her use of quoted speech suggests. What is required is biocommunicability, bringing "the experts" to the fields so that knowledge can be transferred "firsthand." Rather than participating in the production of incommunicability, however,

Luchadoras found Spanish-speaking Latinx physicians who, she reports, engaged in respectful exchanges that enabled farmworkers to converse with the physicians and "to open up and ask questions" in a manner that she described as very spontaneous (*muy natural*). Luchadoras suggests how some activists were able to demedicalize their agendas to prioritize justice in health, even as it indicates the way biocommunicability can continue to structure such efforts.

The pandemic also augmented educational inequities for working-class and racialized populations, especially those living in multigenerational houses packed with "essential workers." My interviews with parents, teachers and administrators from kindergarten through grade 12 (K–12), colleges, and universities and Latinx students revealed how poor internet connections, little access to computers or tablets, lack of quiet space, and vast differences in the support available to people who could not "work from home" mushroomed educational inequities during the pandemic. Research by the Office for Civil Rights of the US Department of Education (2021) provides a broad assessment of these impacts. Many low-income and BIPOC K–12 students and those living with disabilities essentially lost two years of schooling, massively expanding educational injustices. For some, the burdens that constrained efforts to push ahead with educational trajectories included caring for ailing relatives, arranging for medical and other services, and translating for them over the phone or by telemedicine. For families that included undocumented members—who were ineligible for federal COVID-19 relief—the economic effects of the pandemic were often particularly crushing.

Gisselle Rosales, Undergraduate Student, UC Berkeley

I am a first-generation, low-income Latinx student. Both of my parents were born in Mexico. They migrated to the United States when they were very young to work and provide for their families who stayed in Mexico. Since we were very little, our parents always encouraged us to go to school and work hard. I'm very fortunate that due to their hard work and sacrifices I could get a good education and apply to colleges and get accepted to UC Berkeley. In March 2020 I had been at Berkeley for two months already. It was my very first time being away from my parents, so I was homesick a lot. I was starting to have friends and was getting used to being here. I remember talking to one of my friends about COVID-19 and how we didn't think it would get to the United States and spread so quickly. Then a week later, we went on spring break. And we realized we weren't coming back. Suddenly, two weeks away from school turned into months and months away. I ended up leaving Berkeley to go back home, and I remember feeling very stressed because I had to go back to Berkeley to move out of my dorm. At that time, I was very scared of COVID-19. I was scared of getting sick and getting my family sick, because they had to travel with me to pick up my stuff and move out.

Schoolwise, it was very difficult. I'd been surrounded by other students, so we'd study together. Then suddenly I was back home with family. I couldn't really find the time to study because I wanted to help my parents. It was definitely a difficult situation to manage and balance out. I had to babysit my nephew while being on Zoom lectures, because everyone else was working. My nephew was about six months old during that time, so he was very impatient and needed a lot of attention. My sister would ask, "No one can take care of him—are you free?" Even though I had classes, I'd say yes, because there was no one else. So it was just kind of taking things day by day and figuring it out as I went. Many of the times that I was helping out family, I felt guilty that I wasn't doing homework. And when I was doing homework, I was feeling guilty that I wasn't able to be with my family, to help them. I remember sometimes being locked in my room, because I had to do meetings or get stuff done. I could hear them in the background talking, having conversations about their worries. It was difficult to manage being home during the pandemic.

I remember my parents were super worried about finances. My mom cleans houses, and she found that a lot of the time the people that she cleans houses for were canceling on her, so she barely had work. My grandma lives with my aunt, and my aunt works with my mom to clean houses. I remember that they would be very stressed about going to work, because, I mean, you clean houses: you're going into someone's house, and you're touching everything that they touch. So my mother and aunt were very worried that they might get COVID-19 and then pass it on to my grandma. And my grandma is ninety years old right now, so she's at very, very high-risk. And my dad, he fixes cars. People were barely going out during the pandemic, so he also lost a lot of work, because there were barely any cars coming in that he could fix. My sister is a registered nurse. I remember that she was extremely worried about going to work, because she took care of COVID-19 patients. My nephew was only months old, so she was very scared of bringing COVID to the house and maybe getting him sick or getting other family members sick.

I remember my mom calling me a bunch of times worrying that there was, like, no canned food or there was no toilet paper in the stores or napkins. Yeah, I remember she would be like, "How are we going to find stuff? What are we going to do?" So listening to all of that while being over here kind of made me feel powerless, like I couldn't do anything to help them. My mom was dealing with a lot of stress during that time, because she wasn't making a lot of income. I remember her telling me that during this time that she was feeling very tired, physically tired; like, she had no energy to get up and do stuff. When she did have work, she kind of pushed herself to make sure she went, because those were the only days that she could work and earn income. But she continued to tell me that she didn't feel very well. And after a while, she decided to go visit the doctor, and she found out that she had high blood pressure. She had never suffered from high blood pressure before, so I think for her it was very difficult to learn how to manage that.

In a discussion I had with my parents, one of the worries my mom had was that I would be back home and wouldn't be able to focus and get work done. So after talking with my parents, we ultimately came to the decision to have me move back to Berkeley. That's ultimately why I decided to move into a dorm, but with that came other issues. We were told that we couldn't see people who didn't live on the same floor of our building, and we couldn't go outside of the building except to get food or access to emergency services. Although I understood those rules when I signed on to live on campus, I didn't initially think that it would affect me so much. But I remember I barely went outside, and I barely talked to people. That experience was extremely isolating. I was already struggling with depression at that time, so it just kind of made things worse for me. I remember it was very hard for me to focus and get work done. It was tiring, being in this room locked up almost the whole day, every single day, sitting in front of a computer, sitting in front of my desk all day, just going to classes online. It was just very difficult. I can't really express how I was feeling at that time. I remember that one day I just completely broke down and cried on the floor, because I felt like I had no one to talk to. I couldn't go see my friends that often because of the COVID-19 restrictions. I was experiencing a lot of negative thoughts and felt like I was in this hole that I would never get out of. I reached out to my mom a lot of times, but I think it was a very difficult thing to describe to her.

Rosales's poignant account performs a symphony of voices: those of friends, classmates, parents, aunt, sister, and infant nephew, not to mention the way she quotes her own shifting inner speech. A tenor of sacrifice, dedication, and hope regarding gaining admission to UC Berkeley turns to homesickness when she finds herself away from home for the first time in January 2020. Rosales reports that this voice disappeared in only a couple of months as she made friends and adopted the strategy that many first-generation students use to pool knowledge and support: studying together. With the arrival of the pandemic, all of the voices in her narrative symphony are transformed into different inflections of an idiom of distress (Nichter 1981). Rather than being actively, dialogically engaged with them, however, her narrative progressively portrays these other voices as increasingly muted, leaving only her troubled inner speech. Biocommunicability was a constant presence in her narrative as a public health student, even though its role was primarily indirect as the virus and the impact of mitigation measures induced anxiety, economic precarity, and, in the end, a feeling of incarceration ("being locked up"). Rosales never questioned or challenged guidelines—she "understood those rules when signing on to live on campus"—but neither did she foresee their psychologically devastating effects.

At home, Rosales was lucky to have adequate WiFi and a quiet space, which many other working-class Latinx students lacked. Some attended courses on their telephones in front of cafés. Rosales was also fortunate that close family members did not contract COVID-19. In her household, all adults were economically affected by the pandemic, and no one could work remotely. Her account beautifully connects economic inequities with life-threatening health issues as her mother's intense worries about the sudden collapse of the household's income—and the fear of infecting her elderly mother—provided the context in which she first experienced acute symptoms of hypertension. Back home, Rosales immediately reentered the network of care that sustained her family, but other than helping her sister with childcare, she could offer no financial resources to assist a suddenly strapped family. Being forced to continue the same class load from home without the support of peers confronted Rosales with a clash between worlds and competing demands, constructing a collision between conflicting types of ordinary ethics, as emerged in Professor Smith's account. Note that even as these other voices shaped her experience of being home during the pandemic, she seems unable to respond actively to them. In response to her sister's question, "I'd say yes," providing a one-word acceptance of a familial responsibility without articulating her complex feelings or how caring for an infant would jeopardize her class participation. She places her parents' "conversations about their worries" not in active dialogue with her but "in the background." Her mother does call Rosales "a bunch of times" to convey her desperation over the situation and the shortage of goods in stories, but it sparks less a sense of active engagement than one of being "powerless, like I couldn't do anything to help them."

Viewing a conflict between home and school as threatening Rosales's educational success, the parents and daughter continued to position this goal as the priority. Rosales was able to devote all of her time to her studies. Nevertheless, it was harder to find classmates willing to study together and offer emotional support when fellow students were Zoom tiles rather than smiling faces encountered when exiting classrooms. She seemed to become increasingly distanced from potentially supportive voices, even her mother's. Despite their intimacy, conveying the psychological struggles she was experiencing in a college dorm room "was a very difficult thing to describe to her." She was left with her own voice, but even that failed her: not only was she unable to "express how [she] was feeling at that time" when she recorded these reflections in September 2022, but it appears that the only way she could express the depth of her distress at the time was when she "just completely broke down and cried on the floor."

Rosales thus bravely points to the other epidemic: the avalanche of mental health problems that emerged or were exacerbated by fear, loneliness, isolation, and, as Smith and Rosales both beautifully articulate, the impossibility of meeting all of one's obligations. I am pleased to say that Rosales was able to find a way out of the bleak space that she so graphically describes. The Spring 2021 Latinx Autoethnography Collective allowed her and other students to share their stories with peers; they reported feeling a bit less alone during our weekly meetings. We discussed issues related to COVID-19 with Clara Mantini-Briggs on board, and exchanges were dialogic and laterally organized. Returning to in-person classes in the 2021–22 academic year provided Rosales with a much more supportive environment. In spring 2022, her participation in a podcast project directed by Dr. Mantini-Briggs and hosted by UC Berkeley's Latinx Research Center allowed her to share her story publicly. Her remarks are drawn from her contribution to the podcast; with her permission, I use her name. Another participant in the podcast project, Brandon Rubio, commented on the loss of his dream of being at UC Berkeley after working full time to put himself through community college, only to be—he felt—kicked off the space of the campus after a few months. After a year and a half of remote classes—his final semesters—he reported being allowed back onto campus only when he was required to return books to a box in front of a closed library. The COVID-19 pandemic crushed his family's dream of watching his graduation from UC Berkeley.

Complexities and Contradictions of Professional Pandemic Care

I must apologize: I fear that I have created a false impression. I argued in chapter 7 that health professionals attempted to secure a monopoly on the production of knowledge about COVID-19, one that cast laypeople—including those attempting to help figure what the heck was going on—into realms of incommunicability, often stigmatizing ones, such as the categories of "anti-vaxxers" and "conspiracy theorists." At the same time, they largely passed along the burden of care to laypeople, defining care in ways that left out the immense labor laypeople provided to keep family members, friends, and neighbors safe, fed, housed, schooled, and better able to cope with the COVID-19 mental health pandemic. I mentioned that laypeople were largely left on their own with SARS-CoV-2 infections, unless cases were complicated and required professional care, even as I pointed to exceptions I found in the work of community health centers.

If I had not spent hours and hours listening to nurses, physicians, paramedics/firefighters, and public health officials, I might have stopped there, probably losing the trust of my health professional readers. Laypeople would thus lose a crucial opportunity to gain insight into the multiplicity of forms of labor that health professionals provided and the challenges they confronted. Many sources, including mainstream journalists and websites, have described the clinical dilemmas they faced at work. My focus on in/communicability and relations between knowledge production and care open up different angles on how these professionals encountered quandaries, complexities, and contradictions that were often as overwhelming as those faced by laypeople. Unfortunately, during the pandemic, lay versus professional boundaries have often turned into stereotypes and affective relations that range from distanced adulation to failures of empathy to animosity. Here health professionals tell a different story—one that suggests many similarities with what patients and other laypeople faced. Even as they clung to their position as COVID-19 biocommunicability amplifiers, many felt that they, too, were thrust into incommunicability—sometimes, seemingly, by design.

Professionals' accounts generally privilege technology-intensive forms of care, from supplemental oxygen and newly available medications to ventilators and intubation, that, by and large, are available only in the highly specialized clinical settings in which they work. My interviews and ethnographic observations also suggest that these forms of care have engendered reactions from patients and their relatives that range from gratitude to distance, anger, and death threats. In dialogues with a range of professionals, I want to suggest, however, that these contradictions of COVID care have often jeopardized these professionals' belief in themselves, the facilities in which they work, their patients, and the medical attention they can provide. As we know, the pandemic has led far too many health professionals to resign, retire, or move to jobs they hope will free them from work situations that engendered feelings of failure and even despair. Listening to their stories can help get us beyond what, using such labels as "burnout" and "the Great Resignation," has been too quickly summarized, too summarily reduced to forms of individualism associated with resilience and resignation. As these testimonies suggest, there is much more of the story about the pandemic, in/communicability, COVID-19 knowledge and care, and about what is often (and I think mistakenly) labeled anti-science and anti-medicine to be told.

Six Paramedics/Firefighters from a Bay Area Station

CAPTAIN BILL MURPHY: A whole part about reaching to the community is trying to make a connection, to make it feel like they're important, to make them feel like they can trust us whatever the case is. Our driver is a religious man, and he would link with people. He'd see some identifying mark or a cross or something on the wall, and he would stop and pray with them, just to deescalate their situation. We see cues. I might be like, "Hey, Ellie: I see a lot of movies over here. Go give him some movie quotes." Or Lewis, "Hey, there's a lot of music stuff." We each have a little knack for something, right?

Then all of sudden it hits, and everything outside of these walls is stopped, but the bells keep going off. And people are still going to be sick. We've still got to go. Everything changed. I've been doing this since I was nineteen. I'm going to be forty-three. And I hadn't seen that much change in probably fifteen to twenty years of my career. In a week, things changed. It changed so fast that the administration couldn't keep up with it. Rules and regs were changing like two or three times a day. "OK," I thought, "there's so much change going on, we've got to figure this out."

You know the obvious stuff that's going to kill us: on the freeway, in fires on top of a roof, cutting a hole with fire below you—the stuff that's really transparent. But this was, like, we couldn't see it. You didn't know who had it. The challenge is that we don't do things alone, which is good for me, because I'm not a good loner. I'm a twin, so I like being around people. But I was trying not to show that I was worried about going in. So I would gear up and say, "Nah. You guys wait outside. I'm not comfortable sending somebody in. I don't have any kids. I'll go in there. You've got a little kid at home."

ELLIE JONES: And for me, at that time, I was a new medic, so it was, like, definitely kind of turning things upside down. I was the canary going into these houses, because I lived alone with a partner who's also in emergency medical services. I never really felt scared like people with families did.

LEWIS OSMONDSON: The call volume just plummeted. We get a lot of calls for people who can't deal. And then people just *could* deal—they would rather figure stuff out, so we wouldn't get called for a lot of the normal things.

BILL MURPHY: The general public was starting to have a little mistrust in us. I wasn't used to that feeling. We would go places and hear, "Right now we don't want you in here." So the first time in my career you're not welcome. And you're like, "Well, no. You called us. We're here to help you." And they're like, "No, we don't want you in the house." Because they think we have it, we're the ones exposed all over with it. I mean, that was a little switch. That doesn't mean you can't have heart attacks, strokes. The normal human issues were still happening. But people were too scared to call. Sometimes we'd show up and they were *really sick* but would say, "I don't wanna go to the hospital right now, I don't want COVID." I'd say, "But you're having a heart attack. Do you want to die here?"

The community was confused on what to call for. When we did get called, it was often for some kind of COVID-related issue. All of a sudden it was just this kind of crazy, dramatic situation where dispatch would let us know if someone was possibly positive for COVID or was experiencing COVID-like symptoms, and all of our protocols around what we wear on calls completely changed. Up until that point, we'd go in like this [in their firefighter uniforms] to any call and not be too worried about it. Occasionally someone would pick up the flu or something. And then you started becoming afraid of anything you touched, and you didn't know what was going to be the thing that might be what you would take home to your family. I think the issue for us was that if we were just coming in here and interacting, that would have been fine, if that was all it was. But then we all went back home to our families every four-day-off period.

ELLIE JONES: It was definitely pretty isolating. You know, my friends didn't want to see me, like, be anywhere even near me—they didn't want to talk even from outside a bar! And I felt really bad about it.

BILL MURPHY: This house is really good about physical fitness but even more about mental and emotional fitness. We get to know each other here. We trust each other. If we don't take care of each other in the walls here, or the agency as a whole—if we can't shore up the workers to go out and perform—the community sure doesn't care. Just think about it. If you call 911, do you really care about what human comes to help you? You don't think about it as a human who's coming to help you. You think of it as an entity of the fire department, the firefighters, the paramedics. You're not like, "Do you think *they're* having problems, too, when they get here?" When they call 911, they don't care about *my* problems; they don't care about the human who is going to help them. And that's going to be the interesting part about telling stories: there are humans doing all the work on the front lines, even though they've experienced new problems, mental health issues. So sometimes, us talking about it, it feels like it's a relief, you know—you care about it, you're talking to us about it, you're getting our perspective, it kind of feels a little validating. I'd say this is therapeutic.

When I contacted the captain, Bill Murphy, who leads a crew in a Bay Area fire station, he proposed a conversation with all six members of the "house." As we sat around the dining table, it soon became apparent that they had talked about what they wanted to say. Few questions were necessary. They were not about to let the communicative inequities patterned into research interviews or the visitor's professorial status structure what they said or how they organized their remarks. Timothy Tangherlini (1998) carefully documents the importance of narratives in the lives of EMTs and paramedics, a job in which dramatic challenges punctuate long periods of downtime, thus providing lots of opportunities for storytelling. Before I arrived, the crew had discussed which observations to offer and what stories to tell. Rather than allowing me to fit them into my professional norms of narrative elicitation through interview techniques, they politely demanded that I surrender my research, my presence, and my recorder to their narrative practices, which, as in responding to calls, granted the leading and coordinating voice to the captain.

They first taught me about the social organization of the house. One woman and five men spend forty-eight hours together continuously on a shift, sharing meals, conversation, training, and, of course, calls, before returning to their homes for four days off. They are trained as firefighters and paramedics and identify as health professionals. They emphasized that only about 5 percent of calls are related to fires, most are other medical emergencies, including many mental health issues. Beyond an introduction to their lifeworld, this presentation fit a pattern that we have already seen with Smith, Montaño, and, more briefly, Rosales—that of structuring COVID-19 narratives with an initial, pre-pandemic section depicting relatively stable patterns in which actors possessed the knowledge needed to fulfill their roles followed by a pandemic descent into chaos and uncertainty.

The testimony thus continues as Murphy further widens the lens of care as it was extended prior to the pandemic. As trained paramedics, the team was solidly located within biocommunicability, involving precise execution of skills guided by physicians, periodically refreshed in trainings from the doctor who served as the fire district's medical officer. Although laypeople were seen as recipients of interventions, not health education, the team's work opened up complementary communicable circuits. When entering a domestic or other space during an emergency, the crew would find ways of "trying to make a connection." There is an instrumental dimension here, because one goal was to "de-escalate" forms of panic among family members and others on the scene, enabling paramedics to concentrate on providing vital services. It is clear, however, that this "connection" involves focusing on a range of concerns in such situations through what I might call a mode of distributed care. Edwin Hutchins (1995) observes that knowledge is not simply lodged in individual minds but can require know-how distributed across a broader range of people; his example was the operation of a large sailing vessel. In an engine crew, members use dimensions of their individual lives—religion, movies, music—to personalize the care they provided and make the people they encountered "feel like they're important." The crew thus drew on other communicabilities that were part of their off-time repertoires and used them, on an ad hoc basis, in conjunction with the skills they were trained to use as firefighter/paramedics. In suggesting that not all crews share this practice, Murphy pointed to the specific practices of care that the group had collaboratively created, going beyond job requirements and public expectations.

Then COVID-19 transformed the landscape of care. Firefighters/paramedics train constantly, turning skills and regulations into embodied practices to meet specific emergencies. Like a dancer who gets in perfect sync with the

choreographer and other dancers through training and rehearsals, firefighters need to build a communicable network in which education, fire department guidelines, training sessions, and collaboration with fellow crew members during forty-eight-hour periods of continual interaction come together
in ways that are fine-tuned and in keeping with a unique moment and situation and ongoing instructions from the captain. In Pierre Bourdieu's ([1972]
1977) terms, these forms of practice turn bodies, movements, gazes, words,
fires, heart attacks, acute mental illness, and technologies into modernist
symphonies where cacophony and improvisation form part of the music.
As Murphy suggests, the essential practice had not changed substantially in
decades, allowing this synchronization to settle into a durable, embodied,
conscious-cum-unconscious, profoundly ingrained set of dispositions—in
Bourdieu's terms, a *habitus*.

Then, "in a week," this routinized set of affordances became not only insufficient and outmoded but potential sources of danger. New guidelines
became a top-down steady stream, changing "like two or three times a day."
If the biocommunicable basis of paramedic/firefighter care requires training bodies and minds and rehearsing their choreographed synchronizations,
suspending an established habitus plus decreeing new forms of practice
constantly without allowing them to become dispositions produced an experience of incommunicability. Even situations that seemed familiar—heart
attacks, strokes, small fires, and the like—became uncanny, given the possibility that SARS-CoV-2 might be invisibly lurking along the edges. In sync
with Smith's testimony and the interviews with healthcare workers in the
United Kingdom and United States conducted by Block and Vindrola-Padros
(2021), the gaps between training, knowledge, equipment, and shifting relations with people in crisis required constant improvisation, attempting "to
figure this out" anew with each call. The social organization of distributed
care shifted radically: it was no longer the skills and off-duty activities of
crew members that shaped the roles each played. Instead, drawing on intimate knowledge of one another's lives, what counted most was how their
family situations shaped projected futures—the threat of taking COVID-19
home. If possible, only one crew member would enter a dwelling to minimize
the possibility of infection.

The initial part of the narrative points to a repertoire of practices for
quickly devising cartographies of spaces into which firefighters/paramedics
must suddenly insert themselves, including human and human actors, such
as fires, passing vehicles, weapons, unstable structures, and other potentially

threatening elements. Murphy reveals some of the backstage metapragmatic cues he used to mobilize the crew to collectively transform maps into embodied words and actions. Suddenly, their cartographic practices utterly failed. Signaling a major affective reorientation, new domestic or other spaces no longer became opportunities to connect: each call was perceived in terms of its potential for infection. Providing care—a job they still took seriously—was suddenly reduced to identifying what had to be done and wrapping things up as quickly and safely as possible. A change of great significance for my interlocutors was losing their uniforms, a key sartorial symbol of their status and professional identity. Disposable suits were less likely to bring viruses back to the station or to take them out on the next call. The only woman, Ellie Jones, had joined the crew six months earlier. She noted how COVID-19 turned the social organization "upside down" by giving her a lead role on calls because she did not have to worry about infecting family members. Even as she experienced uncertainty and vulnerability, feeling like a canary in a mineshaft, Jones provided a note of bravado, reporting that she "never really felt scared," seemingly unlike her older, more experienced male colleagues. The COVID-19 pandemic fractured gender and seniority hierarchies.

The reactions from the individuals encountered on calls were even more disconcerting for their identities as health professionals. Murphy noted that previously people would call them for nonemergency situations just because they "can't deal" with life. Like other EMTs and paramedics, they talked about people who would dial 911 frequently, drunk, stoned, or just seeking attention. When the pandemic began, the volume of calls plummeted. More strikingly, people's reactions, from fear to hostility, marked a sudden change in how the responders were perceived: less as people who could connect and provide care than as dangerous reservoirs of COVID-19 infection. The first point of patient contact with broader medical systems, they became specters of the microbes waiting to infect them at the other end of the ambulance ride—the dreaded hospital space. Osmondson reported, in an understated fashion, "I wasn't used to that feeling." The disjuncture between calling 911 for help and rejecting the professionals it yielded provided a new sense of uncertainty, a "kind of crazy, dramatic situation," requiring new strategies for dealing with *dis*connection. Suddenly communicable solidarity was out the window, and many people refused the paramedics' care even for such acute and life-threatening conditions as heart attacks and strokes.

This insight takes us beyond issues of improvisation, beyond how they constantly devised new ways to cope with COVID-19 challenges. Rather, they had to ask themselves questions that overturned decades of basic professional assumptions: What is care? Who wants it? Who can provide it? How can an offer of care be interpreted as an intrusion, itself a "risk," even by the person who requested it? Professionals who considered falling through a roof or being hit by a rubbernecker on a freeway as just part of the job suddenly had to ask themselves: What are the costs of giving care for caregivers? And, perhaps more pressingly, for their families? Here we see a basic feature of narrative told by a wide range of people as COVID-19 experiences led them to question and sometimes revise basic perspectives of themselves, the nature of their work, their futures, and the world.

The "house" is a community of care in another sense. Murphy suggested that "firefighters live a double life. How? Because I have a family here that I spend 2,900 hours a year with. Nobody spends time like that." The crew built on this intimacy during the pandemic to deal with the uncertainty, fear, and partial loss of the status of caregivers and its biocommunicable basis. The need to support one another as much in the station as during dangerous assignments was crucial. Murphy stressed the importance of affective connections in the station in contrast to the lack of empathic reciprocity outside; he projected this dimension as shared by other "frontline" workers. Using the rhetorical device of ironically constructing a hypothetical lay voice as sensitively addressing the firefighters'/paramedics' own lives—"Do you think *they're* having problems, too?"—Murphy projects public concern with caregivers' mental health issues as being switched off through the act of dialing 911. In a theme that would emerge repeatedly, Jones suggested that life outside the station was "definitely pretty isolating" because her friends perceived her as a source of infection. They did not want to learn about her "problems" or about how her work had changed. Herein lies yet another failure of care, in this case coming from intimates rather than "the public." Beyond the "house," there seemed to be no back channel for caregivers. Even as they faced fears that received practices could not contain, their powerful closed circuit of decompressive storytelling did not prove sufficient when their identities as care providers were suddenly called into question and they worried about passing their job's most acute danger back to family members. Problem-solvers par excellence, they could not devise a Lockean fix to restore communicability, and their increasingly out-of-touch superiors were of little help. They defined my listening as care, noting that it "kind of feels a little validating" in a new, complex, and unpredictable world of challenges and restricted possibilities for giving and receiving care.

Jana Nagy, ICU Nurse, San Francisco Bay Area

I knew the ICU is for me. I kind of always knew that in nursing school. In the ICU you are assessing and gathering a lot of data and then interpreting it and acting on it in real time. So it's much more interesting. I like puzzles, I guess, or problem-solving, and that's what it is all day, every day. So I moved to the ICU. I got an orientation, just a month. We were just so short-staffed; we had no resources, no breaks. As a new nurse, you want to ask for help a lot, but if your coworkers are spread thin, and they're having to make so many movements, and charge nurses have patients, and it's just totally out of ratio, you feel like an extra burden.

The work stuff brought on heavy anxiety, especially in the beginning. You were hearing the news coming out of Italy; you heard of nurses and doctors sleeping at the hospital. Putting myself in that position, I was, like, "Oh my God. Am I going [to] be sleeping?" In the beginning, you were so nervous all the time, like twelve hours of nerves; that wears you down. I was really stressed about the responsibility I had taken on. I had this oath, and "I'm now a nurse, and I have this responsibility to be a first responder." It was more than I had bargained for. "I'm the only person on a BART [Bay Area Rapid Transit] train, and I don't know if I can touch anything or breathe. I'm just sitting here, just as everybody else is staying home. [*She covers her face with her hands, eyes opened wide.*] I can just feel the quiet on the streets, and I'm just thinking, "What have I done?" So that was the beginning.

Things changed big time in the hospital. Every day you came in to work and there was some new rule, or new policy, or a new way of doing things, like every day. That was so stressful. It was everything from how much PPE to wear to who goes into the rooms. In the beginning, nurses were the only ones who went in the room. We would bring iPads in for the doctors to see. Dietary wouldn't bring the trays. For nurses, it felt like we were just thrown to the wolves. I was so scared. Personal protective equipment was scarce at that time. We were told to bring in our own things, so I'm on the computer buying disposable shower caps. I bought lab chemistry goggles. I'm wearing a shower cap and goggles, so I looked ridiculous. And then I spent, like, $60 buying a paint respirator thing that I never ended up wearing. But you were just scared into "I need to buy this." There were fluctuations in PPE all the time. At this point, we were out of gowns, so we were taking the gown off and hanging it and putting it back on. But to do that and not touch any of the things and stay clean is nearly impossible, because things hit you. Basically, all the things you were taught that were essential you just weren't able to do, like effectively stay clean or sterile. And at that time, I don't think we had a concept of how much transmission was through contact. We were so stressed.

Charles Briggs: How effectively were you able to communicate with patients?

Nagy: It was really difficult. I mean, there's the obvious things like patients that are hard of hearing and read lips, but with the masks it's nearly impossible. A lot of times, I used to yell into these people's ears. Then you add PAPRS [powered air-purifying respirators]; they have this motor, and air is buzzing. So you can sometimes just not hear your patient at all, especially if they're sick and quietly talking. That was definitely really challenging. Then communicating with each other, too, in the room can be difficult if you're both using PAPRS. And then communicating to people outside the room. With COVID isolation, sometimes the doctors are standing outside the room, or the charge nurses, and they're communicating with you. So we would write on whiteboards and hold them up against the window or write right on the window with an erasable marker. Sometimes you avoid going in the room because of all the isolation; you may not go in to tell a patient about something if it's not 100 percent necessary. But that still breaks down those channels of communication, because you're keeping that patient more isolated than you would otherwise. You treat that patient differently.

During the second surge we were so overwhelmed with patients that I had two really sick patients. If a patient's really sick, we should be one to one. You're asking for help, and you can't get it. One patient is having fatal arrhythmias, and I'm having to shock them, and the other patient is desaturating and needs to be intubated immediately, she has COVID. And she has the awareness that she may never come out. I had this emotional thing. I was crying because she had her Bible out and was asking me to pack these things up for her family—the reality of it was palpable. I think people are burned out because when we're short-staffed, you can't get vacations, you don't get a break—you have a twelve-hour crazy day, and you don't get a break. You get to eat when you can in the corner. It's like you don't want to show up the next day.

It's just not fair, not fair working conditions. Patients shouldn't want nurses taking care of them that are overworked and tired and working double shifts and are exhausted and loopy.

I think I did a really good job of compartmentalizing and not feeling the full weight of each individual patient experience. But when I have patients that are at end of life, I definitely cry with the families or to myself, especially during those family end-of-life conversations where they have to make the decision to let people go. I find those really hard. I'm wondering if I have a lot of personal and professional things to feel from these last two years that I haven't quite allowed myself to feel. Because, along with this professional element, there's a whole personal element. For instance, in the beginning I had roommates. And because of all the uncertainty, they didn't know how to handle that I could be bringing the virus into their home while they are just working from home and sheltering in place. So they didn't want to live with me anymore. I did end up having to move out, so I lost my apartment. I was searching for apartments, and people were looking for people that were "COVID safe"; they were posting that kind of thing. In my head, I'm like, "Who's going to want to bring in a nurse at this point?" I ended up moving into a studio. I had to live alone. And some days I'd be driving to work on the empty freeway and be like, "I wish I could just stay at home today." I was mostly nervous for my family and how long I wouldn't be able to see my parents. What I was going through was so hard, I needed support. I needed people and my family. At the beginning of the pandemic to probably mid-April, I literally lived with a burning pain, anxiety pain, in my chest. It was a physical manifestation of the stress. I'd have to, at night, talk myself down. I was so stressed about going to work the next day, I'd say, "Just relax. You need to sleep."

The best way to describe burnout is that it comes from nurses' being trained a certain way, trained to give a certain level of care, but being spread thin or out of ratio—you're not giving a level of care you're trained to give. That's what goes home with you, you replay over, at night, the corners that you had to cut, even though you took an oath not to cut corners. The hospital system is forcing us to risk our own licenses and risk people's safety because of the money. That's sad, and that's what makes it hard to be a nurse right now. For me, I still have a lot to unpack.

Jana Nagy's vivid account highlights many features I encountered in interviews with ICU personnel, particularly nurses, that other researchers cite as common features of pandemic ER and ICU labor. In addition to stress and exhaustion (Craw, Buckley, and Miller-Day 2022), Stephanie Pangborn and her colleagues' (2023) research on frontline healthcare providers echoed issues of the impact on mental health, lack of social support, concerns about infecting family members, and complaints about hospital administrators maximizing profits by overworking staff. At the same time, focusing on how Nagy entextualized these issues can provide us with new insights into what shaped her experience and how it negatively affected her deep commitment to ICU nursing—a topic that is of great concern to the nursing profession and US health care in general.

Nagy's testimony resembles the coming-of-age-in-the-pandemic narratives I often heard while researching a Venezuelan cholera epidemic with Clara Mantini-Briggs (Briggs and Mantini-Briggs 2003). Many doctors and nurses—Clara among them—had completed their training shortly before finding themselves in the middle of a pandemic. After graduating in the spring of 2019 from one of the country's leading nursing schools, Nagy, in her late twenties, struggled to find a job: "No one wanted to hire new nurses at that time because they didn't want to train them." What a different world for nurses today! Nagy worked in a related field of nursing until she could land a job in an ICU in a for-profit health system in August 2020. Finding that "greed" led to inadequate staffing, she moved to a large public hospital in the fall of 2021. The intensity and demands of working in these situations profoundly shaped their professional identities. Nagy is also an excellent exemplar of the ICU and ER nurses and doctors I interviewed in that she was deeply attracted to this highly demanding position. The reasons interviewees gave varied, from "being an adrenaline junkie" to enjoying the intimacy you can build with patients in spaces with low staff-patient ratios and often extended stays to the sense of it being a "team environment" to Nagy's discussion of the intellectual challenges. Such narratives often trace the form of the ritual process that I learned from my beloved teacher Victor Turner (1969), involving a predictable progression from being a neophyte through a liminal stage in which mature members guide them through difficult transitions as their identities, bodies, and natural-cultural relations are transformed to achieving the status they aspire to attain. For Nagy and other professionals whose careers began during the pandemic, the mentorship they expected from experienced nurses was not available, due not simply to the immediate effects of SARS-CoV-2 but also to an avalanche of factors that included ways that health systems attempted to offset lost revenues from other services and often reaped greater profits during a pandemic. This ritual disruption structures her narrative.

Nagy thus confronted a disruption of biocommunicability. As for other health professionals, graduating from nursing school was not enough: on-the-job training and orientation to a particular ICU were crucial. An ICU filled with COVID-19 patients stretched experienced nurses so thin that they had little time to help. There was not enough biocommunicable labor to go around. Having already felt "pretty heavy anxiety" after hearing news reports about the COVID-19 experiences of nurses and doctors in Italy, the gap between what she had learned in school and the labor she had to perform during twelve-hour shifts left her worn down and "nervous all the time." Murphy had a firefighter/paramedic habitus firmly in place before he faced multiple daily changes in "rules and regs." Contrastively, Nagy could not fall back on a solid foundation when her daily return to work faced her with "some new rule, or new policy, or a new way of doing things." Given the lack of additional training, dangerous staffing levels, and lack of time to assimilate new regulations, Nagy felt as if she spent twelve hours a day in an incommunicable world, not to mention the commutes on each side that made her acutely aware of the distance that separated her from the lives of other professionals.

Nagy carefully explained why the care offered in ICUs and COVID-19 wards did not look like the smiling doctors pictured on billboards and in magazine advertisements for physician groups and hospitals. In the ICU, the model of doctor-patient biocommunicability fell to the wayside as doctors and nurses were masked and often wore PAPRs and other PPE, including face plates sometimes, in rooms with noisy air-filtration systems. Some ICU personnel pasted large pictures of themselves with their names on the front of their suits, hoping to lessen the depersonalizing effects of COVID-19 technologies. Nagy honestly reported that these difficulties in speaking with COVID-19 ICU patients could spark reluctance to attempt communication, thereby increasing patients' often fatal descent into incommunicability and affecting the quality of care. As an ICU nursing supervisor noted, the very concept of communication became irrelevant for many COVID-19 patients shortly after they entered the ICU: "Many times, once a person is intubated for COVID, they're going to get some medicine to go to sleep, and they're never going to wake up. That's it. I don't know exactly what the percentages are, but it's a high percentage of people that once they're intubated, they're just not going to survive the illness."

Like other laypeople who adopted an adversarial relationship to health professionals during the pandemic, Frank Miller criticized what he interpreted as an impersonal, uncaring tenor of care afforded acutely ill COVID-19 patients. As she similarly laments the incommunicable chasm separating her from her COVID-19 patients and its adverse effects on care, Nagy challenges the assertion that it is the product of arrogance or disdain. Her vivid account points to the risk of anthropomorphizing acute care as a relationship between two classes of human beings—providers and patients—and thereby missing the central role of technologies and viruses. This feeling of incommunicability extended to colleagues. Nagy reported that "in the beginning, nurses were the only ones who went in the room" with patients. Exchanges between nurses in patients' rooms and physicians and nursing supervisors outside were so problematic that they were often reduced to writing messages on whiteboards or windows. Nagy's account metaphorically crossed species: "It felt like we were just thrown to the wolves."

Accounts by Nagy and other ICU personnel extend an issue that my firefighter/paramedic interlocutors raised: a failure of care *for* health workers. A Mental Health America survey (2020) reported that nurses lacked emotional support. Sitting alone on a BART train going to work reflected a growing sense of isolation and distance from employees—myself included—whose professional privilege and employment allowed them to work remotely. Nagy reported the lack of empathy that often accompanied early efforts to celebrate "essential workers." Perceiving her as an infectious threat rather than a hero, her roommates threw her out during the pandemic; the last person new potential roommates wanted to accept was a nurse. Nagy's days grew longer after she was forced to take a studio apartment in a more distant, low-income city. The complex class positionality of registered nurses is relevant here. Other "essential worker" interlocutors in my research did not report this sort of sanitary profiling and viral segregation. They lived in neighborhoods where practically everyone was classified as an "essential worker." As she rode on BART trains, Nagy did not seem to reflect that grocery store and restaurant workers were also excluded from this "everybody else" who got to stay home.

There was no respite for Nagy's constant feeling of being "stressed out" at work when a twelve-hour shift afforded no breaks, even for meals, and no vacations. She self-diagnosed the effects of her inability to find the forms of self-care she needed: "I literally lived with a burning pain, anxiety pain, in my chest. It was a physical manifestation of the stress." Her rejection of what I would call the pandemic-heroes syndrome articulates what forms of care and appreciation would have mattered: "There were a lot of thank-yous and a lot of food given, so much pizza and whatever. But what we want is better staffing, breaks, pay. We just have to fight so much for the things we want." An ICU nursing supervisor articulated the insensitivity that lay behind pandemic-heroes syndrome and its unanticipated effects:

> At the beginning, in my neighborhood, people were doing the same thing that they were doing everywhere else: banging on pots and pans at eight o'clock at night. It was loud and annoying. I didn't feel honored. I felt just like, "You have no idea what we're going through. This is really hard. And I just want to come home to my neighborhood and have it be quiet and not have to hash out the day again, and your banging on the pots and pans is just making me just go back mentally to the hospital. Please stop it." Nobody else knows what we're doing, and they don't want to know, either. I can tell you: not one friend or family member outside of work has ever asked me, really asked me, "How are you? What exactly is it that you do for a living? How does that look? How does that work? Tell me a little bit about your experiences." They don't want to know.

In their book, sending pizza, banging pots and pans, and noisily holding up signs and cheering outside the hospital performed not care but incommunicability. Mark Nichter (2022, 560) suggests that one reason many ICU and ER health workers often rejected the heroes rhetoric is that they "came to see militarized 'front line' political rhetoric as a ploy to deflect responsibility away from hospital administration for keeping them safe." He also points out that healthcare organizations sometimes muzzled workers who would have liked to tell journalists their stories of insufficient staffing levels and PPE and mistreatment by bottom line-oriented administrators. They were warned that they could lose their jobs (559–60).

Pangborn and her colleagues (2023) suggest that in countering what they perceived as the lack of an effective response to their desires for support, frontline healthcare providers (FHPs) turned to social media to share their experiences and feelings with colleagues. Work that documented the importance of social media to the lives of providers and patients during the pandemic provides an interesting counterweight to the many voices that depict social media as a pandemic villain for promoting "misinformation" and conspiracy theories (see, e.g., Entradas 2022; Romer and Jamieson 2020; Viswanath, Lee, and Pinnamaneni 2020). Pangborn and colleagues report that "Twitter, especially, has become a hub for public dialogues about health: disclosure of personal stories, social support seeking, and community building" (2023, 1509). It became "a space in which FHPs, regardless of role or geographic location, were able to unite in support of one another" (1516). Their analysis of health professionals' posts also suggested that they used Twitter to reach large audiences that included many laypeople in "fulfilling [their] responsibility to educate even within contentious spaces" (1512), mainly to counter "misinformation" (see also Gomez-Vasquez et al. 2022). One interviewee reported that "she received death threats for speaking publicly about her experiences and encouraging adherence to safety measures. She shrugged and said, 'I guess it's considered unprofessional to be scientific at this point.' After investing years in specialized training to perform their essential roles, each interviewee expressed similar frustration that the science upon which their work is grounded had seemingly lost its authority" (Pangborn et al. 2023, 1513). The tweeting health professionals thus attempted to intervene in what they perceived as two distinct realms of lay incommunicability: the failure to listen to their accounts of the emotional, physical, and professional challenges of their work and the rejection of biocommunicability. Pangborn and colleagues report, "One important decision we made . . . was to not write about the very small subset of FHP tweets suggesting COVID-19 was exaggerated or a hoax. Simply put, in good conscience, we could not create more space for discourses that contributed to the onslaught of misinformation, lack of adherence to safety guidelines, and contentious public discourse that exponentially worsened the hardships faced by FHPs during the pandemic" (1510).

The authors, who are communication studies scholars, position themselves affectively alongside the FHPs: "We have been genuinely and deeply affected by [their] lives and stories" (Pangborn et al. 2023, 1510). They join the "combat" against "misinformation" and "conspiracy theories." It would seem as if the real heroes are those—including social scientists—who advance biocommunicability in a struggle against incommunicability. I am struck by the failure to note a fundamental contradiction here. Health professionals, like Nagy and nearly all my interlocutors, rightly believe their family and friends should ask about their experiences. Nevertheless, researchers and their FHP interlocutors do not seem to make space for the same sort of open listening to the perspectives of the Millers, Weavers, and Strongs, to people deemed to exaggerate or perpetuate hoaxes, let alone to go beyond these charged, moralizing stereotypes to parse out the diversity, complexity, and logics of lay responses and what they might add to our understanding of what went wrong in the pandemic.

In a world where everyone wants to hire nurses and ICUs are still understaffed, as current strikes by nurses attest, we need well-trained, dedicated nurses like Nagy. The structure of her narrative is a move from her ideal career and how she envisioned her future through a sudden, seemingly unending present of professional estrangement, labor exploitation, and her status as a witness to how the pandemic exacerbated the demise of failing healthcare systems in the United States, to a begrudging reach toward a distinct, uncertain, far less utopian future. It does not seem to be just the affective load of working with patients as they are dying, which she felt she could handle. For her, at least, the crucial factor behind that much touted—and highly reified—notion of "burnout" lies in the demand that she provide care that did not measure up to biocommunicable standards. What kept her up at night, literally, was not being able to deliver the level of care she was trained to provide in nursing school and the oath she took to translate preparation into practice. The source of the deepest, still unresolved emotional impact and her desire to leave the ICU was being trapped as the only nurse caring for two dying patients. She could not shock one and intubate the other simultaneously. That, she reported, kept her from finding the release she needed after leaving the hospital: "You replay over, at night, the corners that you had to cut." Pangborn and her colleagues report that several providers tweeted how such situations affected their sleep. One wrote, "*I woke up every hour hearing alarms in my dreams of my patients crashing*" (2023, 1512). After three and a half years of facing working conditions that compromised her professional standards, Nagy left the ICU and found a way to use her skills that left her "so much happier."

Nichter (2022) worked closely with health practitioners during the pandemic to support them; his research emerged in tandem with building a coalition to provide PPE, spaces to live while protecting their families, and other resources. He repositions the deus ex machina phrase "burnout" as contained within the radical individualism—one of our most recurrent and virulent legacies of Locke's era—that structures so many interpretations of pandemic experiences. Nichter argues that we should read powerful accounts, such as Nagy's, not as personal narratives of burnout but as idioms of distress.[5] During the pandemic, professionals' accounts turned into signs of moral distress that resulted from facing everyday ethical issues that fundamentally violated the goals that had brought them to their professions; that were inculcated in their training; that were performatively inscribed through their oaths; and that got them out of bed so many mornings when they would have liked to stay home. Other ICU nurses I interviewed similarly denounced the role of greed in creating staffing shortages and worrying that ICU nurses are forced to "risk people's safety." I am not surprised that at Nagy's reporting she "still ha[s] a lot to unpack." I can only hope that our conversation was of value to her in this process.

Valerie Smith, ER Physician, Northern California

I was initially drawn to OB/GYN. I had a couple of early mentors in OB/GYN. The afternoon before I was supposed to leave med school I played a game of Ultimate Frisbee and broke my clavicle, which meant that I couldn't catch babies. So I took the last rotation that was available, which happened to be in emergency medicine, and loved it. I was very surprised that I did love it as much as I did. I think the thing that draws me to the emergency department is the equity of it—anybody can walk in and get care. And that's also what I hate about it. And I like the fact that it's often different things. It's very discreet, very immediate. I liked the excitement of it, too. Now, twenty years later, I'm done with the excitement.

A lot of medicine is based on pattern recognition. At this point, I can scan a waiting room of one hundred people and point out to you the two people there who are going to be in extremis in the next ten to fifteen minutes unless we do something. It's the combination of the way they're holding their body, the respiratory rate, the color of their skin, the very fine sweat that they have on their skin. All of those things go into an algorithm that allows me to rapidly recognize people who were going to be very critically ill shortly. But with COVID, it was just this fear and frustration. I was so scared every day of this thing, because I didn't know this disease. This wasn't anything that I had any frame of reference for. I didn't know what it looked like. I didn't know how patients presented. I didn't know the warning signs.

It's pretty much destroyed us. Early on, we were terrified. And then, the first thing where we were really thrown under the bus was the fact that we weren't given protection; that they just expected us to work. I was told at one point by my chief, early on, "Oh, you know, those masks make patients uncomfortable. You really shouldn't—You're making people uncomfortable wearing those." In my chief's defense, Fauci said something similar really early on, because we honestly didn't really believe that something as low tech as a mask could really be as robustly protective as it is. But it wasn't a statement that aged well. There were four specialties. All the rest of the specialties retreated to their telephone and video visits and got to sit behind screens and sent us all of their patients that they thought might possibly have COVID. They closed down all elective surgery. So it was us, the hospital-based service, anesthesia, and, to a small extent, family practice, some obstetrics that were seeing the *vast* majority of these patients. And we weren't supported by the hospital or by our colleagues at all. There wasn't anybody who volunteered; it was like "whoo" [*shuddering*]. We couldn't sometimes even get consultants to come down to see patients in the ER; they were scared because we had COVID patients down in the ER. They would come up with all sorts of ridiculous excuses not to see a patient. So we really felt abandoned by our colleagues. I spent my nights when I wasn't working online just trying to find a solution, to see who in the world has figured out something that that works, some way to approach this or attack this.

I had this big fear, and I was also terrified of bringing home this virus to Mom and the kids—what effect that would have on them. The cases started ticking up here in March. At the end of March, I got sick with a fever, with what ended up not being COVID. But it was enough of a scare for Mom and me to sit down and decide what we were going to do, which was to partition the household, because it was becoming increasingly clear that this would be a threat to them—to my kids and Mom. So I moved down here to the in-law apartment that's underneath our house, and we closed the door behind me, and we did that for the next ten months. That's one of the hardest things I've ever done, and I think that there is still lingering stuff from that. They're resilient kids, thank God, and my mom is a complete rock star and never, ever, ever complains about anything, but it was really hard on everybody. And it was especially hard not being able to touch them for that amount of time. We eventually came up with a hug door, I put in a plastic temporary door, like they use in construction, and put some Kevlar sleeves in it so at least I could hug them. It was really hard for them, and the girls needed therapy. My son—last night I mentioned that I was coming home at 10 p.m. and then I got stuck at work, and I ended up coming home closer to 11:15. He came down at 10 and was crying and said to his grandmother, "Mom said that she'd be back, and she's not back yet. And I miss her." So I think a lot of that's left over from that time, and definitely it was hard on everybody—and super lonely.

In the late fall, after six months of just going to work and to the grocery store, getting most stuff delivered and not really doing anything besides those things, I had a physician friend visit. She was going to get her own car and then for various reasons didn't and asked me to drive her somewhere. She was wearing a mask, but she changed her mask in my car. We had a lot of smoke and wildfires, and she has severe asthma. She was having a lot of difficulty breathing. So we went to a small get-together that was supposed to be outdoors, but because of the smoke—and the AQI [air quality index] was so high—it was partly indoors and partly outdoors. It was a group of eleven physicians and one nonphysician. The person who had "asthma" [*makes scare quotes with fingers*] did a breathing treatment while she was there. And nine of us got COVID. I was sick for about a month, and that was very scary, like nothing I've ever felt before. It's a ten-day illness, and usually you feel like you have a really bad cold or flu the first three or four days, and then often you get a little break in the middle, and then day seven to ten is when, if you are going to get very sick, you get very sick. And I have asthma. I wrote my will, and that was particularly hard, because I was like, "What if Mom gets this and she dies and I die?" I think it was especially scary because I'm divorced. I called six or seven of my best girlfriends and made them pledge that they would help to raise my children and not let my ex-husband raise my kids—that would not have been a good situation. The idea that because I had taken this risk, because I did not have firm boundaries with this person who then got me sick, because I might, after this extraordinary thing that my family had done and I had done, have to leave them, was just really *awful.*

The coughing finally got better. The oxygen level finally got a bit better. But I'm still not all the way better. I was sleeping with oxygen at night for a couple of months after that. I got better, and then in March I got inexplicably sick again, not for any good reason. It just popped: short of breath out of the blue. I tested for everything. It wasn't COVID again. At that time, I'd been vaccinated. So I don't know when it's going to show up again. I was sick enough to be out of work again for a couple of weeks. And, yeah, so I just feel like I never know when it's going to come back and whether it's going to be as bad as it was.

Most of us were offered vaccination, so there was this brief moment of light at the end of the tunnel: "Maybe this is it!" There was this moment in January or February when we were like, "OK, we might actually be able to see through this." Then it became abundantly clear through the spring and the summer that there were enough stridently anti-vaxx people in the United States especially that we were never going to achieve herd immunity; that this would become endemic. Just the fact that I have to worry about my own safety for the rest of my career has made me feel so completely different. I went so into debt and sacrificed so much personally and have so much to do just to have patients willfully not even care enough to keep their kids safe? That just feels so totally demoralizing. I think I've just seen so much ugliness in terms of human behavior over the last year and a half that I just don't—I've lost a lot of what drew me to medicine, to emergency medicine in particular, which was, "I can help people." These are not people I want to help or who want help. So, yeah. I thought that I would do this for the balance of my life, and now I've been actively planning exit strategies for the last six months.

I suspect it did not take readers long to realize they have just met ER physician Dr. Smith, Professor Smith's daughter. After recounting how an accident forced a career change, she lists the reasons she, surprisingly, fell in love with emergency medicine. The discordant note ("And that's also what I hate about it") provides a narrative preview of the denouement of her story. Smith presents herself as a remarkable embodiment of biocommunicable knowledge, able to pick out signs of impending acute distress from a distance in a crowded ER waiting room. Accordingly, she immediately sensed that the new disease would launch her from a privileged position of biocommunicable clairvoyance into an uncharted incommunicable realm. After watching what was emerging in China, she warned her colleagues that "we were all in unfamiliar territory. We knew we didn't know enough about this. We also knew that our regular channels of peer-reviewed, evidence-based medicine [EBM] weren't going to be able to function in real-time." Here we return to the role of social media in providing health professionals with alternative modes of exchanging observations that had not yet become ratified biomedical knowledge. "Around that time we were starting very rapidly as physicians to build an international community to share information," Smith reported. "A lot of us were joining these large international physician-only groups and sort of sharing information from Singapore, from Australia, from Italy, about how we were taking care of COVID patients, what was working and what wasn't."

Smith worked in an ER that received some of the first US citizens airlifted back from China with COVID-19. She said she knew that "the first thing that it says in the disaster chapter of any emergency medicine textbook is 'do not contaminate your emergency department.'" She protested when these initial patients "were paraded right through our waiting rooms and right past everybody through the interior of our emergency departments" rather than through the outdoor entrance to special negative pressure rooms. Her acute biocommunicable sensibility got "overruled" by hospital administrators invoking nonbiomedical logics: "We don't want these patients to feel uncomfortable. They're just coming back to the United States. We want to make sure that they know we care about them." We hear an echo of the theme introduced by Murphy and Nagy—a failure to consider what constitutes care for caregivers—when Smith remarks that the "parade" left her with "this bottomless feeling of just being like, my God, we're nothing to them. We're nothing to administration. Our lives are not even as important to them as how this is going to look from a [public relations] standpoint." Here a physician returns a crucial gaze to billboards produced by healthcare corporations that project doctors whose smile conveys an inviting, selfless openness to their patients.

By the time we spoke by Zoom in August 2021, Smith had cared for COVID-19 patients for eighteen months. Her sense of confidence had been ruptured by a pandemic incommunicability that many of her colleagues seemed able to keep at virtual arm's length. Medical specializations suddenly were rearranged in two new hierarchies: those that could hide behind screens and telephones and the four specialties whose practitioners were forced to cling to the embodied provider-patient interaction model, even if the verbal component often took place through windows and telephone connections, with PAPRs mediating physical examinations. As EBM biocommunicability fell far short, Smith spent the long nights of her off-duty days trying to establish an online biocommunicable channel in which physicians—and only physicians—shared clinical knowledge.

After her remarkable ability as a doctor-narrator places us in what has become the fearful, "destroyed" in/communicable space of the ER, Smith's account, like that of the epidemiologist-activist Silvia Montaño's in chapter 7, suggests how "the pandemic" gets woven into the fine-grained details of daily life and, specifically, of ongoing familial relations of care. I want to emphasize that the very different forms that COVID-19 assumed as it entered into each person's life—which we could articulate in Veena Das's (2007) terms as a "descent into the ordinary"—were just as valid for health professionals as for laypeople. Note that the depth of this articulation—how daily life transformed the pandemic and how COVID-19 restructured the intimate details of the everyday—was more significant for Dr. Smith than for her mother. Many health professionals, like Smith, shared the terror experienced by "essential workers"—including Rosales's mother and aunt—about COVID-19's refusal to respect boundaries between work and home. What Roman Jakobson ([1957] 1971) refers to as narrated events and narrative events came together as Smith's words—"I moved down here," accompanied by a sweeping gesture—simultaneously positioned her as a storyteller in the unfolding Zoom interview in the space of the basement apartment she occupied during ten pandemic months of isolation. Her gestures also mapped COVID-19 care, the personal challenges and anxieties of health workers, their relations with others, and how they inhabited and crossed multiple spaces.

Even as these two remarkable women and the three children prevented viruses from passing from floor to floor, it would seem—from Dr. Smith's account—that mental health challenges were less respectful of Masonite and plastic boundaries: "It was really hard on everybody." She applauds her mother's "rock star" spirit, but Dr. Smith has a more sober assessment of the impact of the months of separation on her family. The COVID-19 pandemic was not the only palpable onslaught against bodies and minds in the area where she worked at the time. In addition to widespread reactions against police and medical forms of violence against Black lives, wildfires had taken the homes of patients and colleagues in the area where she works. They filled the air with toxic smoke, complicating COVID-19 worries for people, such as Smith, who have asthma, the sorts of comorbidities that Merrill Singer characterized as occasioning syndemics (Singer et al. 2017). After an affective and familial register enables us to picture how a life confined to commuting to a highly stressful job, occasionally going to the grocery store, and glimpsing her children through the window resulted in being "super lonely," Smith shifts back to a biocommunicable register in assessing her actions in hosting a friend and attending a party with fellow physicians not as seeking to address mental health needs but as having "taken this risk and not had firm boundaries." Here her account moves into a remarkable Kleinmanian illness narrative structured as much by clinical profiles of COVID-19 care and complex domestic arrangements as by fragments of the story of a problematic marriage.

Smith suggests—and rightly so—that colleagues and administrators should have extended care to her and other ER staff. We see a glint of mistrust of physicians in the caustic scare quotes around her visiting physician friend's "asthma," the administration's greater concern with public relations than keeping staff safe, and the "ridiculous excuses" that other physicians used to dodge obligations to patients and colleagues. To return to Nichter's (2022) formulation, Smith's story moves from moral distress and outrage to moral injury, the effects of which still lingered after vaccination enabled her to move beyond a pandemic existence consisting of highly stressful work conditions and self-enforced isolation in not quite arm's reach of her family. Smith faced the same sorts of complicated decisions as laypeople in balancing forms of care associated with preventing COVID-19 infection with the mental health impacts of the pandemic. At one point in ten months, it seems, the need for human contact and sociability, so crucial for mental health, outweighed biocommunicable dictates. As she reflected on this encounter, rather than helping herself heal the wounds that still afflicted her mind and body, she judged herself harshly.

Smith initially faced COVID-19 incommunicability, terrified by a disease that could not be contained within her highly developed clinical gaze, a "fear and frustration" amplified by lack of support, not only from her colleagues but from administrators who left her feeling like she had been "thrown under the bus." Her narrative provides not a comforting transition from incommunicability to communicable security but a descent into what seem to be the same sense of uncertainty and precarity regarding post-acute sequelae of COVID-19 as so clearly articulated by Pato Hebert and others who struggled to understand and cope with their own mysterious and lingering COVID-19 repercussions. As I listened to her story, I wished that she might have granted herself more empathy as her illness narrative evaluated how she was infected. Rather than chastising herself for dropping "firm boundaries" associated with COVID-19 biocommunicability, watching her speak from the basement in which she self-quarantined for ten months prompted me to ponder the complex decisions that might have led her to do a complex balancing act between mental health needs on the one hand and constant viral self-surveillance on the other hand. It flashed through my mind that this might have been an opportunity for her to identify with what her patients experienced as their own difficult decisions and how they might have grappled with feelings of guilt, anger, and mistrust. I wanted to ask if this juncture might have led her to feel compassion rather than anger at the "anti-vaxx people" who continued to crowd her ER.

Smith is a remarkably dedicated doctor, daughter, and mother. I hope that she finds a way to reconnect with her sense of "the equity" of the ER and thus with all patients who "can walk in and get care." She, too, asks tough questions: What is care? Who wants it? Who—including the caregivers—deserves it? Perhaps, rather than leaving medicine or the ER, she might enlist us as allies in demanding that "the administration" focus less on "PR" and profit and more on health/communicative justice for providers and patients alike.

Joyce Arden, Infectious Disease Physician and Hospitalist, Montana

I tell people, if you fall and you break your hip, nobody's arguing gravity. But we're arguing the presence of a virus—which is not a force of evil, by the way. It's some RNA and some protein, and it's just trying to make a living like anyone else [*laughs*]. Let's take politics out of that, please. I sort of had a unique position as an infection preventionist and a hospitalist and the only member of the incident command who "wore the blue": you wear the blue as a frontline worker. And I guess you could say I was bilingual—I speak administrative-speak and clinical-speak—so I sort of had that ability to educate. I remember pontificating not in a mean way, but kind of in a joking way. I'd go onto a floor where nurses are and get peppered with one question, another question, another question, another question. One of the things that irritated my husband is I'd be two hours late getting home from my shift not only because I was in meetings with administration but also because I felt like it was time to take that chance to reassure our staff. It was kind of like paint[ing] it for them, and they, in turn, were going to pass that on to their family and friends. I did get on the radio, and I wrote stuff for the local paper. I call it stamping out roaches of misinformation—that's the best way to describe it, just one by one, person by person.

It feels like there was like an exact month where you went from being a hero to a goat. It was the spring after the vaccine was then available very widely. That's when, I would say, not to get too hysterical, the battle lines were drawn between people who were, to put it mildly, vehement in their vaccine refusal and then, by extension, their refusal to acknowledge that this pandemic is real, is not a plot. The vaccine is not injecting DNA material so the government can track you, yada, yada, yada. You've heard every notion known to man. You've heard probably talk about the hydroxychloroquine and then, subsequently, ivermectin. And I would say, October was when ivermectin nearly killed me from a career standpoint [*laughs*].

My colleague and I, one night, were called to a patient's room because there were some friends, family agitating, demanding that we *must* give this elderly unvaccinated person ivermectin on a group phone call with people who identified themselves as the assistant attorney general, active members of the Republican Party, and the acting attorney general.

The ivermectin, my understanding is, got snuck into the patient's room in pills in a [milkshake]. After all my explanations, very learned explanations, about the nature of research and the real ins and outs of the Right to Try Law, the assistant attorney general, who was on that phone, did not understand Right to Try and told me that there would be "real legal ramifications" to refusal. As it turned out, she was correct. At this point, I'm like, "You've got to stand for something. You've got to stand for what you believe in." I was sorry and angry that it became a political thing. I was quite clear that I do not allow politicians or lawyers to dictate my medical care. "And please understand that I know that you don't have the education, training, or experience to tell me how to practice medicine." Part of the issue with the attorney general was that we were, quote, "holding that patient against her will and denying her the right to have visitors." Of course we were. That was our hospital policy since the very beginning: "If you don't like the rules, then go somewhere else. Oh, wait, there's no place else to go. Then you live by our rules." I was angered by the fact that it became a political thing.

And the assistant attorney general was correct in her remarks that "there will be legal ramifications." The attorney general basically sent someone out to arrest us. The attorney general went to our county attorney and said, "Go out and arrest these doctors." And the county attorney said, "I can see no crime that was committed. So, no. I'm not sending the sheriff or the local police department out to the hospital," which is why the brown shirts got called. The best way I can describe it is that the henchmen of the governor's office were sent out. Our chief medical officer said, "I'll go out and talk to law enforcement." My colleague and I were thinking, "You know, maybe we would rather spend a weekend in the clink than get sued for malpractice." It's one thing for doctors and hospitals to have been sued in civil suits, but the whole different next level is to be threatened with criminal action by a governor, as opposed to a lawyer.

At that point, my colleague and I were like, "You know what? Maybe this is not a job for us anymore." And, of course, then we thought better—that we cannot leave our colleagues hanging. We've got to stand for something. But how much longer can I do this? I am quite tired. Over the course of this pandemic, patients and families have assumed more of an adversarial position relative to what one normally understands. If it gets too bad, I'll give my one-year notice. We've already lost nurses. I respect them. It breaks my heart, but I understand their decision. I'd like to think that the staff that remains will be incredibly strong and resilient. Unfortunately, I think a lot of people have been badly injured. On the staff there are quite a few who got COVID, and some are suffering from long COVID. Even if they didn't die or get admitted, they're ill. As far as the hospital goes, I'm afraid that the injuries that have taken over this town and taken over the state are going to leave us ripe for a buyout, a hostile takeover. I don't know that we're going to survive.

Analyzing Dr. Arden's account requires background on Montana, the contours of COVID-19 cases, hospitalizations, and the politics of mitigation measures, particularly masking and vaccinations. This politically heterogeneous state includes vast rural areas often described as "libertarian conservative" Republican, as well as urban areas, such as Helena, the capital, and Missoula, home of the University of Montana, that have more residents who vote Democratic. There are areas with strong Native American nations, from the Crow in the south to the Blackfeet in the north. Nevertheless, many counties report very high percentages of non-Hispanic white people; the figure is over 90 percent for the county where Arden's hospital lies.

Montana was ahead of the curve of COVID-19 policies in two different ways. Democrat Steve Bullock, governor from 2013 to 2021, declared a state of emergency on 12 March 2020 and closed public schools three days later. He issued a stay-at-home order on 26 March, the same day the Montana Hospital Association requested it. In July, Bullock imposed a statewide mask mandate for indoor public spaces and large outdoor gatherings. Thus, Montana not only enacted COVID-19 mitigation measures before many other states but, during the early months of the pandemic, had some of the lowest US rates of hospitalization and death; its first "surge" came in fall 2020. Then things changed dramatically. Endorsed by Donald Trump, Greg Gianforte became Montana's first Republican governor in sixteen years on 4 January 2021. When Gianforte rescinded the mask mandate, Montana's chief medical officer resigned immediately. Gianforte signed a bill limiting the ability of hospitals and other entities to require that employees receive COVID-19 vaccination; businesses were prohibited from requiring that customers be vaccinated. In August, Montana became the first state to ban vaccine requirements for employees—requiring vaccination as a condition for employment became a form of discrimination that violated Montana's human rights laws.

Mask use in this environment was quite uneven. In November 2021 I attended a Catholic mass and an evangelical Christian service; the percentage of congregants who were masked were, respectively, 100 percent and 0 percent (unless you count the ethnographer). Frank Miller had invited me to attend the service at his evangelical Christian church, which had probably been the source of his and his wife's COVID-19 infection and that of the two pastors and most congregants; two died of the disease, one after attending a church event. Although Miller told me I looked "silly" in my mask, I encountered no hostility. It is not the case that all people at evangelical services were unmasked and that all Catholics were observant of masking. Besides the different locations of the two churches—a Catholic congregation in the capital, Helena, and the evangelical church in a small town in a rural area—I found substantial variation among Catholic churches. During an interview, the priest of the entirely masked church suggested that his example of wearing a mask at all times, except during the reading of the Gospel and the homily, "sets an example, it sets a tone, it sends a message, you know," reinforced by months of Zoom masses followed by closing off alternate pews to distance parishioners.

Montana fared well regarding COVID-19 cases and deaths during the first seven pandemic months. The overall statistics for vaccination for the state do not fall too far below national averages, with 51 percent fully vaccinated in Montana on 9 November 2021 and 58 percent nationally. The variability was, however, enormous, say between rural Garfield County, with 25 percent fully vaccinated, versus 67 percent in Missoula County, where the University of Montana is located.[6] This tremendous variation also appeared in other states and, for instance, in coastal versus northern and eastern California counties. Montana's rural population is not homogeneous. I interviewed a friend of Miller's who shared his political and religious views. Nevertheless, the friend had been vaccinated against COVID-19 and described himself as "a great believer in vaccines," adding that he liked going to stores "a lot better when everybody was wearing a mask."

Cases increased massively in the winter of 2021. More than half of the state's hospital beds were filled with COVID-19 patients. Soon critical-care facilities, the ICU, and advanced medical units were nearly full. Oxygen supplies were stretched, and Arden's hospital ran out of COVID-19 specialty drugs, leaving critically ill patients without adequate treatment. As at many hospitals, the morgue was full, requiring freezer trucks in the parking lot. The hospital made a bold move of not just implementing but publicly announcing the imposition of "crisis standards of care," meaning that patients who needed critical services could be turned away or denied essential treatments if, in Paul Farmer's (2020) terms, staff, stuff, space, and systems were unavailable. National Guardsmen helped clean rooms, deliver meals, do laundry, and spend time with patients. In the hospital's announcement, which drew the attention of local and national media, the chief medical officer positioned an exhausted, burned-out staff as facing an increasingly aggressive public.

Like Smith, Arden is both a doctor's doctor and an excellent raconteur. Her knowledge base is broad, including board certification in infectious diseases and several other specialties as well as training in epidemiology. Professionally, she has done it all, from clinical care to public health administration, academic and high-tech medicine, and public health emergency management. In our interview, she walked me unpretentiously through medical history, Foucault, emergency management, immunology, and virology. What had attracted her to Montana a decade earlier, in addition to a shortage of doctors, was a deep engagement with the outdoors and the desire for a work situation that was not overpopulated with overbearing bosses. Being a hospitalist, infectious disease physician, and a key participant in structuring the COVID-19 interagency emergency management response cut into her ability to reserve time for recharging psychic batteries through long hikes and camping. She worked ninety to one hundred hours a week. Unlike most narrators, her story does not begin with a pre-pandemic period of relative certitude and stability. It started right in the middle of conflict and chaos—her lifeworld when we spoke in November 2021.

Arden is a true believer in, and a star of, biocommunicability. She walks the walk, doing clinical rounds, and talks the talk, including spending additional hours speaking with nurses to boost their morale, hoping they will open up a biocommunicable channel to families and friends. Her remarks make it clear that being a strong spokesperson for biocommunicability is a core feature of her identity as a professional. She suggests that being "bilingual"—that is, able to "speak administrative-speak and clinical-speak"—provided her with a perfect position "to educate." I might extend her self-description to call her multilingual, given that she was also fluent in biosecurity-speak, trained in public health and clinical approaches to just such "emergencies" as the pandemic.

My prior interview with the hospital's public relations manager was fascinating and, I learned later, felt cathartic for her. Having decided to put clinicians at the forefront in talking with media and civic groups about COVID-19, the manager often called Arden to speak with reporters and write pieces for the local newspaper. She thus graciously passed along my request to interview members of the hospital staff, leading Arden to contact me. Arden deemed the stakes extremely high for defending physicians' rights to draw on their biocommunicable base in determining patient care. Her dramatic statement that "ivermectin nearly killed me from a career standpoint" was only one of the poetic expressions that emerged in our interview. That a hospital room had been transformed into a site of *political* communicability was apparent when Arden's remote interlocutors identified themselves as elected officials and Republican Party leaders. Never missing a biocommunicable opportunity, Arden offered them "very learned explanations, about the nature of research." She charged "politicians or lawyers . . . [who] don't have the education, training or experience" with trying to pull the biocommunicable rank required to authorize treatments.

Her narrative musters reported speech powerfully. She creates a figure of unshakable biocommunicable authority, which she then occupies, projecting it as the voice that reigns in the hospital and has the power to set rules. By recognizing biocommunicability as the legitimate authority in the hospital, the county attorney became her ally. One contrasting voice was that of "people who were . . . vehement in their vaccine refusal." She analyzes their litany of nonbiomedical views of COVID-19 as devoid of referential content: "Yada, yada, yada." Then comes a voice of right-wing political belligerence, which she fills with the figures of the patient's friends, family, "the assistant attorney general, active members of the Republican Party, and the acting attorney general." Her boundary work (Gieryn 1983) suggests that these voices should be judiciously excluded from spaces where biocommunicability is dominant. She seems to deny the attorney general's voice its legal authority by crossing herself into legal communicability to inform him that he has misinterpreted the Right to Try Act, a Montana law that allows manufacturers to make experimental medications available to terminally ill patients.

The local county attorney agreed that biocommunicability trumps political power regarding patient care, refusing to dispatch police or sheriff deputies to the hospital. Overruling these competing communicable claims, the Montana attorney general sent a state trooper to arrest both infectious disease physicians; the chief medical officer somehow talked him down. State Democratic Party legislators demanded an investigation of the Montana Department of Justice's involvement in the incident, and Republicans agreed. The hospital released a statement that protested that hospital staff had been harassed and threatened by public officials, prompting attention by local and AP journalists. The hospital administration managed to keep Arden's and her colleagues' names out of the press: they lived in a neighboring county where law enforcement would be somewhat less likely, to say the least, to defend them against potential violence. Nevertheless, a far-right website published their names and libelous claims. Her experience moved beyond a transition from moral distress to moral injury, in Nichter's (2022) terms, to one of legal and corporeal vulnerability. She ends her narrative by tracing the limits of the power of her own voice, noting that she had received attacks on right-wing websites and death threats. In the end, the cacophony that emerged during the ivermectin incident seems to threaten the hospital itself. When I spoke with her in late November, Arden thought she would stay on the hospital's staff to support her colleagues, even as she actively contemplated finding a less embattled state to practice medicine and enjoy the outdoors.

Conclusion

Dr. Joyce Arden is a compelling figure—a brave, hardworking, broadly trained physician who sticks by her convictions, colleagues, and hospital. I only hope her hospital, along with Valerie Smith's, and the rest of us can help them return to situations where they feel that their work and lives are valued and that providing care does not turn them into targets for violent speech, gestures, or worse. Even if drawing the line on ivermectin—and interventions by elected officials and state troopers—was the right thing to do, I think we might learn more from Arden's story if we slow it down. I want to do this by placing her in dialogue with Frank Miller.

At first glance, the two share only residence in Montana, a love of the outdoors, and a dislike of domineering bosses, but there is, I think, a whole lot more to it than that. Yes, they are opposites, but that's the point. Each of their stories constructs two sides, where the narrator firmly occupies one space and sees the other figure only from afar. The only context in which they would likely have met is if Miller's COVID-19 had become complicated. He might have ended up in her care. Miller is far too polite and respectful to have "flipped her off" from a hospital bed, as she describes for other patients, but the process of giving and receiving care would likely have been tense. If she had performed "very learned explanations," trying to draw Miller deep into COVID-19 biocommunicability, he probably would have been right out the door, if he was strong enough to walk. Moreover, her efforts would have further confirmed his negative stereotype that health professionals view COVID-19 communicability as their right and duty. However, if the infectious disease in question were something else—a severe infection that followed his knee replacement, for example—their relationship would likely have been relatively smooth and cooperative, and his trust in her diagnosis and treatment plan more forthcoming.

Nevertheless, they need each other. Miller's account requires a figure precisely like Arden, who believes that only people with the proper "education, training, or experience" can appropriately make the rules about COVID care, not politicians or lawyers or, as in Miller's case, retired delivery drivers and contractors. The narrative that Arden builds also needs a figure like Miller, who asserts that paths that lead to decisions about COVID-19 care should not have a single, biocommunicable route and that life experiences and everyday problem solving provide a reasonable basis for sorting out pandemic issues. Indeed, Arden and Miller are perfect for each other, in narrative terms, because both hold firm in their convictions despite the costs: Arden is willing to go to jail to maintain physicians' control over care, just as Miller refuses to contact a physician when he experiences COVID-19 symptoms and declares that if failing to get vaccinated is going to cost him his life, so be it.

You may have noted that their central beef about the course of the pandemic in the United States is the same: how "politics" undermined COVID-19 biocommunicability. Arden, laughingly anthropomorphizing SARS-CoV-2 as "just trying to make a living like anyone else," makes a request: "Let's take politics out of that, please." Miller comments on Trump-bashing by "liberals" in 2020: "It's just politics, leave that part out. Let's get down to the scientific facts of what needs to be done." They define "science" and "politics" in relatively similar ways, except that Arden's notion of science leaves space for uncertainty: she views discarding old hypotheses in the face of new data as good science, not incompetence and prevarication. At root, they both believe that biocommunicability can and must be protected against all other forms of ideological work. In Bruno Latour's ([1991] 1993) sense, they are thoroughly modern, claiming the status of boundary workers trying to separate science and politics. They both decry pragmatic leakages that emerge when people claim that how science is made and circulated should match up at each moment and that what is said should transparently reflect what is done.

That's asking too much for several reasons. First, we need to bring in a part of the Great Divide that Latour misses, too—the Lockean boundary work that confines science and medicine in one "province of knowledge" and puts language and communication in another. The pandemic placed countless viruses, sick bodies, masks, vaccines, news stories, public health pronouncements, websites, social media posts, and electoral contests into competition for attention, dollars, and votes. Accordingly, it was impossible to construct pure scientific and medical objects that only later became communicative "immutable mobiles" (Latour 1988), magically able to move among hospitals, newsrooms, living rooms, pharmaceutical corporations, and political rallies without becoming unstable. They were all mixed up from the get-go.

Second, to echo a theme of this book, ideological labor, metapragmatics, and pragmatics *never* match up perfectly. Ideological models do not map transparently onto the specifics of what is said and done. Things get more complex when you have—as is the case with "doctor-patient interaction," health communication, and COVID-19—competing communicable models, each projected as the only one that should shape and can legitimately interpret pragmatics. Crying incommunicability and blaming it on the other team when things do not match up is an excellent strategy for boundary-work. Still, it simply turns accusations of incommunicability into sources of acrimonious divides that end conversations, prevent cooperation, and multiply and camouflage inequities.

Third, in another lesson from science and technology studies and other research on the more than human, both stories project a zero-sum game with two sets of human players who compete for truth, trust, and ethical standing. A problem here is that there are other key players, including a pesky, confusing little virus that is always looking back and taunting, "Catch me if you can!" not to mention a host of infrastructures, including ones like social media, that enable competing communicabilities to proliferate. Finally, Frantz Fanon, Donna Haraway (1988, 1997), Warwick Anderson (2006), Keith Wailoo (2001), and many others would suggest that leaving race out of the picture (in 2020, no less) constitutes another way of politicizing science. Both Arden and Miller live in counties that are about 90 percent "white alone, not Hispanic or Latino"; neither mentioned that the COVID-19 game was rigged against human players who are not "white alone."

I want to open up a dialogue between Arden and Miller so they can explore the complexities of how they tried to find their way in pandemic worlds. Such a conversation might lead them to discard distanced views of homogeneous opposing actors—arrogant doctors versus anti-vaxx nut heads—who all think and act alike. Perhaps Miller might take Arden back to the dying patient's room and ask a few questions. He might ask her to put the tropes of the Republican Party and the attorney general's office aside for a moment. In keeping with his ongoing critique of the pharmaceuticalization of health, which he shares with many medical anthropologists (Biehl 2007; Dumit 2012), he might argue that focusing so squarely on whether a dying patient received a particular drug (Berlivet and Löwry 2020) begs some critical questions about the authority of EBM, clinical judgment, and lay participation in deciding what constitutes health knowledge and care. Listening to Miller might convince Arden that not all vaccine skeptics lack rationality: his views amount to much more than nonsensical "yada, yada, yada."

Given that he is interested in scientific perspectives and continues to occupy a space with some openness among competing perspectives, she might learn how to go beyond "pontificating" to help Miller in his continuing quest for greater certitude. Arden might better appreciate that the gaps in biomedical knowledge of COVID-19 and fear might have reasonably led laypeople to push back against biocommunicability's demand for a monopoly on pandemic knowledge production as they faced complex issues of prevention and care. The binary she depicts between voices that embody biomedical science and those spouting "every [nonsensical] notion known to man" might not provide an adequate cartography of forms of pandemic knowledge. She leaves out people such as Pato Hebert, who embraced COVID-19 biocommunicability but, when it did not enable him to make sense of his lingering symptoms or figure out what to do, also found it necessary to carefully track what was going on in his body and work with other long COVID patients in developing digital forums for pooling knowledge. Her sensitivity to the plight of long COVID patients, including some of her own colleagues, might seem to prompt openness to laypersons who attempted to coax skeptical doctors into taking them seriously and worked with physicians and scientists to boost research on PASC and develop strategies for coping with its complex, heterogeneous symptoms.

However, having cared for the dying patient, what could Arden tell Miller about the patient's painful struggle to stay alive? As an infectious disease physician, Arden could appeal to Miller's belief in science without politics by describing in detail how human cells react differently to SARS-CoV-2 in bodies that have been vaccinated. Miller might ask Arden if she went beyond the patient's classification as an "elderly, unvaccinated person" to find out who she was, what she was like, and what she did with her life. Who were her children and grandchildren? What did she mean to them? Besides obtaining prescriptions from an outside doctor for ivermectin and hydroxychloroquine and using Republican Party connections, who were those friends and relatives? What forms of care did they provide before she entered the hospital? Was Arden able to ask her what it felt like to be dying and not be able to see them? Did Arden ask the friends and relatives about their fears that she would die without being able to say goodbye? Although these questions would not induce Arden to allow the patient to take ivermectin, they might broaden the discussion.

In the phone call in the patient's room and discussions of the ensuing events, Arden insisted that biocommunicability, defined in terms of COVID-19 protocols, was the only way the conversation—and the story—could unfold. Family and friends demanded that patient-consumer communicability, its symbolic and legal power extended by appealing to Montana's 2015 Right to Try Act and claims for the paramount legitimacy of rights to individual "freedom," should trump biocommunicability. The attorney-general and assistant attorney-general then attempted to reposition the discussion in a different form of communicability—criminal laws that punish mistreatment and unlawful restraint.

The visitation issue, part of complaints by the relatives and Montana elected officials, sparked acrimonious debates in her hospital and in every ICU and COVID ward I researched. It caused friction and pain among patients, their families, and ICU staff members. Some visitors and staff sought to expand definitions of care to include providing emotional support; they saw strict "no visitors" policies as threatening patients' and relatives' emotional well-being. Others angrily insisted, echoing nurse Nagy, that their and their families' health and the possibility of infecting other patients should be the primary consideration. After all, they had to be there twelve hours at a time. Patients' recovery depended on nurses' and doctors' COVID-19-negative status, partly because staffing levels were negatively affected when colleagues needed to go into isolation, let alone when they had to be hospitalized or died. I referred to Cohen's (2020, 543) observation, focused on the fate of the elderly in the pandemic, that care came to be redefined as *not* visiting the vulnerable, a seemingly "perverse" form of care. My interviews suggest that reframing care as not visiting the vulnerable was less a consensus than an active, frequently acrimonious, often painful debate that took place among ICU personnel, as well.

Ultimately, I think everyone lost out in the conversation in the patient's room. The struggle did not change the medical outcome, and I doubt it eased the grieving process for the woman's family and friends. The hospital did not surrender control over treatment protocols. Still, the confrontation left many staff members angry and shaken, fearing subsequent retaliation from the state government, and, in Arden's case, considering leaving the hospital and the state. The attorney general may have scored a few points with conservative voters. Nevertheless, even fellow Republican lawmakers seemed to question the wisdom of going over the heads of doctors, hospital administrators, local officials, and the local sheriff and police—and attempting to criminalize a dispute about care, which echoes current efforts to criminalize providers, patients, family members, and even Uber drivers for abortions.

Ethnographically documenting broader pandemic ecologies of care suggests how bringing different perspectives and forms of care might have kept ivermectin and vaccination from becoming condensed symbols for all sides. Broadening the conversation might have stopped ivermectin and vaccination from becoming so powerful that they could displace other care issues and shut down dialogue, trust, and empathy. We return here to the basic theme of this book: What happens when the medicalization of a situation, seemingly entirely appropriate in debates about treating a dying patient in a hospital, requires positioning biocommunicability as the only (authorized) game in town? Suddenly, everything else just looks like incommunicability. As I examined in chapter 7, knowledge claims that do not bear the stamp of biomedicine and public health consensus get tossed into the same residual bin: anecdotal evidence, conspiracy theory, misinformation, and "emotional" reactions that constitute biocommunicable noise. Herein lies a significant problem with biocommunicability: when it claims to be the only legitimate form of communicability, it produces a moral—and seemingly professional— obligation on the part of doctors, nurses, and public health practitioners to discredit and attempt to eradicate other contenders. Even when healthcare workers who treated COVID-19 patients opened up on a social media platform, telling the stories their family and friends were unwilling to hear, they felt compelled to include this task on the agenda.

In the pandemic, providers did not realize that decades of promoting patient-consumer communicability might subsequently limit the possibility of declaring it off-limits in pandemics. It seemed to come as a surprise that trying to prohibit patient-consumer communicability temporarily would (1) be unsuccessful; and (2) set them up to be perceived as prevaricating, insensitive power grabbers. The heterogeneous roots of patient-consumer communicability prompted diverse forms of resistance to COVID-19 biocommunicability. These ideological differences often converged on a common endpoint: vaccine skepticism or rejection.

Many health professionals also did not realize that patient-consumer communicability had become deeply attached to white supremacy, that it had become one of the significant advantages that white people enjoyed from birth to death simply by virtue of their race. Attempting to extract it from COVID-19 discourse and practices was thus bound to elicit a profoundly adverse reaction from white people who are highly connected to their racialized identities. As the avalanche of COVID-19 coverage in mainstream media and social media exposed the inner workings of science to much more intensive public scrutiny, biocommunicability became a highly visible semiotic, with its hierarchized, top-down, unilinear structure and positioning of laypeople as passive subjects held up for critical inspection. Social media and journalistic attention to biocommunicability's critics also increased the visibility of efforts by people positioning themselves as citizen scientists, particularly on Twitter (Berlivet and Löwry 2020, 529), claiming, like Weaver and Strong, that they were "doing their research," to use the now highly contested phrase. The result was sure to clash with how Miller's pastor summarized the lessons of the pandemic in an interview—"It's all about freedom"—a leitmotif of settler-colonial discourses.

Health professionals could not stop racialized minority communities from perceiving connections between COVID-19 biocommunicability and the painful communicable circuits that recounted experiences engendered by centuries of experimentation on and abuses of Black, Native American, and Latinx bodies, including forced sterilizations (see Laura Briggs 2002). Stories of everyday inequities—problematic access to and low quality of health care and racist treatment by health professionals—also impinged on biocommunicable circuits. I interviewed a hospitalist who treated COVID-19 patients at an Indian Health Service hospital located in the Navajo Nation. She noted in October 2021 that unvaccinated patients continued to fill hospital beds. Identifying as a racialized immigrant community member, she sympathetically recounted conversations with patients and reactions to public presentations in which painful memories of medical experimentation and abuses got connected with fears about COVID-19 vaccines. All in all, this was a train wreck that should have been seen a long way down the tracks.

CONCLUSION

I have developed a decolonial perspective on biocommunicability and in-communicability. Why? A key reason is that my analysis indicates that they provide a fundamental driving force that infuses the medical profession with control over what is deemed legitimate knowledge about health, extending a century-long effort to establish a monopoly by physicians and the capitalist infrastructures that support them over healing in the United States (Brown 1979). Subsequently, patient-consumer communicability played a crucial role in the biomedicalization (Clarke et al. 2003) and pharmaceuticalization (Biehl 2007) of health and in augmenting and naturalizing health inequities. In terms of race, as I have argued, biocommunicability and patient-consumer communicability came to be prominent and quite valuable forms of white social capital. They operate, in Raymond Williams's (1977) terms, as a struc-ture of feeling: not entirely unconscious but more felt than consciously for-mulated. Rupa Marya and Raj Patel (2021, 18) argue that "the history of modern medicine *is* the history of colonialism." Unlike Frantz Fanon, however, they do not diagnose health/communicative inequities as a fundamental part of medicine's continuing coloniality. Here is, if you will, my diagnosis: both of the biocommunicable models that dominate in the United States fundamentally undermine the aspirations of providers, health communicators, and patients. I propose that it is time to move on.

Medicine is by no means the only field that positions dominant communicable regimes as a means of identifying professional vision (Goodwin 1994) and securing authority. I have focused on biocommunicability, but the process is similar in other domains. Excellent work by anthropologists who focus on education suggests that identifying a particular ideological model of speaking, writing, reading, and thinking as required for educational success, constructing Others as incarcerated by competing communicabilities, discrediting or even stigmatizing them, and then using this opposition to assess which children, schools, and regions are successful and which are failures operates analogously (see, e.g., Heath 1983; Rosa 2018; Shange 2019).

Here I want to build on Michel-Rolph Trouillot's (2021) powerful and influential argument regarding how European modernity was constructed as a utopian project by simultaneously crafting what he termed "the savage slot," later elaborated by anthropologists. Producing discourses of Otherness provided an implicit means of enabling "Europe" to cast itself as the locus of the logics and ethics by which "the savage" could become a reality, thereby claiming its own innocence. My discussion of John Locke traced the crucial role of communicability in enabling white, European, elite, nondisabled men to perform their rationality and individual agency and to judge in advance that all others would be stigmatized with varying types and degrees of incommunicability. Building on Trouillot, I would thus suggest that the *incommunicable slot* not only has a centuries-long history in producing colonial inequities and forms of violence but that its negative effects continue to shape the fine details of contemporary life, as witnessed during the pandemic. Racialized medical profiling contributes to the deplorable inequities in the care that Black and Latinx patients receive compared with white people (Smedley, Stith, and Nelson 2003). In short, granting the presumption of biocommunicable competence to white patients and imposing incommunicability on BIPOC patients is a medical, not a "merely communicative," issue. Health/communicative profiling matters.

It is essential to note that these are structural issues, not blanket generalizations that paint all health professionals with the same brush. Critiques by physicians of how capitalist medicine helps produce health inequities and either silence or distort patients' voices are many and important. To cite one leading example, Howard Waitzkin, trained as a physician and a sociologist, has treated patients for more than fifty years. He has worked with social movement organizations and fellow health professionals to create justice-based clinical spaces and has continually drawn on this experience in analyzing the nuts and bolts of clinical medicine and public health, from doctor-patient interaction to ways that international treaties and transnational health corporations thwart the aspirations of patients, doctors, and nurses (Waitzkin 1991, [1983] 2000, 2011; Waitzkin and Working Group for Health beyond Capitalism 2018). Again, one of the major goals of this book is to provide analytical and ethnographic resources to assist health professionals and patients in their efforts to transform dominant regimes of biocommunicability and collaboratively create alternatives.

I have argued that sorting out issues of communicability is crucial for health, healing, medicine, and public health. I want to turn the argument around now to make a slightly different claim for work on communication in general. I hope that linguistic anthropologists and others interested in language and communication issues who have not focused on health or medicine have found valuable insights in the preceding chapters. Just as I have tried to show medical anthropologists and others interested in health how productive it can be to see how ideologies of language and health are coproduced, I hope to have broken down this subdisciplinary boundary in such a way as to de-medicalize linguistic anthropology by showing that the role of in/communicability in producing and naturalizing inequities is crucial for studying language, communication, and interaction in general.

There is often a bias in perspectives on language and communication toward projecting communicability as the standard, presupposed baseline. Ferdinand de Saussure's influential *A Course in General Linguistics* ([1916] 1959, 19) started from the premise that "language exists in the form of a sum of impressions deposited in the brain of each member of a community, almost like a dictionary of which identical copies have been distributed to each individual." In his pathbreaking *Aspects of the Theory of Syntax*, Noam Chomsky (1965, 3) declared that "linguistic theory is concerned primarily with an ideal speaker-listener, in a completely homogenous speech-community, who knows its language perfectly and is unaffected by such grammatically irrelevant conditions as memory limitations, distractions, shifts of attention and interest, and errors (random or characteristic) in applying his knowledge of the language in actual performance." In these remarkably ableist proclamations, communicability became a foundational analytic; incommunicability was, at best, of marginal academic interest.

What might be gained by *starting* with incommunicability and then analyzing how ruptures of understanding and connection are entangled with and help constitute everyday communicative processes? Many dissenting voices have drawn attention to cracks in communicability. Edward Sapir (1921, 38) famously claimed, "Unfortunately, or luckily, no language is tyrannically consistent. All grammars leak." Gregory Bateson (1972) tried to identify the roots of communicative and psychological disorders, focusing on instances where referential content and metacommunicative framing were discordant. Dell Hymes (1974) left room for *in*competence in spaces where shifting languages and codes conflict. John Gumperz (1982) analyzed instances where interlocutors do not share background knowledge and communicative resources.

These and many other examples suggest conducting that ethnographies of incommunicability and using incommunicability as a starting point in building analytics of communication and language would be valuable. Efforts to decolonize the study of language and communication could benefit, I think, from other efforts to discern the colonial legacy of Locke's elevation of communicability as a model for subjectivity, rationality, agency, and social and political order and to propose alternatives. A wonderful example here is the work of Samy Alim (2006). Rather than using linguistics to analyze hip-hop, Alim adopts hip-hop as an analytical point of departure, proceeding to analyze and mediate struggles against linguistic racisms and racial inequities in the streets and the academy. Much more work needs to be done in examining how the effects of Lockean communicability enter into such domains as education, religion, politics, economics, psychology, and psychiatry. Collaborations across subdisciplines might yield a productive anthropology of incommunicability.

Toward a Post-incommunicable World

A major focus of this book has been analyzing how perspectives on and practices of clinical interaction and health communication can create the very incommunicability they are designed to eliminate. As valuable as critique may be in shaking things up, adding yet another tool for diagnosing what is wrong would fall short of making a genuinely meaningful contribution. The interlude presented four examples in which different actors—from healers to choirs and civil rights activists—made significant interventions. My discussion of Pato Hebert's powerful testimony and struggles with long COVID pointed to a third type of communicability—one that is both in dialogue with biocommunicability and seeks to legitimize the efforts of laypeople, particularly patients, to contribute knowledge based on their experience. Many relied on what they learned in the HIV support movement. "Long-haulers" were embraced early on by other communities of patients with autoimmune and other complex illnesses who feel they are not adequately supported by biomedicine. Their experiences point to how such solidarity can advance biomedical research and treatment. Mohan Dutta (2008, 2012) and other critical health communication scholars provide many other examples of "the systemic erasures of subaltern voices from discursive spaces of health communication" (Dutta and Dutta 2013, 14) as well as grassroots efforts to critique biocommunicability, disrupt its production of incommunicable subjects, and craft alternatives. I have stressed that such efforts can take very different forms, from placing radically different communicabilities in dialogue to recognizing the importance of voice, genre, and acoustic materiality to using deep dives into biomedicine by patients and activists to changing the course of research, treatment, and representation. A common thread that runs through them is a brave move—from subtle and harmonious to disruptive and confrontational—on the part of people judged incommunicable.

Promoting a single, one-size-fits-all model would clearly contradict the fundamental argument of this book. However, I think that reflecting on features of the Black Panthers' remarkable project could provide a useful starting point for efforts to transform health care and communication into concrete practices for achieving health/communicative justice. In tune with Latin American social medicine and critical epidemiology (Breilh 2003, 2021), the Panthers emphasized the need to integrate ideological transformation—critiquing hierarchical models based on white supremacy and racial capitalism and developing alternatives—with innovative clinical, political, and media practices to achieve revolutionary changes. Their efforts to democratize health knowledge involved repositioning biocommunicability within a broader range of communicable modalities. They suggest that valuing the lived experience of oppressed and underserved communities provides a crucial basis for facing health problems and challenging established categories of health knowledge and structures of authority.

The examples I outlined in the interlude provide evidence that transforming health communication and health care and strengthening their connection is possible; that the process is complex and precarious; and that such efforts can make significant contributions to the achievement of health, equity, and justice. A major problem here is that dominant scientific, clinical, and public health institutions and universities, primarily located in North America (where I live) and Europe, maintain their dominance both by continually producing what are framed as new and improved models and advertising them in "high-impact" journals and the websites and reports of the World

Health Organization, national and regional centers for disease control and prevention, and dominant nongovernmental health organizations such as the Gates Foundation. Innovative and effective grassroots efforts, by contrast, are seldom documented, often ridiculed and suppressed, rarely celebrated as crucial sources for innovation in global health, and seldom make it onto the pages of the journals frequented by physicians and public health practitioners. By calling attention to their contributions and suggesting why they are so important I hope to have contributed to highlighting them.

I want to offer four suggestions for the form that new transformative efforts might take.

1   To return to the discussion of the Black Panthers, a fundamental goal might be the creation of *incommunicability-free zones*, spaces where confronting health, educational, legal, and other inequities does not create hierarchies of knowledge or stigmatize some participants as being out of the loop, ignorant, irrational, or misguided.

2. I have argued that one of the main things that went wrong in the United States with COVID-19 is that some 99 percent of the population was continually told that it had nothing worthwhile to contribute to making sense of a new, puzzling disease. It is hard to imagine how any type of health communication, from visits to the doctor or nurse-practitioner to global health initiatives, can better the lives of its designated recipients if based on the premise that what they know just doesn't count. Starting from the assumption that all parties have something significant to offer and then placing their perspectives in dialogue is far more likely to result not just in "buy-in" but in perspectives and actions that generate structural change.

3   We need to bury the Lockean legacy, which decrees that communication requires diagnoses of miscommunication and interventions whose ethical value is assured in advance by the claim that they are designed to fix things. Power hierarchies are reinscribed by these instrumentalist logics, and efforts to achieve "efficacy" that do not value justice can exacerbate inequities.

4   These days, we are constantly asked to evaluate, to use standard metrics to assess a visit to the doctor, a bank transaction, a class, or a meal at a restaurant. Metrics, Vincanne Adams (2013, 2016) has argued, form part of what drives the skewed politics of global health. I want to propose a different sort of benchmark. Each clinical encounter, health communication presentation, medical and nursing school class, and grassroots initiative could be evaluated with respect to how it contributes to confronting health/communicative inequities and furthering health/communicative justice.

I have documented the power of the biomedical authority model of communicability, which has a prominent place in all of the countries where I have conducted ethnographic and media research, and of patient-consumer communicability, which is highly visible in the United States and other countries where neoliberalism is dominant. I have suggested that both models negatively affect providers, patients, and public health programs. One crucial problem is that they project laypeople as individuals required to perform their biocommunicable competence to gain health and well-being. The individualism that forms the base of each is "toxic," in Mark Nichter's (2022, 560) terms, and it thwarts precisely the efforts to build collective logics and solutions that social movements and patient-practitioner coalitions identify with lay-activist communicability. My analysis of the COVID-19 pandemic suggests that biosecurity mentalities that stigmatize all departures from unilinear, hierarchically ordered models don't make anyone safer; instead, they squander possibilities for stimulating and valuing all parties' contributions to knowledge production and care. Before yet another pandemic emerges, I hope that the pandemic-industrial-discourse complex will be dismantled. In the United States, rather than saving lives, it made things much worse, and its credibility is now virtually nil. Another problem with allowing biomedical-authority and patient-consumer communicabilities to pass for the only means of structuring health communication is that they are racialized in ways that render them particularly toxic for Black, Latinx, and Native American populations. Decades of promoting patient-consumer self-interest through logics of choice (Mol [2006] 2008) and the rise of white supremacist individualism led to the rejection of calls to protect others, particularly vulnerable strangers, and collectivist appeals that "we are all in this together."

It's time to break the hold of these two dominant models on conceptualizing and practicing health care and global health. The examples in the interlude suggest the value of a range of strategies for democratizing communicability by broadening conceptions of what health knowledge is, who gets to make it, how it circulates, and how it shapes practices inside the clinic and far beyond. We need to get beyond global one-size-fits-all models. When abstract, standardized models dominate practices of speaking and listening, writing and reading, producing and viewing, they make it much more difficult for participants—particularly those in more powerful positions—to attend to what people are actually saying and doing. One thing that is needed is openness, a willingness to make space for exploring new approaches to knowledge and care in each class or practicum, clinical visit, health communication presentation, policy decision, and more.

The COVID-19 pandemic has shown us many things. One is that health-care systems in the United States are fundamentally broken. If we listen care-fully to healthcare workers who are resigning and nurses who are marching in the streets, we can see that the issue is not just pandemic "burnout" but how their efforts over decades to demand better ways of relating to and car-ing for their patients have been crushed by for-profit, bureaucratized health systems. My lay interlocutors—including Frank Miller and others classified as "anti-vaxxers"—are, in their own languages, echoing many of their cri-tiques and searching for new points of departure. They demand that the mul-tiple, including stigmatized and racialized, straitjackets in which lay efforts to contribute to understanding health and well-being be set aside.

Many valuable ways to begin again that emerged during the pandemic are getting lost. Linda Robertson, the food services director at an elemen-tary school in California's San Joaquín Valley, reacted to acute food scar-city among students once the school was closed down. Partnering with state agencies and other sources, she used the cafeteria to produce meals that were distributed on-site. She also worked with school-bus drivers to make the same routes each week with two food service workers on board, dropping off a whole week of breakfasts and lunches for all children right in front of their houses. A school closure thus launched a bold step to address broader food insecurity issues in the valley. Epidemiologist, researcher, and activist Sylvia Montaño amplified the impact on food scarcity of efforts by Robert-son and other food-service employees by mapping these points of food dis-tribution, sharing the list on social media, and sending it to county health and social service agencies and other organizations. My heart fell during my interview with Robertson, however, when she responded to my question in October 2021 as to whether that experience had changed what she is doing in the long run. She reported the school food program had returned to business as usual. The issues here go far beyond COVID-19 and questions of health, even broadly defined. In chapters 7 and 8, I tried to capture some of the in-novative ways that laypeople and health professionals alike expanded defini-tions, visions, and practices of knowledge production and care. Even as we celebrate these and draw out their implications for contexts beyond pandem-ics and health care, it is crucial to recognize how the pandemic deepened inequities of health and health care, education, housing, income, employ-ment, and more. In Hanna Garth's (2021) powerful articulation, we need to prioritize flattening their curves as well.

These problems go far beyond the pandemic. I have traced in these pages a process of personal transformation in which I confronted how my previous work was rooted in attachments to the primordiality of communicability, and thus to whiteness, privilege, and coloniality. By analyzing genealogies of communicability, I hope to have contributed to efforts to confront how racism, racialization, and white supremacy are woven as deeply into academic institutions as the natural/cultural worlds they inhabit. Social scientists can play essential roles in critically engaging the roots of entrenched inequities, drawing attention to how people struggle to confront them and pressing for equitable and just perspectives, policies, and practices. By weaving together perspectives from linguistic and medical anthropology I have analyzed what can be gained by challenging the boundaries of narrow forms of disciplinary training and embracing efforts to decolonize received forms of disciplinary authority. Facing severe restrictions on travel for research and immense challenges in their own daily lives and those of their families and communities, many anthropologists felt compelled to use their particular skills to document, analyze, and write about the pandemic worlds surrounding them. Rather than returning to "the normal," we must find ways to make the insights and experiences that emerged there outlast direct relations to COVID-19 and spark new collaborations and forms of commitment. I can only hope that my modest contributions to these efforts will be of value to readers as they imagine new ways to craft more just and equitable worlds.

INTRODUCTION

1 Bloomberg Quicktake, "CDC Director Says Delta Variant Is Most Infectious Virus of Her Career," YouTube video, June 22, 2021, https://www.youtube.com /watch?v=qxGQgKJsGoM.

2 In using this term, I am cognizant of Eve Tuck and K. Wayne Wang's (2012) important argument that decolonization should be used not "metaphorically" but, rather, strictly in reference to efforts to return lands stolen by settler-colonial regimes. Three factors suggest to me that decolonization is, however, still appropriate as a means of positioning my project. First, I make no attempt here to claim, in their words, a "settler move to innocence" (Tuck and Wang 2012, 10). This project has heightened my own awareness of my positionality within whiteness and privilege. Second, their argument rests on a literalist interpretation of the term *metaphor* and of the discursive and analytic underpinnings of colonialism and oppression, as Tapji Garba and Sara-Maria Sorentino (2020) have pointed out. Indeed, even as Tuck and Wang may break with Locke's theory of land and property, their argument recapitulates his foundational argument about language and communication. In chapter 1 I discuss how deeply Locke's literalist and referentialist perspective on language provides a crucial infrastructure for colonialism and white supremacy. Third, just as land matters, so does life. Here I join with other writers (see, e.g., Marya and Patel 2021) in arguing that the conceptual, material, and institutional underpinnings of health inequities constitute a key site for reproducing colonialism and an indispensable locus of efforts to counter its often lethal effects.

3 Why "inequities" rather than "inequalities"? Identifying *inequalities* involves specifying two phenomena and projecting a relationship between them founded on a presumption of commensurability and an expectation of sameness. The common use of statistics in identifying and interpreting inequalities brings to mind Talal Asad's (1994, 78) remark that "statistics converts the question of

incommensurable cultures into one of commensurable social arrangements without rendering them homogeneous." The language of inequalities accordingly seems to cast differences as exceptional. The term *inequities*, on the other hand, focuses our energies less on observing discrepancies than on analyzing structural factors that produce them, a point that resonates with Latin American social medicine and critical epidemiology (see Breilh 2003).

4   On medicalization—the framing of phenomena as determined by biomedical processes, thus placing their explanation and intervention in the hands of biomedical and scientific professionals—see Zola 1972 but also Fassin 2011.

5   Recent work has emphasized that logics of white supremacy, which pervasively shape policies, institutional practices, and discourses, are global in nature, reaching far beyond the ranks of overtly racist right-wing "extremists," who are similarly found in many countries (Beliso-De Jesús and Pierre 2019).

6   My engagement with Shange's work emerged in a graduate seminar on collaborative, community-driven research. Nate Tilton placed an article by Shange on the syllabus, and our discussion helped push my thinking about race and communicability, for which I thank Cameron Johnson, as well.

7   On ethnographic refusal, also see Ortner 1995.

8   See Brice Heath 1983 and Rosa 2018 for two examples.

9   On this point, see Heller and McElhinny 2017.

10   Carolyn Rouse's provocative study of sickle cell anemia adds to Shange's list. Rouse (2009, 7) suggests that "knowing only a patient's race or ethnicity, even a well-meaning doctor may make presumptions that influence how he or she communicates with and medically treats a patient.... Race emplots individuals in narratives not of their choosing." Black patients' statements about excruciating pain are interpreted as illegitimate requests designed to satisfy drug habits.

11   I owe this articulation to Rachel Lee's fascinating comments on chapter 8 of this book.

12   "Incommunicability" has appeared sporadically in scholarly sources, with a range of meanings. The term, as I use it, does not spring from these sources but from my engagement with work I discuss here.

13   The linguistic anthropologist Krystal Smalls builds on Spillers in analyzing how white bodies, subjectivities, and speech get positioned "as the default Human in our models." She analyzes the resulting "ontological crisis faced by people who encounter their bodies as other than normatively Human" (2020, 242). Bodies and their features shape how signs that move through or in proximity to them get categorized and marked. Work by Kira Hall and Mary Bucholtz (2016) on "embodied sociolinguistics" also provides a point of reference here.

14   Rather than creating fixed binaries, Asif Agha argues that these "figures of personhood" get turned into icons, in Charles Peirce's (1955) terms, enabling them to move frequently across scales as individuals are recruited to stand as their embodiments and vice versa.

15   Note, however, that several health-related chapters appeared in *Case Studies in Language and Social Justice* (Avineri et al. 2019).

16 Here I draw on Gal and Irvine 2019. They carefully distinguish their use of the term from notions of false consciousness, which claim scholarly access to objective structures while criticizing other parties as devising hidden strategies for advancing their self-interest. Gal and Irvine (13–14) instead speak of "ideologizing" and "ideological work," highlighting connections with "power, politics, interest, and social action."

17 Dorothy Roberts's (1997) trenchant analysis of the figure of the bad Black mother whose incommunicability willfully endangers the lives of her children provides an unconscionable baseline for defining the limits of humanity and a key trope of the Moynihan Report's projection of Black culpability for racial inequities and its liberal calls to institutionalize communicability, including through early childhood education.

18 I thank Richard Bauman for emphasizing this point in his reading of an early draft.

CHAPTER 1. THE INCOMMUNICABLE MENACE LURKING WITHIN LOCKE'S CHARTER FOR COMMUNICABILITY

1 For an extensive discussion of Locke's *Essay* and other works that embodied his writing on language and semiotics, see Bauman and Briggs 2003.

2 I use *crisis* here in Janet Roitman's (2014) sense of the term.

3 In *Leviathan*, Thomas Hobbes ([1651] 1968) presented a topology of the uses of speech and corresponding abuses.

4 I thank Richard Bauman for reminding me of this passage.

CHAPTER 2. W. E. B. DU BOIS: INCOMMUNICABILITY AND/AS THE VEIL

1 I thank one of the anonymous reviewers of the manuscript for pressing me to clarify this point.

2 I wish to make it clear that I am not offering any form of evaluation or judgment here of these distinct ways of grieving the death of a child.

3 Here, again, I thank an anonymous reviewer for challenging me to draw out this point.

CHAPTER 3. FRANTZ FANON: DOCTORS, TARZAN, AND THE COLONIAL INSCRIPTION OF INCOMMUNICABILITY

1 I adopt Fanon's term *pidgin*, as used by Richard Philcox in translating *petit-nègre* in referring to how colonial physicians constructed and performed a demeaning speech style that they improperly attributed to colonized patients. To avoid endlessly enclosing the term in scare quotes, I ask readers to remember that I am invoking Fanon's critique of such speech rather than referring to language varieties linguists have often called pidgins (see Hymes 1971).

2 The French text reads: "Vingt malades européens se succèdent: 'Asseyez-vous, monsieur ... Pourquoi venez-vous? ... De quoi souffrez-voùs? ...'—Arrive

un nègre ou un Arabe: 'Assieds-toi, mon brave . . . Qu'est-ce que tu as? . . . Où as-tu mal?'—Quand ce n'est pas: 'Quoi toi y en a? . . .'" (Fanon 1952, 25). Note how this passage pointedly reproduces the use of formal (for "Europeans") and familiar (for "a black man or an Arab") second-person pronouns, drawing attention to the dynamics of power and solidarity later analyzed by Brown and Gilman (1968) 1972.

3 Note that Menéndez (2002, 40) suggests that Fanon's critique extends to ethnographic works as similarly distorting.

4 For scholars who point to Fanon's importance in the history of colonial medicine, see Keller 2007; Manderson 1996; and Vaughan 1991.

5 For the French text of Fanon's reproduction of how colonial physicians use formal second-person pronouns for European patients and the *tu* form, along with other features of pidgin, for colonized patients, see note 2 in this chapter.

6 Fanon parodies how persistent efforts by Algerian patients over multiple visits to speak and gesture "volubly" about their condition are dramatically reduced as "the interpreter (appropriately baffling) translates for us: he says he as a belly-ache" ([1964] 1967, 5).

7 In a later essay, Fanon and Azoulay take a more critical stance on cultural relativism ([2015] 2018, 373).

8 Fanon's allusion is to advertisements for Banania, a banana-favored chocolate drink widely sold in France. Stephan Likosky (2017) documents how images that accompanied the advertisements during World War I portrayed members of the *tirailleurs sénégalais*, Senegalese soldiers who served in the French Army, as childlike grinning men with containers of Banania who seemed to be speaking the line "Y'a bon" (It's good) in the register Fanon calls pidgin.

CHAPTER 5. BIOCOMMUNICABLE LABOR AND THE PRODUCTION OF INCOMMUNICABILITY IN "DOCTOR-PATIENT INTERACTION"

1 However, Steven Epstein (2007) documents how normative whiteness, masculinity, and heterosexuality have been challenged since the 1990s through a politics of "inclusion."

2 I owe this point to my colleague William White (2023).

3 William Hanks (1990) minutely analyzed how indexicality is not rigidly determined by seemingly objective temporal and spatial interactional features. Elinor Ochs (1990) developed the notion of "indirect indexicality," which helps illuminate this interactional and semiotic process.

4 For a general critique of problems in reifying "the context," see Bauman and Briggs 1990, 68.

5 A standard reference point for these terms is Silverstein 1976. Note that John Gumperz (1982) discussed these sorts of metapragmatic features as "contextualization cues."

6 Fisher and Groce's focus is specifically on what they refer to as accounting practices, statements that seem to justify or excuse words and actions. Also see Fisher 1998 on providers' versus patients' questioning strategies.

7 The very concept of "medical translator" fits into the ideological reduction of "a whole family of semiotic processes" (Gal 2015, 226) to what is projected as rendering stretches of referential content portable and yet stable across the borders defined by the "misrecognition of language as autonomous code" (Reynolds and Orellana 2009, 213). See also Díaz-Duque 1998.

8 Children similarly face deep contradictions when they become patients. Ignasi Clemente (2015) documented struggles by children and youth with cancer diagnoses to demand active roles in clinical participation frameworks. Anthony Wright (2019) showed how biocommunicable profiling prompted oncology professionals and arts therapists to reproduce anti-Black stereotypes and adultism in ways that engendered treatment inequities in a pediatric cancer ward.

9 Mishler (1984, 1986) argues for democratizing interviewing practices by challenging interviewer/interviewee power asymmetries.

10 Bauman and Briggs's (1990, 72) call for an ethnography of decontextualization and recontextualization would seem to be still useful in guiding research here.

11 For just a few examples, see Bauman 2004; Hill 1995; and Ochs, Smith, and Taylor 1996. Briggs and Mantini-Briggs (2003, 2016) use these perspectives in analyzing patients' and practitioners' narratives about health and disease, including epidemics.

12 For a further elaboration of this argument, see Briggs and Mantini-Briggs 2016, chap. 5.

13 The distinguished ethnographer Johannes Wilbert has provided extensive documentation of the importance of moriche palms and the *nahanamu* ritual cycle (see esp. Wilbert 1993).

14 Mr. Torres was initiated as a *wisidatu* shaman, and he thus does have some training in dealing with *hebu*. His main specialty, however, is *hoa*, and he does not attempt to remove *hebu* from individual patients.

15 For a detailed analysis of the performance, see Briggs 1996.

16 For additional ethnographies of *wisidatu* healing, see Olsen 1996; Wilbert 1993.

17 Given that he focused on a dictated text (Holmer and Wassén 1947), Lévi-Strauss analyzes a hypothetical case.

18 I thank an anonymous reviewer for Duke University Press for pressing me on this point.

CHAPTER 6. HEALTH COMMUNICATION: HOW
IN/COMMUNICABILITIES JUMP SCALE

Epigraph: "Quotations from Sir Muir Gray," Gurteen Knowledge Community, 2015, http://www.gurteen. com/gurteen/gurteen.nsf/id/ knowledge-and-disease.

1 There are massive literatures on health communication in both communication and public health. With the exception of Mohan Dutta's (2008, 2012) critical, culture-centered approach, which is central to my argument, analyzing

them would take me beyond the scope and the ethnographic orientation in this chapter.

2 For other examples of the now substantial literature on linguistic landscapes, see Blommaert 2013; and Carr 2019.

3 Héctor Becerra, "Program Is Fighting Teenage Pregnancy," *Los Angeles Times*, 8 January 2004, B3.

4 On COVID-19 linguistic landscapes, see also Mundt and Polzenhagen 2022. Dutta 2021 discusses communicative inequities in the pandemic, and Lewis, Govender, and Holland 2021 provide various perspectives on COVID-19 communication early in the pandemic.

5 Denise Nelesen, "Programs Tell Latinos about Diabetes," *San Diego Union-Tribune*, 7 June 2003, E5.

6 On oil camps, see Tinker Salas 2009. Timothy Mitchell (2002) argues that mosquitos were a major problem for British colonialism in Egypt.

7 On the binary between sanitary citizens and insanitary subjects, see Briggs and Mantini-Briggs 2003.

8 Note that this pamphlet was in circulation in 2002. At that time, President Hugo Chávez Frías's efforts to improve the lives of working-class Venezuelans had yet to produce significant results, and the project—Missión Barrio Adentro—that brought free health care to most underserved communities in the country had not yet been enacted (see Briggs and Mantini-Briggs 2009; OPS 2006).

9 I acknowledge my debt to Dr. Clara Mantini-Briggs, coordinator of the National Program for Dengue Fever and National Director of Health Education at the Ministry of Health and Social Development. She shared a copy of the Pedrito pamphlet, and we previously collaborated in analyzing it (see Briggs and Mantini-Briggs 2005).

10 This statement is based on interviews with the public health officials and journalists involved.

11 For a more detailed discussion, see Briggs and Mantini-Briggs 2003.

12 A study conducted during the 1950s–70s by Miguel Layrisse, Johannes Wilbert, and their colleagues placed prepubescent mortality at 50 percent (Wilbert 1980). Research in the northwestern delta in the late 1990s suggested that 36 percent of children died in their first year: see Servicio de Apoyo Local (SOCSAL), "Registro sociodemográfico warao de Punta Pescador," 1998, photocopy. A study of two hundred Orinoco Delta mothers by anthropologists Werner Wilbert and Cecilia Ayala Lafée-Wilbert (2007) determined that nearly 39 percent of their children had died; 78 percent of these deaths occurred before the age of four. More recent findings, compiled from quite a number of regions of the Orinoco Delta, are by Villalba et al. (2013). They found that in 2011, child mortality was approximately 26 percent. Dr. Jacobus de Waard conducted a study of tuberculosis in the Orinoco Delta under the auspices of the Instituto de Biomedicina in Caracas. He reported the figure of 60 percent incidence of tuberculosis in the delta region's population in an interview conducted in Caracas on 2 July 1999.

13 For extensive documentation and analysis, see Briggs and Mantini-Briggs 2003.

14 HIV confessionals can, nevertheless, be highly medicalized. In an excellent discussion of the politics of numbers and "risk" perception in Haitian communities of South Florida, Thurka Sangaramoorthy (2014, 22) reports a patient introducing herself by saying, "I am 400 DC4 count and 250 viral load."

15 Eivind Engebretsen pointed out the importance of evidence-based medicine in the rise of patient-consumer communicability (personal communication with the author, 23 November 2022).

16 Helga Nowotny (1993, 2000) has emphasized the connection between rejecting scientific and medical monopolies on "expert" knowledge and lay moves to evaluate competing sources of facts and claim participation in their production (see also Nowotny, Scott, and Gibbons 2001). Thanks are due to Mark Nichter for a valuable discussion of patient-consumer communicability and sharing his research on Lyme disease.

17 Arline Geronimus (2023) notes that a landmark eight-volume publication by the US Department of Health and Human Services on what were called racial disparities in health prompted decades of calls to eliminate racialized inequities. Largely resting on a "blame narrative" that attributed worse health outcomes for Black Americans to "the effects of their own choices" (5), "the primary recommendation of the report concerned improving individual health behaviors by expanding health education to minoritized individuals" rather than making structural reforms (3). Faulty reasoning, she argues, led to faulty programs and a continuing legacy of racialized health inequities.

INTERLUDE. SOCIAL MOVEMENTS AND
INCOMMUNICABILITY-FREE ZONES

1 This example has scores of parallels in the medical anthropology literature, perhaps most famously in Paul Farmer's (1992) careful study of Haitian and biomedical accounts of the beginning of the AIDS epidemic.

2 There is, of course, a vast literature on this topic. Cindy Patton's *Inventing AIDS* (1990) is one of the most visible.

CHAPTER 7. PANDEMIC ECOLOGIES OF KNOWLEDGE: IN DEFENSE
OF COVID-19 CONSPIRACY THEORIES, SORT OF

1 World Health Organization, "COVID-19 Mythbusters," online slide program, accessed 13 December 2021, https://web.archive.org/web/20200715151718 /https://www.who.int/westernpacific/emergencies/covid-19/information /mythbusters.

2 See, e.g., Proal and VanElzakker 2021. For an earlier study, see Desforges et al. 2014. I thank Megan Moodie for compiling an excellent bibliography on long COVID, and I thank members of the How We Make It: Disability Justice for the

Long Haul group at the University of California, Irvine, Humanities Research Institute for an illuminating discussion.

3 Richard Besser, interview by Daniel Hallin, New York, 3 March 2012, quoted in Briggs and Hallin 2016, 117.

4 Briggs and Hallin (2016) present an outline of these heterogeneous sources.

5 Besser interview.

6 Pato Hebert's website, accessed 15 March 2023, https://patohebert.com/home .html.

7 "About the Patient-Led Research Collaborative," Patient-Led Research Collaborative website, accessed 1 April 2023, https://patientresearchcovid19.com/.

8 See Lowenstein 2022 for a publication that grew out of the Body Politic COVID-19 Support Group.

9 An interview with Miller's brother on 1 March 2022 suggested that his position was rather more complex.

CHAPTER 8. PANDEMIC ECOLOGIES OF CARE

1 For analyses of conspiracy theories, see Barkun 2003; Briggs 2004; Dean 1998; Farmer 1992; Fenster 1999; Hofstadter 1967; Marcus 1999; Scheper-Hughes 1996; and White 2000.

2 Holmes's book describes the situation in Oregon and Washington.

3 The interview was conducted in Spanish. The translation is mine.

4 Reports on COVID-19 conditions in farmworker communities in Bade, Ramirez, and Saxton 2021 and in Ramirez, Mines, and Carlisle-Cummins 2020 provide valuable observations on these issues.

5 For a recent study of how discourses about burnout are woven into the fabric of neoliberal work, see Funahashi 2023.

6 These figures are from the Johns Hopkins University Coronavirus Resource Center, last updated 10 March 2023, https://coronavirus.jhu.edu/region/us /montana.

Aarsleff, Hans. 1982. *From Locke to Saussure: Essays on the Study of Language and Intellectual History*. Minneapolis: University of Minnesota Press.

Açiksöz, Salih Can. 2020. *Sacrificial Limbs: Masculinity, Disability, and Political Violence in Turkey*. Oakland: University of California Press.

Adams, Vincanne. 2013. "Evidence-Based Global Public Health: Subjects, Profits, Erasures." In *When People Come First: Critical Studies in Global Health*, edited by João Biehl and Adriana Petryna, 54–90. Princeton, NJ: Princeton University Press.

Adams, Vincanne, ed. 2016. *Metrics: What Counts in Global Health*. Durham, NC: Duke University Press.

Agar, Michael. 1973. *Ripping and Running: A Formal Ethnography of Urban Heroin Addicts*. New York: Seminar.

Agha, Asif. 2005. "Voice, Footing, Enregisterment." *Journal of Linguistic Anthropology* 15(1): 38–59.

Agha, Asif. 2006. *Language and Social Relations*. Cambridge: Cambridge University Press.

Ahmed, Sara. 2019. *What's the Use? On the Uses of Use*. Durham, NC: Duke University Press.

Ainsworth-Vaughn, Nancy. 1992. "Topic Transitions in Physician-Patient Interviews: Power, Gender, and Discourse." *Language in Society* 21(3): 409–26.

Ainsworth-Vaughn, Nancy. 1998. *Claiming Power in Doctor-Patient Talk*. New York: Oxford University Press.

Alim, H. Samy. 2006. *Roc the Mic Right: The Language of Hip Hop Culture*. New York: Routledge.

Alim, H. Samy, Angela Reyes, and Paul V. Kroskrity, eds. 2020. *The Oxford Handbook of Language and Race*. New York: Oxford University Press.

Alim, H. Samy, John R. Rickford, and Arnetha F. Ball, eds. 2016. *Raciolinguistics: How Language Shapes Our Ideas about Race*. New York: Oxford University Press.

Alim, H. Samy, and Geneva Smitherman. 2020. "Raciolinguistic Exceptionalism: How Racialized 'Compliments' Reproduce White Supremacy." In *The Oxford Handbook of Language and Race*, edited by H. Samy Alim, Angela Reyes, and Paul V. Kroskrity, 472–96. New York: Oxford University Press.

Andersen, Barbara. 2017. "Careful Words: Nursing, Language, and Emotion in Papua New Guinea." *Medical Anthropology* 36(8): 758–71.

Anderson, Warwick. 2006. *Colonial Pathologies: American Tropical Medicine, Race, and Hygiene in the Philippines*. Durham, NC: Duke University Press.

Anschuetz, Kurt F., Richard H. Wilshusen, and Cherie L. Scheick. 2001. "An Archaeology of Landscapes: Perspectives and Directions." *Journal of Archaeological Research* 9(2): 157–211.

Anstey, Peter R. 2011. *John Locke and Natural Philosophy*. Oxford: Oxford University Press.

Appadurai, Arjun. 1988. "Putting Hierarchy in Its Place." *Cultural Anthropology* 3(1): 36–49.

Armada, Francisco, and Carles Muntaner. 2004. "The Visible Fist of the Market: Health Reforms in Latin America." In *Unhealthy Health Policy: A Critical Anthropological Examination*, edited by Arachu Castro and Merrill Singer, 29–42. Walnut Creek, CA: AltaMira.

Arnold, David. 1993. *Colonizing the Body: State Medicine and Epidemic Disease in Nineteenth-Century India*. Berkeley: University of California Press.

Arnold, Lynette. 2020. "Cross-Border Communication and the Enregisterment of Collective Frameworks for Care." *Medical Anthropology* 39(7): 624–37.

Asad, Talal. 1986. "The Concept of Cultural Translation in British Social Anthropology." In *Writing Culture: The Poetics and Politics of Ethnography*, edited by James Clifford and George E. Marcus, 141–64. Berkeley: University of California Press.

Asad, Talal. 1994. "Ethnographic Representation, Statistics and Modern Power." *Social Research* 61(1): 55–88.

Aubrey, Allison. 2020. "CDC: At Least 20 Million Americans Have Had Coronavirus. Here's Who's at Highest Risk." National Public Radio, 25 June 2020. https://www.npr.org/sections/coronavirus-live-updates/2020/06/25/883520249/cdc-at-least-20-million-americans-have-had-coronavirus-heres-who-s-at-highest-ri.

Austin, J. L. 1962. *How to Do Things with Words: The William James Lectures Delivered at Harvard University in 1955*. Edited by J. O. Urmson and Marina Sbisà. Cambridge, MA: Harvard University Press.

Avineri, Netta, Laura R. Graham, Eric J. Johnson, Robin Conley Riner, and Jonathan Rosa, eds. 2019. *Language and Social Justice in Practice*. New York: Routledge.

Bach, Katie. 2022. "Is 'Long Covid' Worsening the Labor Shortage?" Brookings Institution, 11 January 2022. https://www.brookings.edu/research/is-long-covid-worsening-the-labor-shortage.

Bacon, Francis. 1860. "Of the Dignity and Advancement of Learning." In *The Works of Francis Bacon*, vol. 9, edited by James Spedding, Robert Leslie Ellis, and Douglas Denon Heath 13–357. New York: Garrett.

Bade, Bonnie, Sarah Ramirez, and Dvera I. Saxton. 2021. *Always Essential, Perpetually Disposable: California Farmworkers and the COVID-19 Pandemic—*

COFS *Phase Two Preliminary Report*. Santa Cruz: California Institute for Rural Studies. https://cirsinc.org/wp-content/uploads/2021/08/COFS-_Phase-Two -Preliminary-Report.pdf.

Baker, Lee D. 1998. *From Savage to Negro: Anthropology and the Construction of Race, 1896–1954*. Berkeley: University of California Press.

Baker, Stephanie B., Wei Xiang, and Ian Atkinson. 2017. "The Internet of Things for Smart Healthcare: Technologies, Challenges, and Opportunities." *IEEE Access* 5: 26521–44. https://doi.org.10.1109/ACCESS.2017.2775180.

Bakhtin, Mikhail M. 1981. *The Dialogic Imagination: Four Essays*. Edited by Michael Holquist. Translated by Caryl Emerson and Michael Holquist. Austin: University of Texas Press.

Bales, Robert Freed. 1950. *Interaction Process Analysis: A Method for the Study of Small Groups*. Cambridge, MA: Addison-Wesley.

Barilli, Renato. 1989. *Rhetoric*. Translated by Giuliana Menozzi. Minneapolis: University of Minnesota Press.

Barkun, Michael. 2003. *A Culture of Conspiracy: Apocalyptic Visions in Contemporary America*. Berkeley: University of California Press.

Basso, Keith H. 1996. *Wisdom Sits in Places: Landscape and Language among the Western Apache*. Albuquerque: University of New Mexico Press.

Bateson, Gregory. 1972. *Steps to an Ecology of Mind: Collected Essays in Anthropology, Psychiatry, Evolution, and Epistemology*. New York: Ballantine.

Baugh, John. 2003. "Linguistic Profiling." In *Black Linguistics: Language, Society, and Politics in Africa and the Americas*, edited by Sinfree Makoni, Geneva Smitherman, Arnetha F. Ball, and Arthur K. Spears, 155–68. London: Routledge.

Bauman, Richard. 1977. *Verbal Art as Performance*. Prospect Heights, IL: Waveland.

Bauman, Richard. 1992. "Contextualization, Tradition, and the Dialogue of Genres: Icelandic Legends of the *Kraftaskáld*." In *Rethinking Context: Language as an Interactive Phenomonon*, edited by Alessandro Duranti and Charles Goodwin, 125–45. Cambridge: Cambridge University Press.

Bauman, Richard. 2004. *A World of Others' Words: Cross-cultural Perspectives on Intertextuality*. Malden, MA: Blackwell.

Bauman, Richard, and Charles L. Briggs. 1990. "Poetics and Performance as Critical Perspectives on Language and Social Life." *Annual Review of Anthropology* 19:59–88.

Bauman, Richard, and Charles L. Briggs. 2003. *Voices of Modernity: Language Ideologies and Social Inequality*. Cambridge: Cambridge University Press.

Becerra, Hector. 2004. "Program Is Fighting Teenage Pregnancy." *Los Angeles Times*, 8 January 2004, B3.

Beliso-De Jesús, Aisha M., and Jemima Pierre. 2019. "Anthropology of White Supremacy." *American Anthropologist* 122(1): 65–75.

Benjamin, Walter. 1968. *Illuminations*. Edited by Hannah Arendt. Translated by Harry Zohn. New York: Schocken.

Benton, Adia. 2015. *HIV Exceptionalism: Development through Disease in Sierra Leone*. Minneapolis: University of Minnesota Press.

Berlivet, Luc, and Ilana Löwry. 2020. "Hydroxychloroquine Controversies: Clinical Trials, Epistemology, and the Democratization of Science." *Medical Anthropology Quarterly* 34(4): 525–41.

Bhabha, Homi K. 1994. *The Location of Culture*. London: Routledge.

Bianco, Giuseppe. 2012. "The Origins of Georges Canguilhem's 'Vitalism': Against the Anthropology of Irritation." In *Vitalism and the Scientific Image in Post-Enlightenment Life Science, 1800–2010*, edited by Charles T. Wolfe and S. Normandin, 243–67. London: Springer.

Biehl, João G. 2007. "Pharmaceuticalization: AIDS Treatment and Global Health Politics." *Anthropological Quarterly* 80: 1083–126.

Black, Steven P. 2019. *Speech and Song at the Margins of Global Health: Zulu Tradition, HIV Stigma, and AIDS Activism in South Africa*. New Brunswick, NJ: Rutgers University Press.

Block, Ellen, and Cecilia Vindrola-Padros. 2021. "Making Do: COVID-19 and the Improvisation of Care in the UK and US." In *Viral Loads: Anthropologies of Urgency in the Time of COVID-19*, edited by Leonore Manderson, Nancy J. Burke, and Ayo Wahlberg, 303–23. London: UCL Press.

Blommaert, Jan. 2013. *Ethnography, Superdiversity and Linguistic Landscapes: Chronicles of Complexity*. Buffalo, NY: Multilingual Matters.

Bodie, Graham D., Mohan J. Dutta, and Ambar Basu. 2009. "The Integrative Model of E-Health Use." In *Handbook of Research on Distributed Medical Informatics and E-Health*, edited by Athina A. Lazakidou and Konstantinos M. Siassiakos, 104–16. Hershey, PA: Medical Information Science Reference.

Bodner, John, Wendy Welch, Ian Brodie, Anna Muldoon, Donald Leech, and Ashley Marshall. 2021. *COVID-19 Conspiracy Theories: QAnon, 5G, the New World Order and Other Viral Ideas*. Jefferson, NC: McFarland.

Boston Women's Health Collective. 1971. *Our Bodies, Ourselves: A Course by and for Women*. Boston: New England Free Press.

Bourdieu, Pierre. (1972) 1977. *Outline of a Theory of Practice*. Translated by Richard Nice. Cambridge: Cambridge University Press.

Brandt, Allan M. 2022. "The History of Contact Tracing and the Future of Public Health." *American Journal of Public Health* 112(8): 1097–99.

Breilh, Jaime. 2003. *Epidemiología crítica: Ciencia emancipadora e interculturalidad*. Buenos Aires: Lugar Editorial.

Breilh, Jaime. 2021. *Critical Epidemiology and the People's Health*. New York: Oxford University Press.

Briggs, Charles L. 1986. *Learning How to Ask: A Sociolinguistic Appraisal of the Role of the Interview in Social Science Research*. Cambridge: Cambridge University Press.

Briggs, Charles L. 1994. "The Sting of the Ray: Bodies, Agency, and Grammar in Warao Curing." *Journal of American Folklore* 107(423): 139–66.

Briggs, Charles L. 1996. "The Meaning of Nonsense, the Poetics of Embodiment, and the Production of Power in Warao Healing." In *The Performance of Healing*, edited by Carol Laderman and Marina Roseman, 185–232. New York: Routledge.

Briggs, Charles L. 2004. "Theorizing Modernity Conspiratorially: Science, Scale, and the Political Economy of Public Discourse in Explanations of a Cholera Epidemic." *American Ethnologist* 31(2): 163–86.

Briggs, Charles L. 2005a. "Communicability, Racial Discourse, and Disease." *Annual Review of Anthropology* 34:269–91.

Briggs, Charles L. 2005b. "Genealogies of Race and Culture and the Failure of Vernacular Cosmopolitanisms: Rereading Franz Boas and W. E. B. Du Bois." *Public Culture* 17(1): 75–100.

Briggs, Charles L. 2011. "'All Cubans Are Doctors!' News Coverage of Health and Bioexceptionalism in Cuba." *Social Science and Medicine* 73:1037–44.

Briggs, Charles L. 2014. "Dear Dr. Freud." *Cultural Anthropology* 29(2): 312–43.

Briggs, Charles L. 2017. "Towards Communicative Justice in Health." *Medical Anthropology* 36(4): 287–304.

Briggs, Charles L. 2021. *Unlearning: Rethinking Poetics, Pandemics, and the Politics of Knowledge.* Logan: Utah State University Press.

Briggs, Charles L., and Daniel C. Hallin. 2016. *Making Health Public: How News Coverage Is Remaking Media, Medicine, and Contemporary Life.* London: Routledge.

Briggs, Charles L., and Clara Mantini-Briggs. 2003. *Stories in the Time of Cholera: Racial Profiling during a Medical Nightmare.* Berkeley: University of California Press.

Briggs, Charles L., and Clara Mantini-Briggs. 2005. "Hegemonía comunicativa y salud emancipadora: Una contradicción inédita (El Ejemplo del Dengue)." In *Informe Alternativo sobre la Salud en América Latina*, edited by Observatorio Latinoamericano de Salud, Centro de Estudios y Asesoría en Salud, 148–57. Quito: Global Health Watch / CEAS.

Briggs, Charles L., and Clara Mantini-Briggs. 2009. "Confronting Health Disparities: Latin American Social Medicine in Venezuela." *American Journal of Public Health* 99(3): 549–55.

Briggs, Charles L., and Clara Mantini-Briggs. 2016. *Tell Me Why My Children Died: Rabies, Indigenous Knowledge, and Communicative Justice.* Durham, NC: Duke University Press.

Briggs, Laura. 2002. *Reproducing Empire: Race, Sex, Science, and U.S. Imperialism in Puerto Rico.* Berkeley: University of California Press.

Brown, E. Richard. 1979. *Rockefeller Medicine Men: Medicine and Capitalism in America.* Berkeley: University of California Press.

Brown, Roger, and Albert Gilman. (1968) 1972. "The Pronouns of Power and Solidarity." In *Readings in the Sociology of Language*, edited by Joshua A. Fishman, 252–75. The Hague: Mouton.

Buchbinder, Mara. 2015. *All in Your Head: Making Sense of Pediatric Pain.* Oakland: University of California Press.

Buchbinder, Mara. 2021. *Scripting Death: Stories of Assisted Dying in America.* Oakland: University of California Press.

Bucholtz, Mary, and Kira Hall. 2016. "Embodied Sociolinguistics." In *Sociolinguistics: Theoretical Debates*, edited by Nikolas Coupland, 173–97. Cambridge: Cambridge University Press.

Bulled, Nicola. 2015. *Prescribing HIV Prevention: Bringing Culture into Global Health Communication*. Walnut Creek, CA: Left Coast.

Burden-Stelly, Charisse, and Gerald Horne. 2019. *W. E. B. Du Bois: A Life in American History*. Santa Barbara: ABC-CLIO.

Cabalquinto, Earvin Charles, and Tanja Ahlin. 2021. "Care within or out of Reach: Fantasies of Care and Connectivity in the Time of the COVID-19 Pandemic." In *Viral Loads: Anthropologies of Urgency in the Time of COVID-19*, edited by Leonore Manderson, Nancy J. Burke, and Ayo Wahlberg, 344–61. London: UCL Press.

Caduff, Carlo. 2015. *The Pandemic Perhaps: Dramatic Events in a Public Culture of Danger*. Oakland: University of California Press.

Caduff, Carlo. 2019. "Canguilhem's Vital Social Medicine." *History of Anthropology Newsletter* 43. https://histanthro.org/notes/vital-social-medicine.

Caduff, Carlo. 2020. "What Went Wrong: Corona and the World after the Full Stop." *Medical Anthropology Quarterly* 34(4): 467–87.

Canguilhem, Georges. (1965) 2008. "The Living and Its Milieu." In *Knowledge of Life*, edited by Paola Marrati and Todd Meyers, translated by Stefanos Geroulanos and Daniela Ginsburg, 98–120. New York: Fordham University Press.

Canguilhem, Georges. (1966) 1989. *The Normal and the Pathological*. Translated by Carolyn R. Fawcett. New York: Zone.

Canguilhem, Georges. 1994. *A Vital Rationalist: Selected Writings from Georges Canguilhem*. Edited by François Delaporte. Translated by Arthur Goldhammer. New York: Zone.

Canguilhem, Georges. 2012. *Writings on Medicine*. Edited by Stefanos Geroulanos and Todd Meyers. New York: Fordham University Press.

Capps, Lisa, and Elinor Ochs. 1995. *Constructing Panic: The Discourse of Agoraphobia*. Cambridge, MA: Harvard University Press.

Carr, E. Summerson. 2011. *Scripting Addiction: The Politics of Therapeutic Talk and American Sobriety*. Princeton, NJ: Princeton University Press.

Carr, E. Summerson. 2021. "Learning How Not to Know: Pragmatism, (In)expertise, and the Training of American Helping Professionals." *American Anthropologist* 123(3): 526–38.

Carr, E. Summerson, and Michael Lempert, eds. 2016. *Scale: Discourse and Dimensions of Social Life*. Oakland: University of California Press.

Carr, J. R. C. 2019. "Linguistic Landscapes." In *Oxford Bibliographies in Linguistics*, edited by Mark Aronoff, 1–21. New York: Oxford University Press.

Castro, Arachu, and Merrill Singer, eds. 2004. *Unhealthy Health Policy: A Critical Anthropological Examination*. Walnut Creek, CA: AltaMira.

CDC (Centers for Disease Control and Prevention). 2002. *Crisis and Emergency Risk Communication*. Atlanta: CDC.

CDC (Centers for Disease Control and Prevention). (2006) 2007. *Crisis and Emergency Risk Communication: Pandemic Influenza*. Atlanta: CDC.

Chakrabarty, Dipesh. 2000. *Provincializing Europe: Postcolonial Thought and Historical Difference*. Princeton, NJ: Princeton University Press.

Chandler, Nahum Dimitri. 2014. *X—The Problem of the Negro as a Problem for Thought*. New York: Fordham University Press.

Chapin, Macpherson. 1976. "*Muu Ikala*: Cuna Birth Ceremony." In *Ritual and Symbol in Native Central America*, edited by Philip Young and James Howe, 57–65. University of Oregon Anthropological Papers, 9. Eugene: University of Oregon.

Chapin, Macpherson. 1983. "Curing among the San Blas Kuna of Panama." PhD diss., University of Arizona.

Chávez, Leo R. (2008) 2013. *The Latino Threat: Constructing Immigrants, Citizens and the Nation*. Palo Alto, CA: Stanford University Press.

Cherki, Alice. 2006. *Frantz Fanon: A Portrait*. Ithaca, NY: Cornell University Press.

Chomsky, Noam. 1965. *Aspects of the Theory of Syntax*. Cambridge, MA: MIT Press.

Cicourel, Aaron V. 1992. "The Interpenetration of Communicative Contexts: Examples from Medical Encounters." In *Rethinking Context: Language as an Interactive Phenomenon*, edited by Alessandro Duranti and Charles Goodwin, 291–310. Cambridge: Cambridge University Press.

Clarke, Adele. E., Janet K. Shim, Laura Mamo, Jennifer Ruth Fosket, and Jennifer R. Fishman. 2003. "Biomedicalization: Technoscientific Transformations of Health, Illness, and U.S. Biomedicine." *American Sociological Review* 68(2): 161–94.

Clemente, Ignasi. 2015. *Uncertain Futures: Communication and Culture in Childhood Cancer Treatment*. Oxford: Wiley-Blackwell.

Cohen, Lawrence. 2020. "The Culling: Pandemic, Gerocide, Generational Affect." *Medical Anthropology Quarterly* 34(4): 542–60.

Coronil, Fernando. 1997. *The Magical State: Nature, Money, and Modernity in Venezuela*. Chicago: University of Chicago Press.

Corwin, Anna I. 2021. *Embracing Age: How Catholic Nuns Became Models of Aging Well*. New Brunswick, NJ: Rutgers University Press.

Coulthard, Glen S. 2007. "Subjects of Empire: Indigenous Peoples and the 'Politics of Recognition' in Canada." *Contemporary Political Theory* 6(4): 437–60.

Cranston, Maurice. 1957. *John Locke: A Biography*. London: Longmans, Green.

Craw, Erin, Tess M. Buckley, and Michelle Miller-Day. 2022. "'This Isn't Just Busy, This Is Scary': Stress, Social Support, and Coping Experiences of Frontline Nurses during the COVID-19 Pandemic." *Health Communication*. https://doi.org/10.1080/10410236.2022.2051270.

Crowley, Michael, Edward Wong, and Lara Jakes. 2020. "Coronavirus Drives the U.S. and China Deeper into Global Power Struggle." *New York Times*, 22 March 2020. https://www.nytimes.com/2020/03/22/us/politics/coronavirus-us-china.html.

Das, Veena. 2007. *Life and Words: Violence and the Descent into the Ordinary*. Berkeley: University of California Press.

Das, Veena. 2015. "What Does Ordinary Ethics Look Like?" In *Four Lectures on Ethics: Anthropological Perspectives*, by Michael J. Lambek, Veena Das, Didier Fassin, and Webb Keane, 53–125. Chicago: Hau.

Davidson, Brad 2001. "Questions in Cross-Linguistic Medical Encounters: The Role of the Hospital Interpreter." *Anthropological Quarterly* 74(4): 170–78.

Davis, Dána-Ain. 2019. *Reproductive Injustice: Racism, Pregnancy, and Premature Birth*. New York: New York University Press.

Davis, Georgia, and Mark Nichter. 2016. "The Lyme Wars: The Effects of Bio-communicability, Gender, and Epistemic Politics on Health Activation and Lyme Science." In *Diagnostic Controversy: Cultural Perspectives on Competing Knowledge in Healthcare*, edited by Carolyn Smith-Morris, 215–47. New York: Routledge.

Davis, Kathy. 2007. *The Making of Our Bodies, Ourselves: How Feminism Travels across Borders*. Durham, NC: Duke University Press.

Dean, Jodi. 1998. *Aliens in America: Conspiracy Cultures from Outerspace to Cyberspace*. Ithaca, NY: Cornell University Press.

DelVecchio Good, Mary-Jo. 1995. *American Medicine: The Quest for Competence*. Berkeley: University of California Press.

Derrida, Jacques. (1967) 1976. *Of Grammatology*. Translated by Gayatri Chakravorty Spivak. Baltimore: Johns Hopkins University Press.

Derrida, Jacques. (1977) 1988. *Limited Inc*. Edited by Gerald Graff. Translated by Jeffrey Mehlman and Samuel Weber. Evanston, IL: Northwestern University Press.

Desforges, Marc, Alain Le Coupanec, Élodie Brison, Mathieu Meessen-Pinard, and Pierre J. Talbot. 2014. "Neuroinvasive and Neurotropic Human Respiratory Coronaviruses: Potential Neurovirulent Agents in Humans." In "Infectious Diseases and Nanomedicine I." Edited by R. Adhikari and S. Thapa. Special issue, *Advances in Experimental Medicine and Biology* 807:75–96. New Delhi: Springer New Delhi. https://doi.org/10.1007/978-81-322-1777-0_6.

Dewhurst, Kenneth. 1963. *John Locke (1632–1704), Physician and Philosopher: A Medical Biography*. London: Wellcome Historical Medical Library.

Díaz-Duque, Ozzie F. 1998. "Communication Barriers in Medical Settings: Hispanics in the United States." In *Linguistics at Work: A Reader of Application*, edited by Dallin D. Oaks, 86–98. Fort Worth, TX: Harcourt Brace.

Doucet-Battle, James 2021. *Sweetness in the Blood: Race, Risk, and Type 2 Diabetes*. Minneapolis: University of Minnesota Press.

Du Bois, John W. 2007. "The Stance Triangle." In *Stancetaking in Discourse: Subjectivity, Evaluation, Interaction*, edited by Robert Englebretson, 139–82. Philadelphia: John Benjamins.

Du Bois, W. E. B. 1899. *The Philadelphia Negro: A Social Study*. Philadelphia: Publications of the University of Pennsylvania.

Du Bois, W. E. B. (1903) 1990. *The Souls of Black Folk*. New York: Vintage.

Du Bois, W. E. B. 1940. *Dusk of Dawn: An Essay toward an Autobiography of a Race Concept*. New York: Harcourt Brace.

Du Bois, W. E. B. 1995. *W. E. B. Du Bois: A Reader*. Edited by David Levering Lewis. New York: Henry Holt.

Du Bois, W. E. B. (1968) 2007. *The Autobiography of W. E. B. Du Bois: A Soliloquy on Viewing My Life from the Last Decade of Its First Century*. Oxford: Oxford University Press.

Dumit, Joseph. 2012. *Drugs for Life: How Pharmaceutical Companies Define Our Health*. Durham, NC: Duke University Press.

Dutta, Mohan J. 2008. *Communicating Health: A Culture Centered Approach*. Cambridge: Polity.

Dutta, Mohan J. 2012. *Voices of Resistance: Communication and Social Change.* West Lafayette, IN: Purdue University Press.

Dutta, Mohan J. 2021. "Communication Inequality, Structural Inequality, and COVID-19." In *Communicating COVID-19: Interdisciplinary Perspectives,* edited by Monique Lewis, Eliza Govender, and Kate Holland, 85–98. London: Palgrave Macmillan.

Dutta, Mohan J., and Uttaran Dutta. 2013. "Voices of the Poor from the Margins of Bengal: Structural Inequities and Health." *Qualitative Health Research* 23(1): 14–25.

Edwards, Brent Hayes. 2003. *The Practice of Diaspora: Literature, Translation, and the Rise of Black Internationalism.* Cambridge, MA: Harvard University Press.

Ehlen, Patrick. 2000. *Frantz Fanon: A Spiritual Biography.* New York: Crossroad.

Engebretsen, Eivind, and Mona Baker. 2022. *Rethinking Evidence in the Time of Pandemics: Scientific vs. Narrative Rationality and Medical Knowledge Practices.* Cambridge: Cambridge University Press.

Entradas, Marta. 2022. "In Science We Trust: The Effects of Information Sources on COVID-19 Risk Perceptions." *Health Communication* 37(14): 1715–23.

Epstein, Steven. 1996. *Impure Science: AIDS, Activism, and the Politics of Knowledge.* Berkeley: University of California Press.

Epstein, Steven. 1997. "AIDS Activism and the Retreat from the Genocide Frame." *Social Identities* 3(3): 415–38.

Epstein, Steven. 2007. *Inclusion: The Politics of Difference in Medical Research.* Chicago: University of Chicago Press.

Equiano, Olaudah. 1969. "The Life of Olaudah Equiana, or Gustavus Vassa, the African, Written by Himself." In *Great Slave Narratives,* edited by Arna Bontemps, 1–192. Boston: Beacon.

Erickson, Susan L. 2012. "Global Health Business: The Production and Performativity of Statistics in Sierra Leone and Germany." *Medical Anthropology* 31(4): 367–84.

Espiritu, Yen Le. 1992. *Asian American Panethnicity: Bridging Institutions and Identities.* Philadelphia: Temple University Press.

Fanon, Frantz. 1952. *Peau noire, masques blancs.* Paris: Éditions du Seuil.

Fanon, Frantz. (1952) 2008. *Black Skin, White Masks.* Translated by Richard Philcox. New York: Grove.

Fanon, Frantz. (1959) 1967. *A Dying Colonialism.* Translated by Haakon Chevalier. New York: Grove.

Fanon, Frantz. (1961) 1963. *The Wretched of the Earth.* Translated by Constance Farrington. New York: Grove.

Fanon, Frantz. (1964) 1967. *Toward the African Revolution.* Translated by Haakon Chevalier. New York: Grove.

Fanon, Frantz. (2015) 2018. *Alienation and Freedom.* Edited by Jean Khalfa and Robert J. C. Young. Translated by Steven Corcoran. London: Bloomsbury Academic.

Fanon, Frantz, and Jacques Azoulay. (1954) 2018. "Social Therapy in a Ward of Muslim Men: Methodological Difficulties." Pt. 2, chap. 10, in *Alienation and Freedom,* by Frantz Fanon, 353–71. Edited by Jean Khalfa and Robert J. C. Young. Translated by Steven Corcoran. London: Bloomsbury Academic.

Farmer, Paul. 1992. *AIDS and Accusation: Haiti and the Geography of Blame.* Berkeley: University of California Press.

Farmer, Paul. 2004. "An Anthropology of Structural Violence." *Current Anthropology* 45(3): 305–25.

Farmer, Paul. 2020. *Fevers, Feuds, and Diamonds: Ebola and the Ravages of History.* New York: Picador.

Fassin, Didier. (2010) 2012. *Humanitarian Reason: A Moral History of the Present.* Translated by Rachel Gomme. Berkeley: University of California Press.

Fassin, Didier. 2011. "This Is Not Medicalization." In *Drugs and Culture: Knowledge, Consumption and Policy,* edited by Geoffrey Hunt, Maitena Milhet, and Henri Bergeron, 85–93. Farnham, UK: Ashgate.

Faudree, Paja. 2020. "'Making Medicine' with *Salvia divinorum*: Competing Approaches and Their Implications." *Medical Anthropology* 39(7): 582–96.

Fenster, Mark. 1999. *Conspiracy Theories: Secrecy and Power in American Culture.* Minneapolis: University of Minnesota Press.

Ferguson, Charles A. 1975. "Toward a Characterization of English Foreigner Talk." *Anthropological Linguistics* 17(1): 1–14.

Ferguson, James. 1990. *The Anti-politics Machine: "Development," Depoliticization, and Bureaucratic Power in Lesotho.* Cambridge: Cambridge University Press.

Ferreira da Silva, Denise. 2022. *Unpayable Debt.* London: Sternberg.

Fisher, Sue. 1998. "Doctor Talk-Patient Talk: How Treatment Decisions Are Negotiated in Doctor-Patient Communication." In *Linguistics at Work: A Reader of Applications,* edited by Dallin D. Oaks, 99–121. Fort Worth, TX: Harcourt Brace.

Fisher, Sue, and Stephen B. Groce. 1990. "Accounting Practices in Medical Interviews." *Language in Society* 19(2): 225–50.

Foucault, Michel. (1963) 1973. *The Birth of the Clinic: An Archaeology of Medical Perception.* Translated by Alan Sheridan. London: Tavistock.

Foucault, Michel. 1988. "Technologies of the Self." In *Technologies of the Self: A Seminar with Michel Foucault,* edited by Luther H. Martin, Huck Gutman, and Patrick H. Hutton, 16–49. Amherst: University of Massachusetts Press.

Foucault, Michel. 1991. "Governmentality." In *The Foucault Effect: Studies in Governmentality,* edited by Graham Burchell, Colin Gordon, and Peter Miller, 87–104. Chicago: University of Chicago Press.

Freking, Kevin. 2020. "Trump Suggests US Slow Virus Testing to Avoid Bad Statistics." Associated Press, 20 June 2020. https://apnews.com/476068bd60e904830 3b736e9d7fc6572.

Freud, Sigmund. (1900) 1965. *The Interpretation of Dreams.* Translated by James Strachey. New York: Basic Books.

Friend, Juliana Gradeck. 2022. "'Don't Watch This Video!' Online Privacy, Porn, *Sutura,* and Health among Senegal's Digital Dissidents." PhD diss., University of California, Berkeley.

Funahashi, Daena. 2023. *Untimely Sacrifices: Work and Death in Finland.* Ithaca, NY: Cornell University Press.

Gal, Susan. 2015. "Politics of Translation." *Annual Review of Anthropology* 44:225–40.

Gal, Susan, and Judith T. Irvine 2019. *Signs of Difference: Language and Ideology in Social Life*. Cambridge: Cambridge University Press.

Garba, Tapji, and Sara-Maria Sorentino. 2020. "Slavery Is a Metaphor: A Critical Commentary on Eve Tuck and K. Wayne Yang's 'Decolonization Is Not a Metaphor.'" *Antipode* 52(3): 764–82.

Garth, Hanna. 2021. "The 2020 Los Angeles Uprisings: Fighting for Black Lives in the Midst of COVID-19." In *Viral Loads: Anthropologies of Urgency in the Time of COVID-19*, edited by Lenore Manderson, Nancy J. Burke, and Ayo Wahlberg, 91–107. London: UCL Press.

Gascoigne, John. 2009. "The Royal Society, Natural History and the Peoples of the 'New World(s)' 1660–1800." *British Journal for the History of Science* 42(4): 539–62.

Geertz, Clifford. 1973. *The Interpretation of Cultures*. New York: Basic Books.

Geissler, P. W. 2013. "Public Secrets in Public Health: Knowing Not to Know While Making Scientific Knowledge." *American Ethnologist* 40(1): 13–34.

Geronimus, Arline T. 2023. *Weathering: The Extraordinary Stress of Ordinary Life in an Unjust Society*. New York: Little, Brown Spark.

Gershon, Ilana. 2010. *The Breakup 2.0: Disconnecting over New Media*. Ithaca, NY: Cornell University Press.

Gieryn, Thomas F. 1983. "Boundary-Work and the Demarcation of Science from Non-science: Strains and Interests in Professional Ideologies of Scientists." *American Sociological Review* 48(6): 781–95.

Gilroy, Paul. 1993. *The Black Atlantic: Modernity and Double Consciousness*. Cambridge, MA: Harvard University Press.

Goffman, Erving. 1981. "Response Cries." In *Forms of Talk*, 78–123. Philadelphia: University of Pennsylvania Press.

Gómez, Jennifer M. 2015. "Microaggressions and the Enduring Mental Health Disparity: Black Americans at Risk for Institutional Betrayal." *Journal of Black Psychology* 41(2): 121–43.

Gomez-Vasquez, Lina, Enilda Romero-Hall, Nadia Jaramillo Cherrez, Samaha Ghani, et al. 2022. "Keeping Citizens Informed and Engaged during the COVID-19 Pandemic Using #YoMeInformoPMA: A Case from Latin America." *Health Communication* 38(9): 1813–20.

Good, Byron J. 1994. *Medicine, Rationality, and Experience: An Anthropological Perspective*. Cambridge: Cambridge University Press.

Good, Byron J., and Mary-Jo DelVecchio Good. 2000. "'Fiction' and 'Historicity' in Doctors' Stories: Social and Narrative Dimensions of Learning Medicine." In *Narrative and the Cultural Construction of Illness and Healing*, edited by Cheryl Mattingly and Linda C. Garro, 50–69. Berkeley: University of California Press.

Goodwin, Charles. 1994. "Professional Vision." *American Anthropologist* 96(3): 606–33.

Goodwin, Charles. 2010. "Constructing Meaning through Prosody in Aphasia." In *Prosody in Interaction*, edited by Dagmar Barth-Weingarten, Elisabeth Reber, and Margret Selting, 373–94. Amsterdam: John Benjamins.

Goodwin, Charles, and Alessandro Duranti. 1992. "Rethinking Context: An Introduction." In *Rethinking Context: Language as an Interactive Phenomenon*, edited by Alessandro Duranti and Charles Goodwin, 1–42. Cambridge: Cambridge University Press.

Gotkin, Kevin. 2016. "The Norm___ and the Pathological." *Disability Studies Quarterly* 36(1). https://dsq-sds.org/index.php/dsq/article/view/4281/4206.

Gover, Angela R., Shannon B. Harper, and Lynn Langton. 2020. "Anti-Asian Hate Crime during the COVID-19 Pandemic: Exploring the Reproduction of Inequality." *American Journal of Criminal Justice* 45(4): 647–67.

Graham, Laura R. 2011. "Quoting Mario Juruna: Linguistic Imagery and the Transformation of Indigenous Voice in the Brazilian Print Press." *American Ethnologist* 38(1): 164–83.

Gumperz, John J. 1982. *Discourse Strategies*. Cambridge: Cambridge University Press.

Gutiérrez, Ana T. 1998. *Tiempos de guerra y paz: Arnoldo Galbaldón y la investigación sobre malaria en Venezuela 1936–1990*. Caracas: Centro de Estudios del Desarrollo.

Guzmán, Jennifer R. 2020. "Time Discipline and Health/Communicative Labor in Pediatric Primary Care." *Medical Anthropology* 39(7): 609–23.

Han, Clara. 2012. *Life in Debt: Times of Care and Violence in Neoliberal Chile*. Berkeley: University of California Press.

Hanks, William F. 1990. *Referential Practice: Language and Lived Space among the Maya*. Chicago: University of Chicago Press.

Haraway, Donna. 1988. "Situated Knowledges: The Science Question in Feminism and the Privilege of Partial Perspective." *Feminist Studies* 14(3): 575–99.

Haraway, Donna J. 1997. *Modest_Witness@Second_Millennium.FemaleMan© Meets_OncoMouseTM: Feminism and Technoscience*. New York: Routledge.

Harrison, Faye, ed. (1991) 1997. *Decolonizing Anthropology: Moving Further toward an Anthropology for Liberation*. Washington, DC: Association of Black Anthropologists.

Harvey, T. S. 2008. "Where There Is No Patient: An Anthropological Treatment of a Biomedical Category." *Culture, Medicine, and Psychiatry* 32(4): 577–606.

Harvey, T. S. 2011. "Maya Mobile Medicine in Guatemala: The 'Other' Public Health." *Medical Anthropology Quarterly* 25(1): 47–69.

Harvey, T. S. 2013. *Wellness beyond Words: Maya Compositions of Speech and Silence in Medical Care*. Albuquerque: University of New Mexico Press.

Heath, Deborah, Rayna Rapp, and Karen-Sue Taussig. 2004. "Genetic Citizenship." In *A Companion to the Anthropology of Politics*, edited by David Nugent and Joan Vincent, 152–67. Malden, MA: Blackwell.

Heath, Shirley Brice. 1983. *Ways with Words: Language, Life and Work in Communities and Classrooms*. Cambridge: Cambridge University Press.

Heller, Monica, and Bonnie McElhinny. 2017. *Language, Capitalism, Colonialism: Toward a Critical History*. Toronto: University of Toronto Press.

Heritage, John, and J. Maxwell Atkinson. 1984. Introduction to *Structures of Social Action: Studies in Conversation Analysis*, edited by J. Maxwell Atkinson and John Heritage, 1–15. Cambridge: Cambridge University Press.

Heritage, John, and Douglas W. Maynard, eds. 2006a. *Communication in Medical Care: Interaction between Primary Care Physicians and Patients*. Cambridge: Cambridge University Press.

Heritage, John, and Douglas W. Maynard. 2006b. "Problems and Prospects in the Study of Physician-Patient Interaction: 30 Years of Research." *Annual Review of Sociology* 32: 351–74.

Hill, Jane H. 1995. "The Voices of Don Gabriel: Responsibility and Self in a Modern Mexicano Narrative." In *The Dialogic Emergence of Culture*, edited by Dennis Tedlock and Bruce Mannheim, 97–147. Urbana: University of Illinois Press.

Hill, Jane H. 2002. "'Expert Rhetorics' in Advocacy for Endangered Languages: Who Is Listening, and What Do They Hear?" *Journal of Linguistic Anthropology* 12(2): 119–33.

Hill, Jane H. 2008. *The Everyday Language of White Racism*. Chichester, UK: Wiley-Blackwell.

Hobbes, Thomas. (1651) 1968. *Leviathan*. Edited by C. B. Macpherson. Harmondsworth, UK: Penguin.

Hodges, Brian David, and Nancy McNaughton. 2009. "Who Should Be an OSCE Examiner?" *Academic Psychiatry* 33(4): 282–84.

Holloway, Jonathan Scott. 2002. *Confronting the Veil: Abram Harris Jr., E. Franklin Frazier, and Ralph Bunche, 1919–1941*. Chapel Hill: University of North Carolina Press.

Holmer, Nils M., and Henry Wassén. 1947. *Mu-Igala or the Way of Muu: A Medicine Song from the Cuna Indians of Panama*. Göteborg, Sweden: Etnografiska Museet.

Holmes, Seth M. 2013. *Fresh Fruit, Broken Bodies: Migrant Farmworkers in the United States*. Berkeley: University of California Press.

Hubbs, Nadine. 2014. *Rednecks, Queers, and Country Music*. Berkeley: University of California Press.

Hunt, Nancy Rose. 1997. "Condoms, Confessors, Conferences: Among AIDS Derivatives in Africa." *Journal of the International Institute* 4(3): 15–17.

Hurston, Zora Neale. (1935) 1978. *Mules and Men*. Bloomington: Indiana University Press.

Hutchins, Edward. 1995. *Cognition in the Wild*. Cambridge, MA: MIT Press.

Hymes, Dell H., ed. 1971. *Pidginization and Creolization of Languages*. Cambridge: Cambridge University Press.

Hymes, Dell. 1974. *Foundations in Sociolinguistics: An Ethnographic Perspective*. Philadelphia: University of Pennsylvania Press.

Hymes, Dell. 1981. *"In Vain I Tried to Tell You": Essays in Native America Ethnopoetics*. Philadelphia: University of Pennsylvania Press.

Inoue, Miyako. 2003. "The Listening Subject of Japanese Modernity and His Auditory Double: Citing, Sighting, and Siting the Modern Japanese Woman." *Cultural Anthropology* 18(2): 156–93.

Jackson, John L., Jr. 2013. *Thin Description: Ethnography and the African Hebrew Israelites of Jerusalem*. Cambridge, MA: Harvard University Press.

Jaén, Maria Helena. 2001. *El sistema de salud venezolano: Desafíos*. Caracas: Ediciones IESA.

Jakobson, Roman. (1939) 1971. "Signe zéro." In *Selected Writings II*, edited by Roman Jakobson, 211–19. The Hague: Mouton.

Jakobson, Roman. (1957) 1971. "Shifters, Verbal Categories, and the Russian Verb." In *Selected Writings II*, edited by Roman Jakobson, 130–47. The Hague: Mouton.

Jakobson, Roman. 1960. "Closing Statement: Linguistics and Poetics." In *Style in Language*, edited by Thomas A. Sebeok, 350–77. Cambridge, MA: MIT Press.

Jakobson, Roman. (1959) 2012. "On Linguistic Aspects of Translation." In *The Translation Studies Reader*, 3rd ed., edited by Lawrence Venuti, 126–31. London: Routledge.

Juhasz, Alexandra, and Pato Hebert. 2021. "It Could Be So Much Worse." CUNY Academic Works: Publications and Research, 26 January 2021. https://academicworks.cuny.edu/bc_pubs/275/.

Kalocsányiová, Erika, Ryan Essex, and Damian Poulter. 2023. "Risk and Health Communication during COVID-19: A Linguistic Landscape Analysis." *Health Communication*. 38(6): 1080–9.

Keane, Webb. 2016. *Ethical Life: Its Natural and Social Histories*. Princeton, NJ: Princeton University Press.

Keller, Richard C. 2007. "Clinician and Revolutionary: Frantz Fanon, Biography, and the History of Colonial Medicine." *Bulletin of the History of Medicine* 81(4): 823–41.

Kelly, Ann H. 2018. "Ebola Vaccines, Evidentiary Charisma, and the Rise of Global Health Emergency Research." *Economy and Society* 47(1): 135–61.

Kenjar, Kevin. 2020. "Linguistic Landscapes and Ideological Horizons: Language and Ideology in Post-Yugoslav Space." PhD diss., University of California, Berkeley.

Khurana, Mark P., Daniel E. Raaschou-Pedersen, Jørgen Kurtzhals, Jakob E. Bardram, et al. 2022. "Digital Health Competencies in Medical School Education: A Scoping Review and Delphi Method Study." *BMC Medical Education* 22(129). https://doi.org/10.1186/s12909-022-03163-7.

Kleinman, Arthur. 1988. *The Illness Narratives: Suffering, Healing, and the Human Condition*. New York: Basic Books.

Kockelman, Paul. 2007. "Inalienable Possession and Personhood in a Q'eqchi'-Mayan Community." *Language in Society* 36(3): 343–69.

Korsch, Barbara M., and Vida Francis Negrete. 1972. "Doctor-Patient Communication." *Scientific American* 227:66–74.

Kostkova, Patty. 2015. "Grand Challenges in Digital Health." *Frontiers in Public Health* 3(134): 1–5. https://doi.org/10.3389/fpubh.2015.00134.

Krieger, Nancy. 2011. *Epidemiology and the People's Health: Theory and Context*. New York: Oxford University Press.

Kroskrity, Paul V., ed. 2000. *Regimes of Language: Ideologies, Polities, and Identities*. Santa Fe, NM: School of American Research.

Kroskrity, Paul V. 2015. "Discursive Discriminations in the Representation of Western Mono and Yokuts Stories: Confronting Narrative Inequality and Listening to Indigenous Voices in Central California." In *The Legacy of Dell Hymes: Ethnopoetics, Narrative Inequality, and Voice*, edited by Paul V. Kroskrity and Anthony K. Webster, 135–63. Bloomington: Indiana University Press.

Kroskrity, Paul V. 2020. "Theorizing Linguistic Racisms from a Language Ideological Perspective." In *The Oxford Handbook of Language and Race*, edited by

H. Samy Alim, Angela Reyes, and Paul V. Kroskrity, 68–89. New York: Oxford University Press.

Kroskrity, Paul V. 2021. "Covert Linguistic Racisms and the (Re-)Production of White Supremacy." *Journal of Linguistic Anthropology* 31(2): 180–93.

Kuipers, Joel C. 1989. "'Medical Discourse' in Anthropological Context: Views of Language and Power." *Medical Anthropology Quarterly* 3(2): 99–123.

Lacan, Jacques. (1966) 1977. *Écrits: A Selection.* Translated by Alan Sheridan. New York: W. W. Norton.

Lakoff, Andrew. 2017. *Unprepared: Global Health in a Time of Emergency.* Oakland: University of California Press.

Lambek, Michael. 2015. "Living as if It Mattered." In *Four Lectures on Ethics: Anthropological Perspectives*, by Michael Lambek, Veena Das, Didier Fassin, and Webb Keane, 5–51. Chicago: Hau.

Lambert, Helen. 2006. "Accounting for EBM: Notions of Evidence in Medicine." *Social Science and Medicine* 62(11): 2633–45.

Latour, Bruno. 1987. *Science in Action: How to Follow Scientists and Engineers through Society.* Cambridge, MA: Harvard University Press.

Latour, Bruno. 1988. *The Pasteurization of France.* Cambridge, MA: Harvard University Press.

Latour, Bruno. (1991) 1993. *We Have Never Been Modern.* Translated by Catherine Porter. Cambridge, MA: Harvard University Press.

Lee, Nancy Stark. 2007. "Curing Consumers: How the Patient Became a Consumer in Modern American Medicine." PhD diss., University of California, San Diego.

Lévi-Strauss, Claude. (1949) 1963. "The Effectiveness of Symbols." In *Structural Anthropology*, 186–205. New York: Basic Books.

Lewis, Monique, Eliza Govender, and Kate Holland, eds. 2021. *Communicating CO-VID-19: Interdisciplinary Perspectives.* Cham, Switzerland: Palgrave Macmillan.

Likosky, Stephan. 2017. *With a Weapon and a Grin: Postcard Images of France's Black African Colonial Troops in WWI.* Atglen, PA: Schiffer.

Lipsitz, George. 1998. *The Possessive Investment in Whiteness: How White People Profit from Identity Politics.* Philadelphia: Temple University Press.

Livingston, Julie. 2012. *Improvising Medicine: An African Oncology Ward in an Emerging Cancer Epidemic.* Durham, NC: Duke University Press.

Lock, Margaret. 1993. *Encounters with Aging: Mythologies of Menopause in Japan and North America.* Berkeley: University of California Press.

Locke, John. (1690) 1959. *An Essay Concerning Human Understanding.* New York: Dover.

Locke, John. (1690) 1960. *Two Treatises of Government.* New York: New American Library.

Locke, John. (1695) 1714. "The Reasonableness of Christianity, as Delivered in the Scriptures." In *The Works of John Locke*, vol. 2, 471–541. London: John Churchill.

Locke, John. (1706) 1966. *Of the Conduct of the Understanding.* Edited by Francis W. Garforth. New York: Teachers College Press.

Lowenstein, Fiona, ed. 2022. *The Long COVID Survival Guide: How to Take Care of Yourself and What Comes Next.* New York: Experiment.

Macey, David. 2000. *Frantz Fanon: A Biography.* New York: Picador.

Macpherson, C. B. 1962. *The Political Theory of Possessive Individualism: Hobbes to Locke*. Oxford: Oxford University Press.

Maldonado-Torres, Nelson, Mireille Fanon Mendès France, Shahnaaz Suffla, Mohamed Seedat, and Kopano Ratele. 2021. "Fanon's Decolonial Transcendence of Psychoanalysis." *Studies in Gender and Sexuality*: 22(4): 243–55.

Manderson, Leonore. 1996. *Sickness and the State: Health and Illness in Colonial Malaya, 1870–1940*. New York: Cambridge University Press.

Marcus, George E., ed. 1999. *Paranoia within Reason: A Casebook on Conspiracy as Explanation*. Chicago: University of Chicago Press.

Marya, Rupa, and Raj Patel. 2021. *Inflamed: Deep Medicine and the Anatomy of Injustice*. New York: Farrar, Straus and Giroux.

Marriott, David. 2018. *Whither Fanon? Studies in the Blackness of Being*. Palo Alto, CA: Stanford University Press.

Marsilli-Vargas, Xochiquetzal. 2022. *Genres of Listening: An Ethnography of Psychoanalysis in Buenos Aires*. Durham, NC: Duke University Press.

Mattingly, Cheryl. 1998. *Healing Dramas and Clinical Plots: The Narrative Structure of Experience*. Cambridge: Cambridge University Press.

Mattingly, Cheryl, and Linda Garro, eds. 2000. *Narrative and the Cultural Construction of Illness and Healing*. Berkeley: University of California Press.

Mazzarella, William. 2019. "The Anthropology of Populism: Beyond the Liberal Settlement." *Annual Review of Anthropology* 48:45–60.

McCullouch, Jock. 1983. *Black Soul, White Artifact: Fanon's Clinical Psychology and Social Theory*. Cambridge: Cambridge University Press.

Meek, Barbra A. 2006. "And the Injun Goes 'How!' Representations of American Indian English in White Public Space." *Language in Society* 35(1): 93–128.

Meek, Barbra A. 2013. "The Voice of (White) Reason: Enunciations of Difference, Authorship Interpellation, and Jokes." In *Persistence of Language: Constructing and Confronting the Past and the Present in the Voices of Jane H. Hill*, edited by Shannon T. Bischoff, Deborah Cole, Amy V. Foundation, and Mizuki Miyashita, 339–63. Amsterdam: John Benjamins.

Mendenhall, Emily. 2022. *Unmasked: COVID-19, Community, and the Case of Okoboji*. Nashville: Vanderbilt University Press.

Menéndez, Eduardo. 2002. "El malestar actual de la antropología o de la casi imposibilidad de pensar lo ideológico." *Revista de Antropología Social* 11:39–87.

Menéndez, Eduardo L. 2009. *De sujetos, saberes y estructuras: Introducción al enfoque relacional en el estudio de la salud colectiva*. Buenos Aires: Lugar Editorial.

Menéndez, Eduardo L., and Renée B. Di Pardo. 1996. *De algunos alcoholismos y algunos saberes: Atención primaria y proceso de alcoholización*. Mexico City: Centro de Investigaciones y Estudios Superiores en Antropología Social.

Mental Health America. 2020. "The Mental Health of Healthcare Workers in COVID-19." Accessed 23 June 2022. https://mhanational.org/mental-health-healthcare-workers-covid-19.

Metzl, Jonathan M., and Helena Hansen. 2014. "Structural Competency: Theorizing a New Medical Engagement with Stigma and Inequality." *Social Science and Medicine* 103:126–33.

Meyers, Todd. 2019. "A Living Room." *History of Anthropology Newsletter* 43. https://histanthro.org/notes/living-room.

Miserandino, Christine. 2003. "The Spoon Theory." Accessed 1 May 2023. https:// web.archive.org/web/20191117210039/https://butyoudontlooksick.com/articles /written-by-christine/the-spoon-theory/.

Mishler, Elliot. 1984. *The Discourse of Medicine: Dialectics of Medical Interviews.* Norwood, NJ: Ablex.

Mishler, Elliot. 1986. *Research Interviewing: Context and Narrative.* Cambridge, MA: Harvard University Press.

Mitchell, Timothy. 2002. *Rule of Experts: Egypt, Techno-politics, Modernity.* Berkeley: University of California Press.

Mol, Annemarie. (2006) 2008. *The Logic of Care: Health and the Problem of Patient Choice.* New York: Routledge.

Molina, Natalia. 2006. *Fit to Be Citizens? Public Health and Race in Los Angeles, 1879–1939.* Berkeley: University of California Press.

Moran-Thomas, Amy 2019. *Traveling with Sugar: Chronicles of a Global Epidemic.* Oakland: University of California Press.

Moynihan, Daniel P. 1965. *The Negro Family: The Case for National Action.* Washington, DC: US Department of Labor.

Mundt, Neele, and Frank Polzenhagen. 2022. "Corona in the Linguistic Landscape." In *Pandemic and Crisis Discourse: Communicating COVID-19 and Public Health Strategy*, edited by Andreas Musolff, Ruth Breeze, Kayo Kondo, and Sara Vilar-Lluch, 135–65. London: Bloomsbury.

Myers, Todd. 2019. "A Living Room." *History of Anthropology Newsletter* 43. Accessed 13 July 2022. https://histanthro.org/notes/living-room/.

Mykhalovskiy, Eric, and Lorna Weir. 2004. "The Problem of Evidence-Based Medicine: Directions for Social Science." *Social Science and Medicine* 59(5): 1059–69.

Nading, Alex M. 2014. *Mosquito Trails: Ecology, Health, and the Politics of Entanglement.* Berkeley: University of California Press.

Nelson, Alondra 2011. *Body and Soul: The Black Panther Party and the Fight against Medical Discrimination.* Minneapolis: University of Minnesota Press.

Nguyen, Vinh-Kim. 2010. *The Republic of Therapy: Triage and Sovereignty in West Africa's Time of AIDS.* Durham, NC: Duke University Press.

Nichter, Mark. 1981. "Idioms of Distress: Alternatives in the Expression of Psychosocial Distress: A Case Study from South India." *Culture, Medicine, and Psychiatry* 5(4): 379–408.

Nichter, Mark. 2008. *Global Health: Why Cultural Perceptions, Social Representations, and Biopolitics Matter.* Tucson: University of Arizona Press.

Nichter, Mark. 2013. "The Rise and Transformation of Evidence-Based Medicine." *American Anthropologist* 115(4): 647–49.

Nichter, Mark. 2022. "From Idioms of Distress, Concern, and Care to Moral Distress Leading to Moral Injury in the Time of COVID. *Transcultural Psychiatry* 59(4): 551–67.

Nichter, Mark, and Jennifer Jo Thompson. 2006. "For My Wellness, Not Just My Illness: North Americans' Use of Dietary Supplements." *Culture, Medicine, and Psychiatry* 30: 175–222.

Nowotny, Helga. 1993. "Socially Distributed Knowledge: Five Spaces for Science to Meet the Public." *Public Understanding of Science* 2(4): 307–19.

Nowotny, Helga. 2000. "Transgressive Competence: The Narrative of Expertise." *European Journal of Social Theory* 3(1): 5–21.

Nowotny, Helga, Peter Scott, and Michael Gibbons. 2001. *Re-thinking Science: Knowledge and the Public in an Age of Uncertainty.* Cambridge: Polity.

Ochs, Elinor. 1990. "Indexicality and Socialization." In *Cultural Psychology: Essays on Comparative Human Development,* edited by James W. Stigler, Richard A. Shweder, and Gilbert Herdt, 287–308. Cambridge: Cambridge University Press.

Ochs, Elinor. 2015. "Corporeal Reflexivity and Autism." *Integrative Psychological and Behavioral Science* 49(2): 275–87.

Ochs, Elinor, Ruth C. Smith, and Carolyn E. Taylor. 1996. "Detective Stories at Dinnertime: Problem Solving through Co-narration." In *Disorderly Discourse: Narrative, Conflict, and Inequality,* edited by Charles L. Briggs, 95–113. Oxford: Oxford University Press.

Ochoa, Marcia. 2014. *Queen for a Day: Transformistas, Beauty Queens, and the Performance of Femininity in Venezuela.* Durham, NC: Duke University Press.

Ødemark, John, and Eivind Engebretsen. 2022. "Challenging Medical Knowledge Translation: Convergence and Divergence of Translation across Epistemic and Cultural Boundaries." *Humanities and Social Sciences Communications* 9(71). https://doi.org/10.1057/s41599-022-01088-6.

Office for Civil Rights, US Department of Education. 2021. *Education in a Pandemic: The Disparate Impacts of COVID-19 on America's Students.* Washington, DC: US Department of Education.

Olsen, Dale A. 1996. *Music of the Warao of Venezuela: Song People of the Rain Forest.* Gainesville: University Presses of Florida.

OPS (Organización Panamericana de la Salud). 2006. *Barrio Adentro: Derecho a la salud e inserción social en Venezuela.* Caracas: OPS.

Ortner, Sherry B. 1995. "Resistance and the Problem of Ethnographic Refusal." *Comparative Studies in Society and History* 37(1): 173–93.

Pandolfo, Stefania. 2010. "Clad in Mourning: Violence, Subjugation and the Struggle of the Soul." *Review of Women's Studies* 6:25–39.

Pangborn, Stephanie M., Brandon C. Boatwright, Caleigh L. Miller, and Madelyn N. Velting. 2023. "'I Don't Feel Like a Hero': Frontline Healthcare Providers' Social Media Storytelling during COVID-19." *Health Communication* 38(8): 1508–18.

Paredes, Américo. (1978) 1993. "On Ethnographic Work among Minority Groups: A Folklorist's Perspective." In *Folklore and Culture on the Texas-Mexican Border,* edited by Richard Bauman, 73–110. Austin: Center for Mexican American Studies, University of Texas, Austin.

Parkin, David. 2013. "Medical Crises and Therapeutic Talk." *Anthropology and Medicine* 20(2): 124–41.

Parsons, Talcott. 1951. *The Social System.* Glencoe, IL: Free Press.

Patton, Cindy. 1990. *Inventing AIDS*. New York: Routledge.

Peirce, Charles S. 1955. "Logic as Semiotic, the Theory of Signs." In *Philosophical Writings of Peirce*, edited by Justus Buchler, 98–119. New York: Dover.

Peña-Guzmán, David M. 2018. "Dossier Georges Canguilhem: Canguilhem's Concepts." *Transversal* 4:27–46.

Perez Hattori, Anne. 2004. *Colonial Dis-Ease: US Navy Health Policies and the Chamorros of Guam, 1898–1941*. Honolulu: University of Hawai'i Press.

Perley, Bernard C. 2011. *Defying Maliseet Language Death: Emergent Vitalities of Language, Culture and Identity in Eastern Canada*. Lincoln: University of Nebraska Press.

Phillips, Steven, and Michelle A. Williams. 2021. "Confronting Our Next National Health Disaster: Long-Haul COVID." *New England Journal of Medicine* 385:577–79.

Pigg, Stacy Leigh. 2001. "Languages of Sex and AIDS in Nepal: Notes on the Social Production of Commensurability." *Cultural Anthropology* 16(4): 481–541.

Posnock, Ross. 1998. *Color and Culture: Black Writers and the Making of the Modern Intellectual*. Cambridge, MA: Harvard University Press.

Pritzker, Sonya. 2014. *Living Translation: Language and the Search for Resonance in US Chinese Medicine*. Oxford: Berghahn.

Proal, Amy D., and Michael B. VanElzakker 2021. "Long COVID or Post-acute Sequelae of COVID-19 (PASC): An Overview of Biological Factors That May Contribute to Persistent Symptoms." *Frontiers in Microbiology* 12:698169. https://doi.org/10.3389/fmicb.2021.698169.

Qu, Yan, Adam J. Saffer, and Lucinda Austin. 2023. "What Drives People Away from COVID-19 Information? Uncovering the Influences of Personal Networks on Information Avoidance." *Health Communication* 38(2): 216–27.

Rabinow, Paul. 1992. "Artificiality and Enlightenment: From Sociobiology to Biosociality." In *Incorporations*, edited by Jonathan Crary and Sanford Kwinter, 234–52. New York: Zone.

Rabinow, Paul. 1994. "Introduction: A Vital Rationalist." In *A Vital Rationalist: Selected Writings from Georges Canguilhem*, edited by François Delaporte, translated by Arthur Goldhammer, 11–23. New York: Zone.

Ramirez, Sarah M., Richard Mines, and Ildi Carlisle-Cummins. 2020. *Always Essential, Perpetually Disposable: Initial Impact of the COVID-19 Pandemic on California Agricultural Workers—COFS Phase One Report*. Santa Cruz: California Institute of Rural Studies. https://cirsinc.org/wp-content/uploads/2021/08/CA-COFS-Phase-One-Final-Report.pdf.

Redfield, Peter. 2013. *Life in Crisis: The Ethical Journey of Doctors without Borders*. Berkeley: University of California Press.

Reid, Roddey. 1997. "Healthy Families, Healthy Citizens: the Politics of Speech and Knowledge in the California Anti-secondhand Smoke Media Campaign." *Science as Culture* 29:541–81.

Reid, Roddey. 2004. "Tensions within California Tobacco Control in the 1990s: Health Movements, State Initiatives, and Community Mobilization." *Science as Culture* 13(4): 515–37.

Reid, Roddey. 2005. *Globalizing Tobacco Control: Anti-smoking Campaigns in California, France, and Japan.* Bloomington: Indiana University Press.

Reynolds, Jennifer F., and Marjorie Faulstich Orellana. 2009. "New Immigrant Youth Interpreting in White Public Space." *American Anthropologist* 111(2): 211–23.

Rhodes, Jane. 2007. *Framing the Black Panthers: The Spectacular Rise of a Black Power Icon.* New York: New Press.

Robbins, Dennis, and Patrick Dunn. 2019. "Digital Health Literacy in a Person-Centric World." *International Journal of Cardiology* 290:154–55.

Roberts, Dorothy. 1997. *Killing the Black Body: Race, Reproduction, and the Meaning of Liberty.* New York: Vintage.

Rogers, Katie. 2020. "Trump Now Claims He Always Knew the Coronavirus Would Be a Pandemic." *New York Times,* 17 March 2020. https://www.nytimes.com/2020/03/17/us/politics/trump-coronavirus.html.

Rogers, Katie, Lara Jakes, and Ana Swanson. 2020. "Trump Calls It the 'Chinese Virus': Critics Say That's Racist and Provocative." *New York Times,* 19 March 2020. https://www.nytimes.com/2020/03/18/us/politics/china-virus.html.

Roitman, Janet. 2014. *Anti-crisis.* Durham, NC: Duke University Press.

Romanell, Patrick. 1958. "Locke and Sydenham: A Fragment on Smallpox (1670)." *Bulletin of the History of Medicine,* 32(4): 293–321.

Romer, Daniel, and Kathleen Hall Jamieson. 2020. "Conspiracy Theories as Barriers to Controlling the Spread of COVID-19 in the US." *Social Science and Medicine* 263. https://doi.org/10.1016/j.socscimed.2020.113356.

Rosa, Jonathan. 2018. *Looking Like a Language, Sounding Like a Race: Raciolinguistic Ideologies and the Learning of Latinidad.* New York: Oxford University Press.

Rosa, Jonathan, and Nelson Flores. 2020. "Reimagining Race and Language: From Raciolinguistic Ideologies to a Raciolinguistic Perspective." In *The Oxford Handbook of Language and Race,* edited by H. Samy Alim, Angela Reyes, and Paul V. Kroskrity, 90–107. New York: Oxford University Press.

Rose, Nikolas. 2007. *The Politics of Life Itself: Biomedicine, Power, and Subjectivity in the Twenty-First Century.* Princeton, NJ: Princeton University Press.

Rouse, Carolyn Moxley. 2009. *Uncertain Suffering: Racial Health Care Disparities and Sickle Cell Disease.* Berkeley: University of California Press.

Rouse, Carolyn Moxley. 2021. "Necropolitics versus Biopolitics: Spatialization, White Privilege, and Visibility during a Pandemic." *Cultural Anthropology* 36(3): 360–67.

Sackett, David L., Sharon E. Straus, E. Scott Richardson, William Rosenberg, and R. Brian Haynus. 2000. *Evidence-Based Medicine: How to Practice and Teach EBM.* 2nd ed. New York: Churchill Livingstone.

Sacks, Harvey. 1984. "On Doing 'Being Ordinary.'" In *Structures of Social Action,* edited by J. Maxwell Atkinson and John Heritage, 413–29. Cambridge: Cambridge University Press.

Sacks, Harvey, Emanuel A. Schegloff, and Gail Jefferson. 1974. "A Simplest Systematics for the Organization of Turn-Taking for Conversation." *Language* 50(4): 696–735.

Sandoval, Chela. 2000. *Methodology of the Oppressed.* Minneapolis: University of Minnesota Press.

Sangaramoorthy, Thurka. 2014. *Treating AIDS: Politics of Difference, Paradox of Prevention*. New Brunswick, NJ: Rutgers University Press.

Santa Ana, Otto. 2002. *Brown Tide Rising: Metaphors of Latinos in Contemporary American Public Discourse*. Austin: University of Texas Press.

Sapir, Edward. 1921. *Language: An Introduction to the Study of Speech*. New York: Harcourt, Brace.

Sauer, Carl O. 1925. "The Morphology of Landscape." *University of California Publications in Geography* 2(2): 19–53.

Saussure, Ferdinand de. (1916) 1959. *A Course in General Linguistics*. Edited by Charles Bally and Albert Sechehaye. Translated by Wade Baskin. New York: McGraw-Hill.

Saxton, Dvera I. 2021. *Devil's Fruit: Farmworkers, Health, and Environmental Justice*. New Brunswick, NJ: Rutgers University Press.

Schegloff, Emanuel A. 1992. "On Talk and Its Institutional Occasions." In *Talk at Work: Interaction in Institutional Settings*, edited by Paul Drew and John Heritage, 110–34. Cambridge: Cambridge University Press.

Scheper-Hughes, Nancy. 1996. "Theft of Life: The Globalization of Organ Stealing Rumors." *Anthropology Today* 12(3): 3–11.

Schieffelin, Bambi B., Kathryn A. Woolard, and Paul V. Kroskrity, eds. 1998. *Language Ideologies: Practice and Theory*. New York: Oxford University Press.

Seymour, Cheryl K., Carrie Griffin, Seth M. Holmes, and Carlos Martinez. 2018. "Structural Differential—a 32-Year-Old Man with Persistent Wrist Pain." *New England Journal of Medicine* 379(25): 2385–88.

Shah, Nayan. 2001. *Contagious Divides: Epidemics and Race in San Francisco's Chinatown*. Berkeley: University of California Press.

Shange, Savannah. 2019. *Progressive Dystopia: Abolition, Antiblackness, and Schooling in San Francisco*. Durham, NC: Duke University Press.

Sherzer, Joel. 1983. *Kuna Ways of Speaking: An Ethnographic Perspective*. Austin: University of Texas Press.

Silverstein, Michael. 1976. "Shifters, Linguistic Categories, and Cultural Description." In *Meaning in Anthropology*, edited by Keith H. Basso and Henry A. Selby, 11–55. Albuquerque: University of New Mexico Press.

Silverstein, Michael. (1987) 1996. "Monoglot 'Standard' in America: Standardization and Metaphors of Linguistic Hegemony." In *The Matrix of Language: Contemporary Linguistic Anthropology*, edited by Donald Brenneis and Ronald K. S. Macaulay, 284–306. Boulder, CO: Westview.

Silverstein, Michael. 1993. "Metapragmatic Discourse and Metapragmatic Function." In *Reflexive Language: Reported Speech and Metapragmatics*, edited by John Lucy, 33–58. Cambridge: Cambridge University Press.

Silverstein, Michael. 2003. "Indexical Order and the Dialectics of Sociolinguistic Life." *Language and Communication* 23(3–4): 193–229.

Simpson, Audra. 2014. *Mohawk Interruptus: Political Life across the Borders of Settler States*. Durham, NC: Duke University Press.

Singer, Merrill, Nicola Bulled, Bayla Ostrach, and Emily Mendenhall. 2017. "Syndemics and the Biosocial Conception of Health." *Lancet* 389(10072): 941–50.

Smalls, Krystal A. 2020. "Race, Signs, and the Body: Towards a Theory of Racial Semiotics." In *The Oxford Handbook of Language and Race*, edited by H. Samy Alim, Angela Reyes, and Paul V. Kroskrity, 233–60. New York: Oxford University Press.

Smedley, Brian D., Adrienne Y. Stith, and Alan Nelson, eds. 2003. *Unequal Treatment: Confronting Racial and Ethnic Disparities in Health Care*. Washington, DC: National Academies Press.

Snow, Catherine E., and Charles A. Ferguson, eds. 1977. *Talking to Children: Language Input and Acquisition*. Cambridge: Cambridge University Press.

Sobo, Elisa J., and Elżbieta Drażkiewicz. 2021. "Rights, Responsibilities, and Revelations: COVID-19 Conspiracy Theories and the State." In *Viral Loads: Anthropologies of Urgency in the Time of COVID-19*, edited by Leonore Manderson, Nancy J. Burke, and Ayo Wahlberg, 67–88. London: UCL Press.

Sointu, Eeva. 2016. "'Good' Patient/'Bad' Patient: Clinical Learning and the Entrenching of Inequality." *Sociology of Health and Illness* 39(1): 63–77.

Solomon, Miriam. 2015. *Making Medical Knowledge*. Oxford: Oxford University Press.

Spillers, Hortense J. 1987. "Mama's Baby, Papa's Maybe: An American Grammar Book." *Diacritics* 17(2): 64–81.

Sunder Rajan, Kaushik. 2006. *Biocapital: The Constitution of Postgenomic Life*. Durham, NC: Duke University Press.

Syndenham, Thomas. 1666. *Methodus curandi febres, propriis observationibus*. London: J. Crook.

Talmor, Ruti. 2022. *Pato Hebert: Lingering*. Claremont, CA: Kallick Gallery, Pitzer College.

Tangherlini, Timothy R. 1998. *Talking Trauma: Paramedics and Their Stories*. Jackson: University Press of Mississippi.

Tapia, Ruby C. 2011. *American Pietàs: Visions of Race, Death, and the Maternal*. Minneapolis: University of Minnesota Press.

Taussig, Karen-Sue, Rayna Rapp, and Deborah Health. 2003. "Flexible Eugenics: Technologies of the Self in the Age of Genetics." In *Genetic Nature/Culture: Anthropology and Science beyond the Two-Culture Divide*, edited by Alan H. Goodman, Deborah Heath, and M. Susan Lindee, 58–76. Berkeley: University of California Press.

Taussig, Michael. 1980. "Reification and the Consciousness of the Patient." *Social Science and Medicine* 14(1): 3–13.

Taylor, Janelle S. 2011. "The Moral Aesthetics of Simulated Suffering in Standardized Patient Performances." *Culture, Medicine, and Psychiatry* 35(2): 134–62.

Ticktin, Miriam. 2011. *Casualties of Care: Immigration and the Politics of Humanitarianism in France*. Berkeley: University of California Press.

Timmermans, Stefan, and Marc Berg. 2003. *The Gold Standard: The Challenge of Evidence-Based Medicine and Standardization in Health Care*. Philadelphia: Temple University Press.

Timmermans, Stefan, and Emily S. Kolker. 2004. "Evidence-Based Medicine and the Reconfiguration of Medical Knowledge." *Journal of Health and Social Behavior* 45:177–93.

Tinker Salas, Miguel. 2009. *The Enduring Legacy: Oil, Culture, and Society in Venezuela*. Durham, NC: Duke University Press.

Tomlinson, Barbara, and George Lipsitz. 2019. *Insubordinate Spaces: Improvisation and Accompaniment for Social Justice*. Philadelphia: Temple University Press.

Trnka, Susanna. 2021. "Be Kind: Negotiating Ethical Proximities in Aotearoa / New Zealand during COVID-19." *Cultural Anthropology* 36(3): 368–80.

Trouillot, Michel-Rolph. 2021. "Anthropology and the Savage Slot: The Poetics and Politics of Otherness." In *Trouillot Remixed: The Michel-Rolph Trouillot Reader*, edited by Yarimar Bonilla, Greg Beckett, and Mayanthi L. Fernando, 53–84. Durham, NC: Duke University Press.

Tuck, Eve, and K. Wayne Yang. 2012. "Decolonization Is Not a Metaphor." *Decolonization: Indigeneity, Education, and Society* 1(1): 1–40.

Turner, Victor. 1969. *The Ritual Process: Structure and Anti-structure*. Chicago: Aldine.

Urciuoli, Bonnie. 1996. *Exposing Prejudice: Puerto Rican Experiences of Language, Race, and Class*. Boulder, CO: Westview.

Ureña, Carolyn. 2019. "Decolonial Embodiment: Fanon, the Clinical Encounter, and the Colonial Wound." *Disability and the Global South* 6(1): 1640–58.

Van Ryn, Michelle, and Jane Burke. 2000. "The Effect of Patient Race and Socioeconomic Status on Physicians' Perceptions of Patients." *Social Science and Medicine* 50(6): 813–28.

Vaughan, Megan. 1991. *Curing Their Ills: Colonial Power and African Illness*. Palo Alto, CA: Stanford University Press.

Villalba, Julián A., Yushi Liu, Mauyrui K. Alvarez, Luisana Calderon, et al. 2013. "Low Child Survival Index in a Multi-dimensionally Poor Amerindian Population in Venezuela." *PLOS ONE* 8(12): 1–13.

Viswanath, K., Edmund W. J. Lee, and Ramya Pinnamaneni. 2020. "We Need the Lens of Equity in COVID-19 Communication." *Health Communication* 35(14): 1743–46.

Vološinov, V. N. (1929) 1973. *Marxism and the Philosophy of Language*. Translated by Ladislav Matejka and I. R. Titunik. New York: Seminar.

Wagner, Anna, and Doreen Reifegerste. 2023. "'The Part Played by People' in Times of COVID-19: Interpersonal Communication about Media Coverage in a Pandemic Crisis." *Health Communication*. 38(5): 1014–21.

Wailoo, Keith. 2001. *Dying in the City of the Blues: Sickle Cell Anemia and the Politics of Race and Health*. Chapel Hill: University of North Carolina Press.

Waitzkin, Howard. 1991. *The Politics of Medical Encounters: How Patients and Doctors Deal with Social Problems*. New Haven, CT: Yale University Press.

Waitzkin, Howard. (1983) 2000. *The Second Sickness: Contradictions of Capitalist Health Care*. Rev ed. Lanham, MD: Rowman and Littlefield.

Waitzkin, Howard. 2011. *Medicine and Public Health at the End of Empire*. Boulder, CO: Paradigm.

Waitzkin, Howard, and Working Group for Health beyond Capitalism. 2018. *Health Care under the Knife: Moving beyond Capitalism for our Health.* New York: Monthly Review Press.

White, Luise. 2000. *Speaking with Vampires: Rumor and History in Colonial Africa.* Berkeley: University of California Press.

White, William A., III. 2023. *Segregation Made Them Neighbors: An Archaeology of Racialization in Boise, Idaho.* Lincoln: University of Nebraska Press.

Wilbert, Johannes. 1980. "Genesis and Demography of a Warao Subtribe: The Winikina." In *Demographic and Biological Studies of the Warao Indians,* edited by Johannes Wilbert and Miguel Layrisse, 13–47. Los Angeles: UCLA Latin American Center.

Wilbert, Johannes. 1993. *Mystic Endowment: Religious Ethnography of the Warao Indians.* Cambridge, MA: Center for the Study of World Religions, Harvard University.

Wilbert, Werner. 1996. *Fitoterapia Warao: Una teoría pneumica de la salud, la enfermedad y la terapia.* Caracas: Instituto Caribe de Antropología y Sociología.

Wilbert, Werner, and Cecilia Ayala Lafée-Wilbert. 2007. "Los Warao." In *Salud Indígena en Venezuela,* edited by Germán Freire and Aimé Tillett, 331–96. Vol. 2. Caracas: Gobierno Bolivariano de Venezuela, Ministerio del Poder Popular para la Salud.

Wilce, James M. 2009. "Medical Discourse." *Annual Review of Anthropology* 38: 199–315.

Wilderson, Frank B., III. 2010. *Red, White, and Black: Cinema and the Structure of U.S. Antagonisms.* Durham, NC: Duke University Press.

Williams, A. N. 2005. "Physician, Philosopher, and Paediatrician: John Locke's Practice of Child Health Care." *Archives of Disease in Childhood* 91(1): 85–89.

Williams, Raymond. 1977. *Marxism and Literature.* Oxford: Oxford University Press.

Woolhouse, Roger. 2007. *Locke: A Biography.* Cambridge: Cambridge University Press.

World Health Organization (WHO). 2020. "Managing the COVID-19 Infodemic: Promoting Healthy Behaviours and Mitigating the Harm from Misinformation and Disinformation." World Health Organization, 23 September 2020. https://www.who.int/news/item/23-09-2020-managing-the-covid-19-infodemic -promoting-healthy-behaviours-and-mitigating-the-harm-from-misinformation -and-disinformation.

Wright, Anthony. 2019. "The Promise of Poison: Life in the Field of Pediatric Cancer Treatment." PhD diss., University of California, Berkeley.

Wynne, Brian. 1992. "Misunderstood Misunderstanding: Social Identities and Public Uptake of Science." *Public Understanding of Science* 1(3): 281–304.

Yates-Doerr, Emily 2019. "Whose Global, Which Health? Unsettling Collaboration with Careful Equivocation." *American Anthropologist* 121(2): 297–310.

Zentella, Ana Celia. 2003. "José Can You See: Latin@ Responses to Racist Discourse." In *Bilingual Games: Some Literary Investigations,* edited by Doris Sommer, 51–66. New York: Palgrave Macmillan.

Zola, Irving Kenneth. 1972. "Medicine as an Institution of Social Control." *Sociological Review* 20(4): 487–504.

Body Politic COVID-19 Support Group, 179, 183, 282n8
body schema, 68
borders of communicability and incommunicability, 110
Boston Women's Health Collective, 138
boundary-work, 3, 10, 39, 63, 165, 168, 251–53, 255–59; challenged, 155; between communication and medicine, 2–3, 4–5, 17, 29–30, 36, 81, 258; between professional and lay health knowledge, 165
Bourdieu, Pierre, 55, 193, 232
Boyle, Robert, 30
Brandt, Alan, 201
breakthrough: into communicability, 101; into performance, 94
Breilh, Jaime, 72–73, 269, 276n3
Briggs, Laura, 263
Broussais, Victor, 73
Buchbinder, Mara, 15
Bucholtz, Mary, 276n13
Bulled, Nicola, 141
Bullock, Steve, 253
Burden-Stelly, Charisse, 47
Burke, Jane, 16, 86
Burkina Faso, 135
"burnout," 228, 237, 243, 272, 282n5
Bustos, Roselia, 218–22

Cabalquinto, Earvin, 168
Caduff, Carlo, 77, 161, 162, 169, 170, 172
California, 19, 88, 112, 113, 114, 116, 185, 192, 208, 209, 211, 213, 217, 218, 244, 254, 272
Canguilhem, Georges, 22, 36, 71–78, 89, 94, 95, 98, 103, 111, 182
cannibalism, 65, 66, 68
capitalist medicine, 42, 105, 137, 142, 155, 238; as producing health inequities, 266
carcerality, 8, 61
care: as *autoatención*, 95; failures of for caregivers, 230, 248; criminalization of, 251–53, 255–56, 262; definitions of transformed in pandemic, 229, 231–34; lay views of, 187; narration and, 97–98; "perverse" forms of, 261; physicians' control over, 251–62; as structuring experiences in the pandemic, 217
care technologies, 226
Carr, E. Summerson, 15, 16, 145
case definitions, 146
"cheat and abuse of words," 34
cell phones, 15, 183, 194
censorship claims, 213
Centers for Diseases Control and Prevention (CDC), 2, 5, 134, 161, 165–66, 169, 172–73, 174, 179, 181, 183, 188, 189
Chakrabarty, Dipesh, 65

challenges to "expert" authority, 84
Chandler, Nahum, 43–44, 47, 50
chanting, 99
Chartier, Émile, 71
charts, 96
Chávez Frías, Hugo (president of Venezuela), 19, 131, 280 n8
Chávez, Leo, 112, 113
chicken pox, 149
chief medical officer, 252, 256
child birth, 102
childcare: increased burdens during pandemic, 204, 223, 225–26
child mortality, 18, 21, 49, 126, 280n12
children, 30, 35, 55, 117–24, 127, 266, 277n17, 279n8; effects of pandemic on, 245; as translators, 92–93
China, 155, 247; as deliberately causing the pandemic, 210
"Chinese virus," 174, 211
cholera, 18, 19, 124–32, 145, 146, 147, 149–51, 175, 238
Chomsky, Noam, 267
Christianity, 15, 32, 92, 151, 188, 212, 253, 254
chronic diseases, 22, 39, 71, 73, 77, 78, 88, 111, 172, 179, 180, 183, 198
chronotopes, 132, 169, 170, 207, 215, 216
churches, 156; pandemic and, 187, 188, 191, 193, 204, 215, 253–54
Cicourel, Aaron, 14, 86
citizen scientists, 138, 263
civil rights activists, 268
Clarke, Adele, 137, 140
Clarke, Edward, 37, 265
classification, 7, 33, 165, 211
Cleaver, Eldridge, 155
Clemente, Ignasi, 279n8
clinical medicine: colonial surveillance and, 62; communicability in Fanon's practice and, 64; encounters, phases of, 83; presentations, 96; as producing incommunicability, 65, 71–78; power asymmetry in, 85 racial violence and, 60
clinical trials, 153, 154
CNN, 208, 212
code-switching, 55, 133, 145
Cohen, Lawrence, 216, 261
colonialism, 21, 81, 91, 103, 105, 111, 129, 131, 134, 140, 143, 147, 151, 155, 175, 265, 266, 268, 273, 275n2; in Algeria, 69; comic books and, 65; Fanon's analysis of, 53–70; language hierarchies and, 129–30; pandemics and, 175; as shaping communicability, 38; slavery and, 34; stereotypes and, 69; violence of, 69; whiteness and, 35
colonial mimicry, 57, 58, 69, 104
commensurability, 133, 185, 275–76n3

communicability, 1–4, 32, 163, 213, 220, 221; in Africa, 134–35; authority and, 12; competing forms of, 4, 5, 6, 146; conflated with pragmatics, 163; as embodied by lay people in pandemic, 219; failure, 5, 76, 83, 104, 145; as foundational ontology, 44; medical profiling and, 92, 93; nosologies of, 76; pandemic disruptions in, 229, 231–34; solidarity, 232; as space of revolutionary transformation, 69; subject production and, 50; switching, 145; symbolic domination and, 17, 70, 91, 101; whiteness and, 40, 262–63

communicable: assemblages, 125; citizenship, 131; competence, 104; humility, 103; stereotypes, 58, 86, 93, 105, 131; subjects, 11, 46

communication studies, 242

communicative inequities, 8, 12, 16–17, 26, 98, 230, 259, 265

communicative incompetence, 16

community-based, 175, 181

community gardens, 217n62

community health centers, 200

comorbidities, 249

competence orientation in medicine, 84

complementary and alternative medicine, 137

computers: pandemic life and, 206, 222

Comte, Auguste, 73

concepts, 72

confessional technologies, 60–61, 92, 134–35, 201, 281n14

conspiracy theories, 19, 165, 166–68, 242, 282n1; Chinese roots of COVID-19 and, 210; COVID-19 and, 187, 191–92, 251; 5G cell towers and, 166–67; heterogeneity of, 194, 212; as reductionist label, 165–67, 171; vaccine as changing DNA, 211

contact tracing, 200–201

contextualization, 73, 88–89, 278n5

contractors, 258

contradictions: biocommunicable, 63

conversation analysis, 16, 82

coproduction, 32, 81, 94

corona virus, 184

Coronavirus Task Force, White House, 174, 189

Coronil, Fernando, 116

Corwin, Anna, 15

cosmopolitanism, 42

coughing, 245

Coulthard, Glen, 67

COVID-19 care: in emergency rooms, 200, 202, 203, 244–45, 246–51; in ICUs, 203, 235–43, 254, 261; interpreted as state intervention, 185–93, 251–63; provided by laypeople, 24, 177–84

COVID-19 narratives, 176–84, 231

COVID-19 pandemic, 1–2, 5–6, 19, 23, 25, 161–263, 243, 255; as augmenting inequities, 6, 19, 25, 114, 168, 169, 170, 199, 222, 223–27, 263; cultural production and, 177–84; debates about lethality,

187; debates among scientists, 191; effects on other health conditions, 224; as exposing scientific practices, 262; gender and, 209; health communication, 113–14; initial perceptions of, 218, 222; origin stories, 174; politics and, 185–86; pulmonology symptoms, 179; social media and, 162; spatialization of, 1, 170; specialty drugs, 254; temporalities, 1, 170; theories of transmission, 1, 168–69; as transforming fundamental conceptions of work, 234; variants, 1, 2, 162, 169, 170, 209. See also conspiracy theories

COVID-19 vaccination breakthrough cases, 169, 176–77

creativity, 5, 15, 24, 25, 144, 180, 197, 199, 213

credibility, 188, 189

Crisis (NAACP magazine), 42

crisis and emergency risk communication, 142, 165, 172–73, 189

crisis standards of care, 170, 254

critical epidemiology, 72–73, 269, 277n3

Cuba, 147, 155

culturalist logics, 48, 114–16, 126, 221

cultural relativism, 61, 278n7

dance: health communication and, 152

Das, Veena, 97, 248

Davis, Dána-Ain, 16

Davis, Georgia, 139

Davis, Kathy, 138

death threats, 228, 242, 257

decolonial, 265

decolonization, 10, 20, 69, 70, 99, 265, 268, 273, 275n2

decolonizing: anthropology, 3, 273; the study of language and medicine, 3, 10, 20, 99, 265, 268

decontextualization, 33, 85, 129

dehydration, 125

delivery drivers, 258

Delta Amacuro, 18–19, 92, 125–32, 146, 149–51

DelVecchio Good, Mary-Jo, 84, 105

demedicalization, 156, 198, 216

dementia, 15, 64, 103

Democratic Party, 210

democratization of science, 191

democratizing health knowledge, 269, 270

dengue fever, 116–24

dental care, 198

depression, 198, 214, 216, 224

deprovincialization, 65, 77

Derrida, Jacques, 33, 166, 167

Descartes, Renée, 29, 37, 71

descent into the ordinary, 248

diabetes, 17, 88, 111, 114–16

diagnosis, 21, 77, 82, 83, 87, 90, 257; colonial medicine and, 60, 62, 64, 66, 69; Fanon's method of, 54; of incommunicability, 32, 35; political, 155

hoarotu, 99
Hobbes, Thomas, 29, 277n3
Holmes, Seth, 217, 282n2
Homeland Security, 172
H1N1 ("swine flu") pandemic of 2009, 2, 161, 169, 172, 173
Horne, Gerald, 47
hospital administrators: failure to protect employees in pandemic, 241, 244–45, 247–48; as muzzling employees, 241; profit orientations, 238, 243, 250
hospitalists, 251, 255, 263
hospitals: debates over excluding visitations during pandemic, 252; perceived as sources of infection, 233; racialized health inequities and, 48; restrictions on visitation during pandemic, 214; transformed by pandemic, 235
hospital services: shifting during the pandemic, 244
House (TV series), 109
house cleaners, 223, 225
housing, 19, 20, 48, 77, 131, 139, 145, 156, 199, 217, 221, 272
Hubbs, Nadine, 96, 145, 185
humanitarianism, 59, 135, 136
Hume, David, 29
humor, 173
Hunt, Nancy Rose, 134
Hurston, Zora Neale, 47
Hutchins, Edwin, 231
Huygens, Christian, 30
hydroxychloroquine, 251, 260
hygiene, 69, 70, 193
Hymes, Dell, 94, 101, 268
hypertension, 225

ideological labor, 81, 89, 111, 175, 259
ideologies of science, 190–91
idioms of distress, 14, 225, 243
ignorance, 95, 165, 168
"illiterate" people, 30
illness narratives, 14, 93–98, 178, 187; of COVID-19, 176–77, 245–46, 249; in health communication, 134
immigration: communicability and, 139; policies, 107; status, 199
immobility, 4
immunology, 153, 255
immutable mobiles, 258
imperialism, 42, 51
improvisations, 202, 203, 206, 232, 233
incident command, 251
income, 272
incommunicability: definition of, 9, 12, 17, 181; as classifying good versus bad patients, 91; colonialism and, 64, 77; as confirming white

physicians' authority, 63; as constructed in health communication, 109–47; "crises" of, 31; decolonial, 69; as foundational analytic, 10, 267; inhabitation of, 8, 31, 50, 68, 75, 76, 94–95;laypeople's accounts of, 95; loss of the self and, 66, 67; as marginalized in linguistic theory, 267; medical practice as producing, 58, 75; medical technologies and, 236, 239; modes of writing and, 45; pandemic's divisive effects and, 259; in physicians, 62; as positioning white readers, 45, 54, 56–57; scholarly uses of term, 276n12; stereotypes of patients as, 16, 58, 86, 93, 114–16, 156; subjects, 12, 20, 122, 140, 144, 269; in whites, 50
incommunicability-free zones, 25, 156, 157, 270
indexicality, 39, 278n3; linguistic racism and, 175
indexical order, 89, 92, 106, 107, 189
Indian Health Services, 263
indigeneity, 9–10, 13
individualism, 171, 243; in medicine and public health, 33; toxic, 271
individualization, 77
infantilization, 56, 120, 167
infant mortality: in Black populations, 48
infectious disease physicians, 251, 255, 260
influencers, 172
influenza, 176, 187, 229
infodemic, 5, 162, 190
information: constructions of, 144, 165–66, 219
infrastructures: communicable, 133, 259. *See also* public health infrastructures
inner speech, 217, 225
innovation: in COVID-19 care, 24, 197–03
Inoue, Miyako, 12, 56, 104, 105
insecticides, 116
insomnia: as symptom of long COVID, 178–79, 184
Instagram, 181
Institute of Medicine, 86
instrumentalism, 51, 58, 64, 75, 76, 104, 108, 143, 270
insurance companies, 86, 96, 106, 141
integrative critical transformation, 154–57
intensive care units (ICUs), 6, 235–43
interaction: research on, 82–83
International Monetary Fund, 123
internet, 162, 199, 206; inequities in access to, 141, 222, 225; used by physicians for guidance on COVID-19, 245
interventionism, 108; incommunicability as requiring, 31, 38, 40, 51, 57
interviews, 95–98, 230; critiques of, 96
intonation, 77, 98, 133
intubation, 236, 239
invisibility, 67, 96
Irvine, Judith T., 91, 277n16

isolation, 191, 202, 204, 207, 249; as experienced by health professionals, 230, 234, 237, 240
isolation: of COVID-19 patients, 249; of students living on campus, 224, 225, 226
Italy, 235, 239, 247
iteration, 167
ivermectin, 251–52, 257, 259, 260, 262
Ivory Coast, 135

Jackson, John, 8
Jakobson, Roman, 34, 59, 94, 248
Japanese Americans, 175
Jefferson, Gail, 82
job loss, 199
Johns Hopkins University Coronavirus Research Center, 1, 169, 282n6
Johnson, Cameron, 276n6
jokes, 15, 151, 152
Jones, Ellie, 228–34
journaling: during the COVID-19 pandemic, 181, 182
journalists, 6, 8, 51, 96, 124, 125, 137, 153, 161, 180, 181, 191
Journal of the American Medical Association, 191
Juhasz, Alexandra, 180, 182
justice, 269; imagined spaces of, 47; social, 17, 155. *See also* health/communicative justice

Keller, Richard, 59
Kenjar, Kevin, 112
Khurana, Mark, 142
Kleinman, Arthur, 14, 93–98
knee replacement, 257
knowledge/communication binary, 110
knowledge exchange, 199
knowledge translation, 106, 188
Kockelman, Paul, 99
Korsch, Barbara M., 83
Kostova, Patty, 141, 142
Krieger, Nancy, 17
Kroskrity, Paul, 4, 13
Kuipers, Joel, 14
"kung flu," 174

labor, 61
laboratories, 3, 110, 155
laborers, 30, 35, 39
labor market, 169
lab results: as evidence of incommunicability, 93; digital health and, 142
Lacan, Jacques, 34, 55
Lafée-Wilbert, Cecilia Ayala, 280n12
Lakoff, Andrew, 161
laments, 18, 78
landscapes, 88, 183; linguistic, 112–16, 280n2, 280n4

language: barriers, 199; as a province of knowledge, 29–30, 32
language ideologies, 4, 13, 32, 33, 54–57, 64, 188, 175, 267; in health communication, 133–34; personalistic, 46; referentialist, 45–46, 133, 275n2
Latin American social medicine, 72–73, 269, 276n3
Latinx, 6, 11, 182; biomedical-authority communicability and, 140; health inequities, 16, 19, 222–27; patients, 86, 266; physicians, 221; populations, 271; students, 114, 222–27
Latinx Research Center, 19, 226
Latour, Bruno, 188, 190–91, 258
lay-activist communicability, 134, 139, 153–54, 163, 164, 177–84, 271
lay contributions to COVID-19 knowledge, 164, 181–84, 195, 212–13
lay forms of health labor. *See autoatención*
lay perceptions of COVID susceptibility, 209
laypersons: as coproducers in health knowledge, 24, 94. *See also* communicability
lay reception: of health knowledge, 188
Lee, Rachel, 276n11
leisure, 31, 39, 206
Lévi-Strauss, Claude, 33, 102, 183, 279n17
liberals, 9, 211, 258
Likosky, Stephan, 278n8
liminality, 238
Lingering (art exhibition by Pato Hebert), 183
linguistic anthropology, 4, 11–13, 54, 57, 64, 73, 87, 88, 89, 96, 97, 112, 129, 132, 141, 267; vis-à-vis medical anthropology, 3, 10–18, 98, 135, 136, 151, 175, 267–68, 273, 276n13
linguistic profiling, 6, 13, 14, 16–17, 113
linguistic racism, 12–13, 33, 81, 130, 175, 268; in health communication, 127–32; in medical encounters, 54–70
linguistics, 29, 267–68
Lipsitz, George, 139, 157
listening: constructions of, 82
listening subjects, 12, 56, 104
Livingston, Julie, 202
lockdowns, 170, 223
lockdown warriors, 162, 171
Locke, John, 11–12, 20–21, 25, 29–40, 55, 76, 78, 83, 93, 94, 111, 116, 133, 163, 165, 166, 168, 188, 258, 266, 268, 270, 275n2, 277n1; on cannibalism, 66; on communicative failure, 83; as disabled, 20; legacy of, 111, 116, 133, 145, 270; on performativity, 67–68; as physician, 20–21, 36–37; slavery and, 34, 50; *Two Treatises of Government*, 35, 37, 275n2; vis-à-vis Frantz Fanon, 55, 57, 66, 67; vis-à-vis W. E. B. Du Bois, 41, 42–43, 45, 46, 47, 49, 50
logics of choice, 271
logocentrism, 33
London, 32, 39, 114

loneliness: during pandemic, 249

long COVID, 24, 168, 169, 177–84, 195, 245, 253, 260, 268, 281n2; activists, 176–84, 195; as affecting healthcare professionals, 246, 250, 253; biomedical authority communicability and, 177–84; emergence of concept, 178; social media and, 178; solidarity among patients, 179

Long COVID Survival Guide, The (Lowenstein), 176

long-haulers, 178, 268

Los Angeles, 177, 183

Los Angeles Times, 113

Lowenstein, Fiona, 176, 181n8

low-income populations, 132, 134, 199

Lowry, Ilana, 163, 259

Luchadoras del Campo, 218, 219–22

lupus, 179, 183, 184

Lyme disease, 139, 281n16

Macey, David, 55, 62

Macpherson, C. B., 32

magazines, 65

malaria, 18, 116

Malcom X, 25

Maldonado-Torres, Nelson, 55

malpractice, 252

mandates, 170, 193, 194, 201, 202, 211, 253

Mantini-Briggs, Clara, 14, 18, 19, 92, 131, 149, 200, 226, 238, 279n11, 279n12, 280n9

Mao Zedong, 155

Mariusa, 99, 103

Marriott, David, 60, 63

Marya, Rupa, 265, 275n2

masks, 3, 5, 6, 24, 162, 170, 172, 174, 183, 185, 186, 188, 192, 194, 199, 201, 202, 210, 245–46, 253–54, 258; "conspiracy theorist" acceptance of, 209, 211, 212; as impeding provider-patient communication, 236, 239; mandates, 253; as symbol of the pandemic, 180; value initially underestimated by health professionals, 244

materiality, 8, 97

mathematical mapping, 170

Mattingly, Cheryl, 14, 16, 97

Mayan, 15, 99, 136, 146

Maynard, Douglas, 83, 85

Mazzarella, William, 185

McElhinny, Bonnie, 276n9

measles, 149

media: harassment of health professionals and, 256; incommunicability and, 43; linguistic racism and, 65; as racialized, 21; as source of COVID-19 knowledge, 201

media coverage of health, 13; of cholera epidemic, 124, 131–32; of COVID-19, 185–86, 188, 212; of HIV/AIDS, 153; patients' perceptions of symptoms and, 177, 179

media ideologies, 15

medical: associations, 183; education, 16, 22, 93; histories, 89, 255; interpretation, 61–62, 91–93; knowledge and communicability, 36–37; knowledge of COVID-19; knowledge gaps, 260; medical-industrial system in US, 155; nosology and incommunicability, 59; profiling, 6, 14, 16–17, 38, 48, 58, 92, 111, 182, 221, 266; racism, 58; schools, 3, 14, 25, 76, 82, 105, 106, 142; semiology, 5

medical anthropology, 16–17, 54, 132, 194, 259, 281n1; vis-à-vis linguistic anthropology, 3, 10–18, 98, 135, 136, 151, 175, 267–68, 273, 276n13

medicalization, 140, 276n4; versus incommunicability, 262

Medicare and Medicaid, 141

Medina, José, 100–102

Meek, Barbra, 13, 66

memorial services, 199

Menéndez, Eduardo, 56, 73, 85, 95, 97, 98, 136, 146, 193, 202, 278n3

mental health, 69, 72, 231; in pandemic, 198, 224, 225, 226, 249, 250

Mental Health America survey, 240

mentorship, 238, 244

metaphysics, 50

metapragmatic control, 91, 92

metapragmatic regimentation, 173

metapragmatics, 89, 90, 92, 103, 259

metrics, 145, 270

Metzl, Jonathan, 106

Meyers, Todd, 73

Mickey Mouse, 65

microbiome/virome communities, 184

middle class, 119–23, 124–25, 145

Middle East Respiratory Syndrome coronavirus (MERS-CoV), 172

militaries, 62, 127, 134, 161, 174; military medicine, 127–32, 134

Miller, Frank, 24, 184–93, 200, 203, 208, 212, 239, 242, 253, 257–61, 272

Miller, Linda, 208, 212

Ministry of Health and Social Assistance, Venezuela, 117, 124

miscommunication, 25

Miserando, Christine, 184

Mishler, Elliot, 85, 279n9

"misinformation," 5–6, 19, 95, 162, 165–67, 171, 168, 178, 181, 190, 194, 250, 262; as biocommunicable target, 242; healthcare professionals' effects to counter, 251; as residual category, 262; social media and, 241–42

misrecognition, 58

Mission Barrio Adentro, 19, 280n8

Missoula, Montana, 253, 254

mistrust, 250

Mitchell, Timothy, 280n6

mitigation measures, 6, 164, 211, 209, 218; critiques of, 169, 170; as designed by and for middle-class professionals, 199; differential impact on essential workers, 199; as racialized, 113–15, 170

mobility, 4, 132

Mol, Annemarie, 271

molecular mimicry, 184

Molina, Natalia, 49, 175

monoglot standard, 11

monopolies: communicable, 23; 259–63, 265

Montana, 19, 24, 170, 185, 198, 200; anti-mandate legislation, 253; assistant attorney-general, 251, 256; Democratic party, 256; as focus of COVID-19 coverage, 255; healthcare professionals in, 251–62; politics of masking in, 254; predominantly white population, 253; rates of vaccination, 254; Republican party in, 256, 260

Montaño, Sylvia, 213–17, 231, 248, 272

Moodie, Megan, 281n2

moral distress, 243, 249, 257

moral injury, 249, 257

Moran-Thomas, Amy, 17

more-than-human research, 259

morgues, 254

moriche palms, 99, 279n13

mosquitos, 116–24

mothers: as target of health communication, 119–23, 124, 125

mourning, 47, 68; in pandemic, 199, 215

multiculturalism, 9

multigenerational households, 197, 203, 222

multilingualism, 11, 64, 77, 112, 255

multimodality, 97, 114

multiple: laterally organized communicabilities, 149–51

multiple sclerosis (MS), 179, 183

Murphy, Bill, 228–34, 239

music, 15, 18, 45–47, 65, 66, 102, 151–53, 228, 231, 232

myalgic encephalomyelitis / chronic fatigue syndrome (ME/CFS), 179, 183

Mythbusters (WHO website), 166–68, 175, 190

myths, 18, 165–67, 173, 211

Nabsanuka Clinic, 101

Nading, Alex, 117–18

Nagy, Jana, 235–43, 261

nahanamu ritual, 150, 279n13

narrated events, 94, 248

narrating class, 96, 145, 185

narrative events, 248

narratives: as archives of lay care, 97; clinical practice and, 93; as controlled by physicians, 105; in health communication, 119, 120; landscapes and, 88; social lives of, 96–97

National Association for the Advancement of Colored People (NAACP), 42

National Guard: role in pandemic, 255

National Liberation Front (FLN), 59

Native American nations, 176; in Montana, 253

Native Americans, 6, 11, 65, 175, 271; biomedical-authority communicability and, 140; COVID-19 vaccination and, 176; in pandemic, 199

nativism, 107

natural history, 35

naturalization, 2, 4, 11, 12, 13, 17, 30, 38, 54, 59, 84, 85, 89, 130, 131,140, 265, 267

Navajo Nation, 175, 263

negative pressure rooms, 247

Negrete, Vida Francis, 83

Nelson, Alan, 16, 86

Nelson, Alondra, 154–57

neoliberalism, 123, 137, 143, 163

Nepal, 133–34, 135, 146

neurological problems, 184

New England Journal of Medicine, 106, 191

new materialism theory, 49

New Mexico, 19

New Negro Movement, 42

news coverage, 104, 139, 165, 171; of cholera epidemic, 124, 125, 131; of COVID-19 pandemic, 2, 177, 181, 185–86, 188, 194, 193, 200, 208, 210, 212, 213, 214–17, 235, 239, 258, 259; of HIV/AIDS pandemic, 134

newsletters, 110, 153

Newsom, Gavin, 218, 220

newspapers, 61, 66, 124, 125, 139, 156, 255; of Black Panther Party, 156; physicians writing for, 251

Newton, Isaac, 30

New York Times, 2, 208, 212

New York University, 180, 182

Nguyen, Vinh-Kim, 134–35

Nicaragua, 117–18

Nichter, Mark, 14, 125, 137, 139, 191, 241, 243, 249, 257, 271, 281n16

non-biomedical healers, 18

noncompliance, 60, 83, 93, 95

nongovernmental organizations (NGOs), 15, 110, 135, 136, 144, 145, 146, 220, 270

nonhumans, 88

nonknowledge, 165

normal, the, 22, 71–78, 86, 87, 94; COVID-19 and, 170, 182, 205, 273

Normal and the Pathological, The (Canguilhem), 71, 72, 73, 77

normalization, 75–76, 95

normativization, 75, 104, 105, 108

North African Syndrome, 57

North America, 269

nosology of incommunicable pathologies, 32, 33

Nowotny, Helga, 281n16

nurse-patient communication, 236, 239–40
nurses, 16, 18, 19, 24, 60, 70, 82, 89, 91–92, 98, 102,
103, 110, 114, 131, 149, 153; class positionality of,
240; coping with patients' deaths, 236–37, 243;
demands in pandemic on, 235–43; future of
profession, 237, 238, 242–43; in pandemic, 164,
184, 198, 202, 203, 212, 223, 227, 235–41, 242–43,
251, 252, 255, 261, 262, 267, 272; staff shortages of,
235–43; as translators, 92;
nursing schools, 82, 235, 238

oaths: taken by health professionals, 243
Obama, Barack, 173
OB/GYN, 244, 245
objectification, 67, 73, 84
Ochoa, Marcia, 122
Ochs, Elinor, 14, 278n3
Ødemark, John, 11, 105, 137, 188
online funerals, 199
ontologies, 4, 32, 33, 36, 44, 74, 143, 276n13
ordinary ethics, 208, 225, 226
Orellana, Marjorie Faulstich, 92, 279n7
origin of COVID-19 pandemic: debates regarding,
210
origin stories, 31, 33
Osmondson, Lewis, 228–34
otherness, 266
over-reassurance, 172–74
Owen, Johnnie, 186, 192, 200
oxygen, 254; therapy, 245

pain, 75, 77, 86, 88, 99
palimpsests, 88
pamphlets: in health communication, 110, 111,
117–24, 127–32, 143, 146, 280n80
pandemic: biocommunicability, 165–68; as blurring boundaries between work and home, 248;
as coming-of-age experience, 238; ecologies
of care, 202–3, 262; ecologies of knowledge,
164–95; false alarms, 172; fatigue, 5, 162; heroes
syndrome, 240–41; incommunicability, 248; as
transforming fundamental concepts of work, 250
pandemic-industrial-discourse complex, 161, 163,
165, 197, 271
pandemic inequities: biocommunicable roots of,
199
Pandolfo, Stefania, 66, 68
Pangborn, Stepanie, 238, 241, 243
Papua New Guinea, 91–92
paramedics. See firefighter/paramedics
Paredes, Américo, 96
Parkin, David, 14
Parsons, Talcott, 88
passive lay receivers, 6, 24, 138, 139, 141, 143, 164,
165, 171, 172, 191, 194, 197, 212, 213, 263
Patel, Raj, 265, 275n2

pathological, the, 73–78
pathologization: of alternative communicabilities,
38; of incommunicability, 37, 76, 104; of patient-
activist organizations, 183
patient-advocacy groups, 138, 179, 183
patient-centered medicine, 76
patient-consumer communicability, 6, 261, 271;
anti-vaxxers and, 171; as complexly interwoven
with biomedical authority communicability,
171–72; connections to white supremacy, 262;
as displacing biomedical authority in pandemic,
261; heterogeneous roots of, 137, 138, 171–72,
262; as key modality for performing identities,
172; in pandemic, 171–72, 192–93, 262
Patient-Led Research Collaborative for long
COVID, 179, 183
patient organizations, 183
Patton, Cindy, 281n2
Paxlovid, 200
Pedrito, 120–24
peer review, 191, 247
Peirce, Charles S., 276n14
Peña-Guzmán, David, 72
performance, 94
performative acts: racist, 66–68
performativity, 67, 68, 77
Perley, Bernard, 13
perlocutionary effects, 66
personalism, 13, 33
personal protective equipment (PPE), 197, 215, 217,
220, 235, 239, 241, 243; as impeding communication in clinical settings, 236, 239; shortages
of, 197, 217, 220, 235–36, 241, 243–44. See also
gowns; masks; powered air-purifying respirators
(PAPRS)
Peru, 124
pharmaceutical corporations, 134, 137, 186, 193, 259
pharmaceuticalization, 137, 258, 265
pharmaceuticals, 172, 193
phatic uses of language, 34
Philadelphia, 48
philosopher-physicians, 20, 21, 22, 29–40, 53–70,
71–78, 116, 163
philosophy of science, 72
photography, 125, 180, 183
physician-patient communication. See doctor-
patient communication
physician-patient interaction. See doctor-patient
communication
physicians: Black, 69; colonialism and, 55–65;
failures of self-awareness, 63; heterogeneity in
perspectives, 86; as media spokesperson, 255
"pidgin" (petit-nègre): Frantz Fanon on, 55–59,
63–64, 66, 69, 105, 113, 277n1
Pierre, Jemima, 276n5
Pigg, Stacy Leigh, 132–34

Trump, Donald, 162, 186, 189, 210, 213, 253; as anti-masker, 174; bashing of, 258; COVID-19 vaccine development and, 210; patient-consumer communicability and, 192; supporters of, 164, 188, 195, 208; violation of CDC pandemic communicability, 173–75, 190

trust, 60, 61, 64, 104, 135, 150, 186, 187, 190, 192, 210, 212, 227, 228, 257, 259, 262; in COVID-19 discourse, 184, 188, 189, 219; between health professionals, 230; transformed into mistrust in pandemic, 164, 170, 175, 184, 188, 189, 200, 201, 210, 229, 233

truth, 30, 35, 43, 92, 179, 186, 187, 210, 259
tuberculosis, 18, 48, 126, 145, 280n12
Tuck, Eve, 275n2
Turner, Victor, 238
Twitter, 174, 190, 241–42, 243, 263
Two Treatises of Government (Locke), 35, 37

uncanny, 194, 232
uncertainty, 35, 46, 63, 173, 188, 195, 209, 218, 250, 258; about long COVID, 169, 183, 250; experienced by health professionals, 198; in pandemic, 1, 169, 195, 209, 218, 231, 233, 234, 236, 237, 243
undocumented migrants, 221, 222
unemployment benefits, 221
United Farm Workers (UFW), 219
universals, 77
University of California, Berkeley, 11, 19, 114, 218, 222, 223, 224, 225, 226, 227
University of Montana, 254
unprecedented: COVID-19 pandemic as, 141, 163, 205
unsanitary subjects, 48, 118, 125, 129–32
Ureña, Carolyn, 62
utilitarianism, 37, 38, 56, 57, 102, 104

vaccination, 18, 153, 167, 175, 184, 194, 198, 202, 210, 251, 254, 262; as condensed symbol, 262; farmworkers and, 106–7, 113–16, 219, 220, 221; for healthcare workers, 246, 249; legislation opposing vaccine mandates, 253; online scheduling of, 141, 199, 221; racialized minority populations and, 175–76, 263
vaccine-breakthrough cases, 169, 176–77
vaccine hesitancy and refusal, 5, 6, 24, 162, 164, 170, 172, 186–92, 194, 200, 201, 202, 208, 210–11, 251, 256, 258, 260, 262; biocommunicability and, 6
vaccine shortages, 199
VanElzakker, Michael, 184, 281n2
Van Ryn, Michelle, 16, 86, 156
variants: of COVID-19, 2, 162, 169, 170, 209
Veil, the, 21, 42–47
Venezuela, 6, 18–19, 238, 280n8; cholera and, 124–32; dengue fever and, 116–24; health communication in, 116–32

Ventura County, California, 113–15
Villalón, María Eugenia, 129
Vindrola-Padros, Cecilia, 197, 201–2, 232
violence: biocommunicable, 38, 110–11; committed by police, 156, 249; domestic, 198, 221; against health workers, 256–57; linguistic, 56, 63–64, 65–70, 109; racialized, 6, 7, 8, 21, 34, 35, 43, 45, 47, 54, 59, 62, 65–70, 140, 175, 249, 266; reproductive, 156
viral transmission: views of, 186–87, 190
virology, 153, 255
Viswanath, K., 162, 191
vocables, 101, 102
voice, 269; in illness narratives, 225
voice quality, 102
voice timbre, 77
Vološinov, V. N., 217
vomiting, 128, 129

Waard, Jacobus de, 280n12
Wagner, Anna, 212
Wailoo, Keith, 259
Waitzkin, Howard, 16, 85, 87–90, 107, 142, 266–67
wakes, 198
Wakuhana, 149–51
Walensky, Rochelle, 2
Wang, K. Wayne, 275n2
war, 69
Warao language, 18, 92, 101, 127, 130, 151
Washington, Booker T., 42
Weaver, Polly, 208–13, 242, 263
websites, 3, 132, 138, 141, 144, 166, 177, 199, 201, 212, 227, 256–57, 258, 269
well-being, 37, 87, 93, 110, 137, 138, 272
White, William, 278n2
white listening subjects, 12, 56
whiteness, 145, 273; communicability and, 35; linguistic inequities and, 11–13; patient-consumer communicability and, 139–40, 262–63
white privilege, 7, 12, 139, 145, 273, 275n2; during COVID-19 pandemic, 207, 212; HIV/AIDS epidemic and, 154
white social capital, 265
white supremacy, 3, 6, 10, 11, 20–21, 35, 70, 96, 265, 269, 271, 275n2, 190, 273; as attached to patient-consumer communicability, 262; communicability and, 33, 35, 38, 40, 44, 51, 81, 262–63, 269, 273; W. E. B. Du Bois's critique of, 5; global nature of, 276n5; the politics of refusal and, 44; racist compliments and, 68
whooping cough, 149
Wilbert, Johannes, 279n13, 279n16, 280n12
Wilbert, Werner, 129, 280n12
Wilce, James, 14
Wilderson, Frank, 8
wildfires, 246, 249
Williams, A. N., 36, 39

Williams, Raymond, 265
wisidatu healer, 99–102, 149–51, 279n16
witchcraft, 69
women, 12, 61, 65, 77, 112, 124, 138, 139, 154, 209,
    210, 218; as incommunicable, 30, 35, 39; unpaid
    labor of care and prevention, 116–25
Woolhouse, Roger, 36, 37
work: as focus of clinical encounters, 87–89.
    See also labor
Working Group for Health beyond Capitalism,
    142, 267
workshops, 110, 111, 132, 135
worksites, 87–90, 164
World Bank, 123
World Health Organization (WHO), 5, 23, 132, 162,
    166–68, 169, 174, 183, 190, 211, 269

World War II, 134, 175
Wretched of the Earth, The (Fanon), 62, 69,
    155
Wright, Anthony, 279n8

Yates-Doerr, Emily, 91
yellow fever, 120, 124
"Yellow peril" discourses, 175
yoga, 138
YouTube, 3, 192, 212, 213

Zentella, Ana Celia, 113
zero-sum logics, 10, 259
Zola, Irving Kenneth, 140, 276n4
Zoom, 19, 205, 206, 223, 226, 248, 249, 254
Zulu, 151

Printed and bound by CPI Group (UK) Ltd, Croydon, CR0 4YY

09/06/2025

14685752-0001

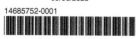